For Churchill Livingstone:

Commissioning editor: Alex Mathieson
Project development manager: Valerie Dearing
Project manager: Derek Robertson
Page make-up: Gerard Heyburn

Current Issues in Community Nursing 2

Specialist Practice in Primary Health Care

Edited by

Jenny Littlewood BSc(Hons) PhD RHV
Director of Health Research, Faculty of Health,
South Bank University, London, UK

Foreword by

Baroness Cumberlege
House of Lords, London, UK

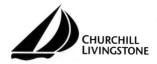

CHURCHILL
LIVINGSTONE

EDINBURGH LONDON NEW YORK PHILADELPHIA ST LOUIS SYDNEY
TORONTO 1999

CHURCHILL LIVINGSTONE
An imprint of Harcourt Publishers Limited

© Harcourt Publishers Limited 1999

🌧 is a registered trademark of Harcourt Publishers Limited

First published 1999

ISBN 0 443 05981 0

British Library Cataloguing in Publication Data
A catalogue record for this book is available from the
British Library

Library of Congress Cataloging in Publication Data
A catalog record for this book is available from the Library
of Congress

Note
Medical knowledge is constantly changing. As new information
becomes available, changes in treatment, procedures,
equipment and the use of drugs become necessary.
The editor, contributors and the publishers have, as far as it
is possible, taken care to ensure that the
information given in this text is accurate and up to date.
However, readers are strongly advised to confirm that the
information, especially with regard to drug usage, complies
with the latest legislation and standards of practice.

Printed in China

Contents

Contributors

John Albarran BSc(Hons) MSc PGDip in Advanced Nursing Practice
PGDipEd RN DipN(Lond)
Senior Lecturer, Faculty of Health and Social Care, University of
the West of England, Glenside Campus, Bristol

After qualifying as a nurse at the Queen Alexandra Hospital in Portsmouth, John
worked in a variety of critical care settings before taking the post of Charge
Nurse in a Renal/Intensive and Coronary Care Unit at Southmead Hospital,
Bristol. In 1993, John moved into education and is currently a Senior Lecturer in
Critical Care Nursing and is also a member of the Editorial Advisory Board for
the journal *Nursing in Critical Care*. John has published on a range of subjects
including providing sexual advice for patients following AMI, political
awareness in nursing and the history of specialist and advanced nursing
practice. His research interests relate to factors influencing a patient's decision to
seek assistance when suffering chest pain, and how patients and their partners
adapt to living with an automated implantable cardiac defibrillator. His first
book, written with Theresa Price and entitled *Managing the Nursing Priorities in
Intensive Care,* was published this year.

Owen Barr BSc(Hons) PGDip Coun Ad DipEd RGN RNMH CNMH
Lecturer in Nursing – Learning Disabilities, School of Health
Sciences, University of Ulster, Coleraine, Northern Ireland

Owen started his nursing career within the general nursing arena in Ireland. After
qualifying as an RGN, he undertook further nurse education in Exeter to obtain
an RNMH before returning to Northern Ireland. For 12 years, he worked within
this aspect of nursing, initially in hospital and then as a Community Nurse for
people with learning disabilities, before obtaining a series of nurse education
posts. He has a firm belief in the rights of people with learning disabilities to
access high quality health and social services, and views community nurses as
integral in making this reality. Owen has been the option leader since 1994 for the
only CNLD course in Ireland, delivered at the University of Ulster. He also
regularly provides input relating to the services for people with learning
disabilities and community care issues into social work courses.

Linda Burke MAEd BA RGN PGDipEd
Senior Lecturer, School of Health and Social Care, South Bank
University, London

Having worked for several years as an oncology nurse, Linda moved to South Bank
University as a Senior Lecturer and then as Course Director to the BSc (Hons)

Nursing Studies Course. In 1993, she completed an MA in Educational Studies for Health Care Professionals, in which she explored the implementation of Working Paper 10, and is now following this up with doctoral research into the development and management of education consortia. She teaches health policy to a range of nursing students, including those undertaking specialist community practitioner courses and community nurses practising at D and E grades.

Edna Elias RGN RM NDN CertCPT HECert
Specialist Nurse, Breast Care, King's Healthcare NHS Trust, London

Following extensive community health education experience, Edna has focused on the promotion of breast screening advice and breast cancer prevention, particularly for black and minority ethnic groups, in which area she is currently pursuing her doctorate. She organises the biannual National Conference on Breast Cancer for nurses, and was the nurse representative for South Thames Region on the National Committee for Breast Screening services. She is currently undertaking a Department of Health funded project which is looking at the attitudes and beliefs of African and Afro-Caribbean women concerning breast cancer.

Debbie Harris MScNursStud RGN DipNursEd RCNT
Senior Lecturer, School of Health and Social Care, South Bank University, London

Debbie has worked within pre-registration programmes for several years, teaching in what is now the College of Health Studies in London and at the South Bank University in areas related to the theory and practice of nursing. She is a member of the BSc(Hons) Nursing Studies Course and Course Director of the MSc Nursing Studies Programme. She teaches both pre- and post-registration students with regard to professional development and the implications of PREP.

Jenny Littlewood PhD BSc(Hons)Psychol HV
Director of Health Research, Faculty of Health, South Bank University, London

For the past 10 years, Jenny has included comparative health care (anthropology) in her studies in nursing, as well as health psychology. She is involved in the use of cognitive mapping in health care, and is researching comparative health care. She has published extensively including in *Anthropology and Medicine, Journal of Child Health* and *Journal of International Nursing Studies.*

Nizam Mohammed MBA MSc BEd CIM DipN(Hons) CertEd RMN RGN RCNT RNT
Principal Lecturer at Kingston University and St George's Hospital Medical School in Healthcare Management and Research

After qualifying at Broadmoor and the Royal Berkshire Hospitals, Nizam qualified in general and psychiatric nursing. He has been seconded to the United

Nations Relief and Works Agency, Gaza, with Save the Children Fund to develop a pre-registration nursing curriculum, and Ghana, where he undertook research in training needs analysis. He is currently researching for his doctorate – the perception by professionals of the rights of the mentally disordered offender.

Sotirios Plakas MSc BANurs

After qualifying in Nursing at the Technological Educational Institution (TEI) in Athens, Greece, Sotirios was awarded a 6 months' grant from the EU and worked in the ICU (NDU) at Chelsea and Westminster Hospital, London. He completed his master's degree at the University of Wales College of Medicine, Cardiff, and is currently a PhD student at the South Bank University, London. His research is looking at the families of critically ill patients. He has worked for more than 5 years as a Staff and Charge Nurse in ICU.

G. Hussein Rassool MSc BA RN FETC RCNT RNT CertEd
Senior Lecturer and Course Director for the post-registration ENB courses in Substance Misuse and Addictive Behaviour in the Department of Addictive Behaviour, St George's Hospital Medical School, London and is also involved in a similar course at the Maudsley Drug Unit

Hussein has spoken about and written extensively for national and international audiences on addiction nursing. He is a member of the Editorial Board of the *Journal of Advanced Nursing*, and is News Editor of that journal.

Mary Saunders MSc BA RGN RHV NDN Cert DipN(Lon) DipNEd DNT
Senior Lecturer, School of Health and Social Care, South Bank University, London

Mary has considerable experience as a specialist practitioner working for a number of years in the community as a health visitor, district nurse and palliative care specialist. She has taught pre- and post-registration nursing and is currently coordinator of the Health Studies course.

Lynette Stone CBE BA RN RM(NSW) DMS
Nursing and Business Development Manager for the Dentistry and Dermatology Group at Guy's and Thomas' Hospital Trust, London

Following her appointment as Sister in the Department of Dermatology at St Bartholomew's Hospital and the Clinical Manager for St John's Institute of Dermatology, Lynn consolidated her interests by being the inaugural chairman of the British Dermatological Nursing Group, is a member of the steering committee of the Skin Care Campaign and is the Nurse Advisor to the All Party Parliamentary Group on Skin. She has lectured nationally and internationally, and has published extensively on issues concerned with dermatological nursing.

Mark Whiting MSc BNursing PGDip(Ed) RSCN RGN RHV DN RNT
Senior Lecturer, Community Children's Nursing, South Bank
University, London

Initially appointed to a small team of CCNs working in Brent in 1985, Mark
undertook a national survey of Community Children's Nursing service
provision as part of his MSc studies at King's College in 1988. As paediatric
service manager, he was responsible for the introduction of CCN services in
Waltham Forest in the early 1990s, and then returned to clinical practice as team
leader with the Paediatric Home Care Team in Paddington in 1993. Mark moved
into education in 1995, initially as a lecturer/practitioner, but more recently as a
full time lecturer in community children's nursing.

Claire Whittle BSc(Hons) MSc RGN RNT
Senior Curriculum Tutor – Taught Higher Degrees, School of
Health Services, The University of Birmingham

After qualifying at The Queen Elizabeth Hospital, Birmingham, Claire
developed her post-registration experience in acute and critical care nursing. She
has spent 18 years in both nursing and nurse education. Her research interests
are related to advancing nursing practice and she is now Senior Curriculum
Tutor for Taught Higher Degrees at The University of Birmingham. She has
recently visited the USA to examine health assessment and advanced nursing
practice.

Foreword

For decades, community nursing was carried out with quiet dedication, was taken for granted and was confined to very specific treatments and care – it was simply nursing outside hospital. Health visiting was a specialty in its own right but even those closely involved could never be sure what health visitors did or achieved.

This has changed. Community nurses – health visitors, community psychiatric nurses, school nurses, district nurses – are in the forefront of health care, and the development of their roles formed the basis of the first volume of *Current Issues in Community Nursing*.

In this volume, issues in specialist practice are addressed. Nurses working alongside the core primary health care team are appreciated by patients and seen by many as the vital component in keeping them out of hospital. The principles and foundations of community nursing have not changed but the remit has, and this is highlighted in the book.

Specialist and advanced practitioners are now able to prescribe. In many fields they have learned new skills and are pushing forward the frontiers of health care, enabling sophisticated treatments to be carried out in patients' homes. This requires confidence, knowledge, practice based on evidence, and continual evaluation.

The new requirements concerning Clinical Governance will mean that those working in the community will have to keep their practice up to date. A better-informed population will ensure that they do so. With information readily available through the internet and other multimedia sources, community practitioners will have to build different relationships with their patients and local communities. This means stronger partnerships and less command and control. Many people will be expected to be active partners in care, whether they be patients or carers.

The Government sees the core members of the primary health care team and specialist nurses as a powerful force to help address risky behaviour in adolescents and other age groups. They are crucial in contributing to the care of people with chronic disorders such as diabetes, asthma or skin conditions such as psoriasis. Specialists in primary care have a particular role in the rehabilitation of elderly people or those who have had severe mental illness.

The strong focus on mental health and the determined resolution to tackle many challenging and extremely difficult issues will be through National Service Frameworks, initially setting standards for the care of those with mental health problems and elderly people (and later for all other client groups), and will require well-educated specialists. With increasing numbers of adults and children, who may be critically ill, disturbed mentally ill offenders, people with addictions, or people with severe and unremitting learning difficulties, being cared for in their homes, the nurse's role in advocacy will become central.

Primary Care Groups, and later Trusts, will give an even stronger voice to those working outside hospitals. With heavy responsibilities for commissioning services and influencing local health improvement programmes, specialists (the subject of this volume) and community nurses have never been more influential.

This well-researched book could not be more timely and relevant for those working in the field. It is an excellent tool and contains many useful insights. I commend it to you.

1999   Baroness Cumberlege

1

Specialist and advanced nursing practice: the debate

John Albarran   Claire Whittle

INTRODUCTION

The role of health care workers in the community is increasingly evolving; this has been as a consequence of many factors including National Health Service (NHS) mandates, professional initiatives, patterns of health and population profiles, as well as due to the rapid discharge of patients from hospital or from long-term institutions. Nurses are one group that have responded to these challenges by broadening and developing their clinical and theoretical expertise, in order to provide sophisticated and cost-effective quality patient-centred care. Further, the opportunities created by these changes have also enabled nurses to effectively identify and address the needs of individual patients or to overcome factors which may influence the health status of a targeted or deprived group by innovative approaches (Thomas 1997, Twinn et al 1992). In other areas community nurses, owing to their unique background, have either provided strategic advice on setting and planning the purchasing of local health services, or have contributed to shaping health care policy (Goodwin 1992). In addition, as a result of the proliferation of scientific knowledge, NHS reorganisations and reforms, as well as increases in patient dependency, have forced nurses to redefine their role and examine their practice in a climate of shifting priorities and competing demands. This expectation has been in part steered by the regulating body which has provided a new structure for promoting clinical expertise, which equally recognises that developing the frontiers of nursing practice is inextricably linked with the concepts of specialist and the advanced nurse practitioner (UKCC 1990a, 1994a).

The purpose of this chapter is to critically examine the debates surrounding professional, specialist and advanced nursing practice as related to community practice. In the first instance, the text will provide a brief historical account of the emergence of a clinical framework. The discussion will then review the preparation required for nurses to progress from the newly qualified stage through to the level of advanced practitioner. However, with regard to the debates and conflicts, this investigation reveals that the core themes centre on whether the role of the nurse practitioner fulfils the Council's requirements. Other controversies relate to the use of existing terminology, the educational preparation of nurses to reach these levels of practice, the ability to exercise autonomy and the integration of these clinicians into the patient environment. Each of these areas will be discussed in turn and possible solutions will be suggested as relevant.

BACKGROUND

To understand the impetus which has led the profession to the point of official recognition that specialist and advanced practice nurses provide a distinctly sophisticated level of patient care, it is necessary to have a grasp of the historical context. Castledine (1991a) has provided an outline of the four major influences; only an overview is included here but a more detailed discussion can be found elsewhere (Albarran & Fulbrook 1998).

The expansion and the development of medical specialisms and specialist hospitals, for example, emphasised the importance of obtaining clinical skills and academic knowledge relevant to the particular field of practice. Simultaneously, with the rapid progression of medical technology, nurses began to assume a broad range of skills and expertise which were previously in the domain of medicine. Nursing responsibilities and skills both expanded and extended into various areas, including urethral catheterisation, venepuncture, monitoring infant development, cervical smear tests, and immunisation. There was also role extension into areas of continuing care involving asthma, diabetes and hypertension clinics. With these developments came the widespread introduction of stoma, nutrition, rheumatology, breast care and diabetes nurses who provided a service both in the hospital and community settings. Those appointed tended to be supervised by medical staff and, because of the narrow focus of their role, became technically competent in their prescribed tasks and responsibilities which had been traditionally performed by physicians (Castledine 1986). In many instances, so-called specialist nursing roles arose as a result of medical pressure and health service reforms (Head 1988, Sargeant 1985), whereas at hospitals such as the Marsden, nurses were encouraged to study beyond registration and broaden the remit of the nursing role to encompass research and educational functions, as well as be much more patient-focused (Tiffany 1984). These post holders were described as clinical nurse specialists (CNS), a term and role which was well established in North America and is strongly linked to the concept of advanced nursing practice (Castledine 1992). For Wilson-Barnett (1985), the purpose of having advanced nursing roles was to improve the well-being of patients and to overcome the deficiencies in the health service. Implied here was that nurses needed to be equipped with the additional range of skills which would enable them to improve standards of practice and to develop nursing frontiers, and by further implication this required a specific level of practitioner.

During this period of change, British nursing also witnessed a number of clinical and academic initiatives which can be conceived as instrumental in imploring recognition of nursing expertise and the value of advanced clinical practice. For example, Manchester University was one of the first to introduce joint appointments and a masters' programme in clinical nursing. Furthermore, through this initiative and the introduction of the nursing process and nursing models, the visibility of nursing practice and contributions to patient care began to accumulate.

In other areas, new spheres of practice were being pioneered; examples of this are the Burford Clinical Nursing Unit (Pearson

1983) and Tameside Nursing Development Unit (Wright 1986). In addition, the integration of primary nursing as a system of organising patient care, nursing development units, the dynamic standards project (RCN 1990) and the named nurse concept began to highlight how practice could make a difference to a patient's experience, and helped to transform the delivery of nursing care (Wright 1992). Many of these developments had an impact on the political agenda (Wright 1992) but more significantly they 'accentuated the growing strength and scope of clinical practice and nurtured a vision of wider possibilities for practitioners' (Albarran & Fulbrook 1998).

Many of these clinical innovations have been realised, owing to the vision of a few who have sought to broaden nursing practice and to stretch professional boundaries (Castledine 1991a, Pearson 1983, Stilwell 1982, Wright 1986). However, it has long been claimed that to strengthen the standing of clinical practice and to forge new frontiers in patient care depends on retaining experts at the bedside. Furthermore, their academic preparation should enable nurses to deliver care which is underpinned by nursing philosophy and a wide theoretical base (Castledine 1991b, Pearson 1983).

Within community care, nurses were also extending their roles into diverse fields, namely psychiatric nursing and oncology (Black & Simon 1980, Castledine 1991a, Graves & Nash 1991). Community developments also witnessed the emergence of the nurse practitioner in primary care, whose role evolved to manage the complex health care needs of patients and often in an independent capacity. As a result, these individuals began to challenge intraprofessional boundaries (Burke-Masters 1986, Stilwell 1982). Such nurses were able to assess physical and psychological health status, diagnose, refer patients, prescribe or adjust medications and provide complete episodes of care. Clinical posts have since been implemented to provide a service where none existed before, or to promote effective use of resources; the most frequent areas for this include paediatric care, accident and emergency, and nurse-led clinics.

The concept of a clinical nurse consultant/specialist in this country had been advocated by the Royal College of Nursing (RCN 1975). As far back as 1975, the RCN argued that the profession needed clinical leaders to improve falling standards and promote an understanding of nursing core values within the health care system. It was proposed that for these practitioners to be effective in their field of practice, they should possess further educational preparation to fulfil the requirements of the post which 'should attract salary recognition consistent with the level of responsibility and the high degree of expertise' (RCN 1975).

Ironically, these roles were attempting to celebrate clinical practice and retain experts at the bedside but instead were viewed as a threat by many senior sisters (Albarran & Fulbrook 1998). Political and professional factors have equally contributed to the belief that expertise amongst practitioners is variable and that this should be acknowledged. For example, the Royal Commission on the NHS (DHSS 1979) indicated that there should be an improved career structure and financial rewards for clinical staff but that these should be offered according to the development of expertise and on the basis of increased responsibility for decision-making.

A more recent document from the RCN (1988) tried to define the specialist nurse amidst the growing proliferation of roles and misuse of the title. It was suggested that specialists had a wealth of experience and knowledge; additionally 'specialist practice involves a clinical and consultative role, teaching, management, research and the application of relevant nursing research. Only if a nurse is involved in all these is she a specialist nurse' (RCN 1988).

With reference to the profession, the Code of Conduct (UKCC 1984) and the Scope of Professional Practice (UKCC 1992b) have stressed the increased responsibility and accountability that nurses have towards delivering excellence in patient care. In addition, the Scope of Professional Practice (1992b) has empowered nurses to expand and adjust the margins of their practice only if it can be demonstrated that the expansion of the role is in the interest of the patient's well-being. Collectively, these changes and advances in clinical practice, as well as reforms within nurse education (for example Project 2000, UKCC 1986), led to recognition that it was necessary for nurses to develop further roles and structures that would enhance 'care provision and realise the potential of clinical practice' (DoH 1989c). However, recently there has been an acceptance that pre-registration educational programmes have only furnished nurses with the skills and knowledge to perform to a particular level of competency and failed to equip them to respond to shifting changes in health care, with the delivery of care being fragmented and task-centred (Briggs 1997).

In addressing the ever changing health needs of patients, it seems that a major contention has emerged over which strategic approach to take. One solution seems to continue: to institute new expanded roles for nurses that involve assuming a broad range of medical tasks, presumably to meet the shortfall in medical personnel resulting from the reduction in junior doctors' hours (Briggs 1997, DoH 1989c, McSweeney 1996, NHSE 1996c). However, the profession has promoted the notion of a clinical career structure for developing nurses into specialist and advanced practitioners, as a means of dealing with the complexity of health care needs of a rapidly changing society (UKCC 1990a, 1994a). This latter view has been espoused in response to the growing impact that clinicians have had on the theoretical and practice base of nursing (Castledine 1991a). In addition, many of the initiatives cited have also drawn attention to the conviction that nursing expertise in the management of patient care varies (Benner 1984, McMurray 1992).

Nurses are not interchangeable; indeed the education, clinical experience and skills of practitioners mean that individuals practise at varying levels (Benner 1984). Moreover, an individual's level of competency develops according to length of experience until the stage of expert is reached. Over this time it is claimed, a nurse's practice becomes highly perceptive and creative, clinical judgements become refined as well as accurate, and the individual is able to diagnose, synthesise and suggest a range of innovative options to problems (Benner 1984, Calkin 1984, McMurray 1992). However, despite the acceptance that patients with unique needs require the clinical expertise of specially prepared nurses, guaranteeing this may be largely determined by sociopolitical, economic and professional factors.

PREPP RECOMMENDATIONS

The introduction of the post-registration education and practice project identified the need for, and endorsed the implementation of, a clinical career structure (UKCC 1990a). This, according to Castledine (1992), was the first indication of official recognition of advanced practice by the profession. For Castledine (1992), this acceptance was overdue, stating 'that the political and professional road to identification of advanced practice has been a continual uphill struggle'. To accommodate the changes in practice and education, the PREPP (UKCC 1990a) report aimed to provide a rational and cost-effective framework for post-registration education and practice. It was also proposed that modern health care called for nurses, midwives and health visitors to be prepared in a way which was relevant and sensitive to the current needs of patients and to shifting patterns of health. Following their proposal (UKCC 1990a), there was a period of extensive consultation (Cole 1991) and debate, lasting nearly 4 years, but the recommendations were finally accepted in 'The Future of Professional Practice' document (UKCC 1994a). The Council's standards for education and practice following registration (UKCC 1994a) included three major sets of requirements:

• standards for a period of support for newly registered practitioners, under the guidance of a preceptor
• standards for maintaining effective registration
• standards for post-registration education.

Relevant to this discussion are the standards for post-registration education. The introduction of PREPP (UKCC 1990a) confirmed amongst other things that clinical expertise varies according to an individual's development. The report thus advocated a career structure which would demarcate this difference in expertise, but equally would enable newly registered nurses to proceed in their careers to consultant level, with their development linked to specific academic achievements. The rationale behind this strategy, it seems, was to provide nurses with a clinically based, academically credible pathway for future progression, and thus reduce the ad hoc pre/post-registration educational provision that has resulted in nurses taking courses that duplicate previous study and are unrecognised by other professionals (Albarran & Whittle 1997). Following a period of consultation, the three areas of practice initially proposed were later changed to include *professional, specialist* and *advanced* levels of practice (UKCC 1994a).

Professional nursing level of practice

The stage defined as professional practice concerns the period after registration in which newly qualified nurses consolidate their training. With experience of nursing patients in a clinical environment, nurses develop competence and may begin to accept greater responsibility. In particular, the professional level of practice means that a newly qualified nurse continues to develop confidence and competence in planning care for a range of clinical situations (McGee 1993). In addition, the individual will be expected to acquire further specialist competencies, knowledge and attitudes in order to deliver safe, holistic and effective patient care. However, to meet the unique specialist health care needs of patients in the community requires further educational preparation of the nurse. The nurse would also be required to maintain a professional profile which should reflect individual development and achievement (UKCC 1994a). It is speculated that the majority of nurses may not wish to go beyond this level; others will seek to broaden their practice and knowledge by the acquisition of specific courses and thus are likely to move on from the 'professional' level.

Specialist nursing level of practice

The Council (UKCC 1994a) has stated that 'whilst pre-registration nursing education provides practitioners with the knowledge, skill and attitudes to give safe and effective care, professional practice alone following registration is not enough to meet additional specialist needs'. Thus, for nurses at diplomate level wishing to achieve specialist status, continued direct patient care in a defined area of practice as well as undertaking a specialist course rated at first-degree level will be compulsory (UKCC 1994a).

Educational programmes leading to a specialist community health care nursing qualification have to be approved by a National Board and the length of the programme must be a minimum of an academic year, 32 weeks full time or the part-time equivalent. The programmes should prepare nurses to develop knowledge and skills in the following broad areas:

* clinical nursing practice
* care and programme management
* clinical practice leadership
* practice development.

Apparently this preparation will assist in differentiating professional level nurses, in that at the specialist stage practitioners will be able to demonstrate refined analytical thinking. Moreover, the course content will be structured to equip nurses to exercise higher levels of discretion in decisions regarding patient care provision so that they can be more effective in serving the interests of the public (UKCC 1994a). However, owing to the divergence of needs within the community and for nurses to be able to function effectively, it is impractical for them to be multi-skilled; thus specific programmes will prepare practitioners to meet the specialist needs of patients or client groups.

The new educational standards and structure created a new unified discipline of specialist community health care nursing practice which comprises:

- general practice nursing
- community mental health nursing
- community mental learning disabilities nursing
- community children's nursing
- public health nursing/health visiting
- occupational health nursing
- nursing in the home/district nursing
- school nursing.

Many of the competencies would be transferable and form part of a core which the specialist community health care nurse should demonstrate. In particular, it is expected that the ability to monitor and improve standards of care through the supervision of practice, clinical nursing audit, developing and leading practice, contributing to research, teaching and supporting professional colleagues will be within the specialist nurse practitioner (SNP) remit. Specialist practitioners will equally play a vital role in many ways, such as providing the supporting structure between the professional and advanced level nurses, as well as leadership in the clinical field and development of other staff.

The discipline of community health care nursing was created to integrate existing strengths of practice, in order to meet the broad range of health care needs within community settings. Equally, it has been reasoned that the new approach had a definitive contribution to make to the *care* and *health* of patients, their families and the whole of society (UKCC 1994a). Billingham & Boyd (1996) and Hyde (1995), however, would suggest that these claims are based on invalid assumptions as in the past community disciplines have mistrusted each other and maintained interprofessional rivalries. It is more likely that the views above reflect the combined remit of community health nursing, but not of every practitioner because 'a common focus which binds all eight named specialist ... nurses is hard to find' (Hyde 1995, p. 23).

To avoid undervaluing prior learning and experiences, those with traditional district nursing courses will be eligible to register as specialist practitioners providing that the individuals can satisfy all of the Council's criteria. In particular, to achieve specialist practice status, the educational programmes previously undertaken must meet with degree-level academic standards. The Council has also indicated that a nurse does not automatically fulfil the criteria of specialist practitioner by virtue of working in a specialist area (UKCC 1994a). This distinction aims to define a specific level of nursing practice and to reduce the misuse of specialist's titles which followed health service reorganisations in the 1980s.

However, the UKCC (1996c) has recently made some transitional arrangements regarding the specialist practitioner title and the specialist qualification. Those currently practising who seek to use the title of 'specialist nurse practitioner' can do so, providing their education and learning from practice reflects the relevant criteria. This strategy has been designed to ensure that practice nurses are not disadvantaged in the transitional period, which began on 1 October 1998. Following this date, nurses wishing to register as specialist practitioners need to undertake a validated programme of education to the standards set by the Council and approved by the National Boards. In this way, the clinical career structure also serves to assure protection for the public, since specialist qualifications will be registerable (UKCC 1994a).

Advanced nursing level of practice

At the outset, the Council indicated that advanced nurse practitioners will be involved in direct patient care, adjusting the boundaries for the development of practice, pioneering new roles responsive to changing needs and with advancing clinical practice, research and education (UKCC 1994a, 1996c). The Council did make clear that advanced nursing practice (ANP) 'is not an additional layer of practice superimposed on specialist nursing practice. It is, rather, a description of an important sphere of professional practice ....' Presumably, as a result of this and extensive consultations within the profession, the term ANP has been abandoned and the title Nurse Consultant has been adopted as it is viewed as a more embracing ideal (UKCC 1996c).

It is foreseen that nurses at this level will be developing the delivery of nursing practice, identifying areas for professional research and implementing research-based protocols. Their practice will be autonomous and directed at developing and pushing forward the frontiers of nursing, health visiting and midwifery practice, as well as contributing to regional, national and international policy-making (UKCC 1996c). It is assumed that advanced nurse clinicians will demonstrate high levels of clinical leadership, provide expert advice through a consultancy role and instigate practice initiatives which are responsive to both consumer and organisational needs. This suggests that they must possess a number of skills. One study identified that these included decision-making based on specialised knowledge, diagnostic and therapeutic skills, advanced communication and problem-solving attributes, acting as a resource and conducting and facilitating research projects (Hunsberger et al 1992). Sparancino (1992) views the advanced nurse as possessing a high level of autonomy and being particularly skilled in conducting comprehensive assessments, diagnosis and formulating decisions for a range of clinical situations, and doing so by incorporating a range of variables into his or her judgements and actions. Heffline (1992) considers that the subroles of change agent, coaching and being a catalyst are vital competencies to the effectiveness of the ANP. Patterson & Haddad (1992), in contrast, suggest that ANPs demonstrate distinct attributes such as approaching problems with a vision, risk-taking, flexibility, articulateness, proactivity and leadership skills. Moreover, it is claimed that these characteristics are critical in distinguishing the ANP. With this background, these nurses are expected to be involved in a number of activities, including publishing articles and delivering conference papers, active in policy-making and possibly holding an honorary lectureship.

Many models suggest that advanced practitioners fulfil clinical, teaching, research, leadership and consultancy roles (Albarran & Whittle 1997). Curiously, these elements were absent in the Council's discussions, even though they are established functions of advanced nursing practice. The Council, by not being prescriptive in the way advanced practice develops, presumably allows for roles to evolve according to local circumstances and need. Conversely, it may be because the profession is still 'uncertain about what advanced practice really is' (Castledine 1991b), or because 'the meaning of advanced practice in the current literature is defined by broad generalisations' (Patterson & Haddad 1992). Other difficulties seem to persist over interpretation of the concepts, standards, related functions, skills and characteristics (Castledine 1996b, Davies & Hughes 1995, Luft 1997, Murray & Thomas 1997). This inevitably presents problems with regard to communicating the ideas to individual practitioners as well as in designing programmes of education that capture the different facets and competencies expected of these levels of practice, a view supported across the Atlantic (Davies & Hughes 1995).

With regard to the distinct value of SNPs and ANPs, numerous studies provide evidence of how these nurses provide care that is comprehensive, high quality and cost-effective (Modica et al 1991, Price et al 1992, Safriet 1992, Wilson-Barnett & Beech 1994). Successful patient outcomes in the fields of diabetic, paediatric, oncology and cardiopulmonary care have been attributed to the unique contribution of these nurses.

A study by Wade & Moyer (1989), for example, examined the role and function of these nurses within diabetic care. Their analysis suggests that the strategies implemented by this calibre of nurse contributed to a reduced length of hospital stay and to fewer admissions to hospital. Moreover, diabetic patients and families who had access to these nurses tended to become more knowledgeable, proficient in self-care and confident. Wade & Moyer (1989) also report that specialists in diabetes were regarded as a valuable resource by patients and their families, and such findings have been described with other patient groups (Layzell & McCarthy 1993).

Lipman (1986) equally suggested that newly diagnosed diabetic children who were educated by a clinical nurse specialist (CNS) in combination with staff nurses, were discharged on average 2.2 days earlier than children taught solely by staff nurses. This it may be reasoned assisted in reducing the amount of psychological distress for the patient and family, and thereby influenced recovery. Moreover, this study also highlights how a unified approach enhances the overall management of patients. The reduction of the mean length of inpatient stay following the introduction of paediatric community nurses has also been evaluated. In this project, Hughes (1993) highlights how the implementation of specific nursing strategies enabled sick children to be discharged earlier, thereby reducing inpatient costs, and ensured that the transition of patients from the hospital to the home environment was smooth and uncomplicated.

Arguably, the preparation of SNPs and ANPs enables them to manage complex health needs and make a difference to the quality of care experienced by both children and adults. For example, research conducted by Alexander et al (1988) demonstrated that the involvement of a CNS in a respiratory centre resulted in a significant increase in the knowledge base of children and families living with asthma. This in turn enabled the patient to gain independence and the family a sense of control. In contrast, Box (1993) describes how patients with cystic fibrosis were able to receive high intensive care nursing whilst at home, owing to the expertise of the nurses. Additional benefits included the opportunity for the domestic situation to be assessed as well as for the patient, nurse and family relationship to develop. The evaluation of the programme identified that the role of clinical experts was therapeutically significant for the recipients of nursing.

McCorkle and colleagues (1989) conducted a random clinical trial to assess the effects of home nursing care for patients with progressive lung cancer. Subjects in this study were assigned either to CNSs in oncology nursing, home helpers or to receive standard care. The results indicated that care provided by a CNS was associated with statistically significantly less symptom distress and greater independence than in the other groups. In addition, those nursed by a CNS had lower hospital admission rates. McCorkle et al (1989) concluded that CNSs have the requisite knowledge and the skills which enable them to instigate interventions which prevent symptoms and complications in a way that makes a critical difference to patients' well-being.

Kegal (1995) likewise has described how ANPs can refine the management of patients with heart failure. In terms of the role of advanced nurse practitioners in the community, it appears that it is their exceptional knowledge of cardiovascular disease and clinical skills which enables them to promote the quality and efficiency of patient care through the coordination and provision of services both in the hospital and home settings. This may be through the provision of 'high-tech' continuity of care, monitoring clinical progress, reinforcing health education messages regarding diet and fluid management, evaluating responsiveness to drug therapy and adjusting this accordingly, emotional support, encouraging independence and liaison with relevant services.

From the studies outlined above, various themes can be identified that relate to the role of specialist and advanced clinicians. It would appear that the length of stay in the hospital setting can be reduced and with it come improvements that are not merely financial, for example impact with early recovery, support in adjusting and confidently coping with an acute or long-term illness. Furthermore, patients and families involved in care can, with the assistance of community nurses, acquire a deeper understanding and with it a greater empowerment in achieving independence according to their abilities. Nurses can bring a wide base of knowledge and skills and use assets to enhance the assessment of and delivery of care to their patients (Robinson et al 1995). Robinson et al (1995) highlight that this level of expertise should be able to assure the smooth transition between the hospital and community settings. This process must not be seen as being from hospital to community. With the developments in care and treatment now enabling greater life expectancies, as in cystic fibrosis, the movement between hospital and community settings is two ways and should be based on models of collaboration and continuity. Nurses operating at these levels should also be able to implement policies that optimise intraprofessional communication, develop cost-effective patient-centred care and redefine the margins of professional practice. It goes without saying that, to make a significant and realistic impression about the value of nurses at this level, more substantive evaluative research is required, which may include a range of methodologies as well as meta-analyses – as without this form of empirical testimony, convincing the profession and others will be a major obstacle.

DEBATES ON SPECIALIST AND ADVANCED NURSING PRACTICE
The role of the nurse practitioner

Controversy over notions of specialist and advanced nursing practice have, to some extent, been attributed to the imposition of many clinical roles which interface with medicine. Nursing as a whole has had to adapt and change to growing social, professional and economic pressures within the last two decades. These pressures have resulted in a variety of roles being adopted by nurses within the community which, even 10 years ago, may have been thought to be unimaginable. This movement to previously uncharted areas of practice has obviously raised the question of the level of knowledge at which nurses are performing, and what practitioners should adopt in terms of the specialist and advanced framework. One such role is the *nurse practitioner* (NP). The term would seem to fit adequately the nurse practising in the community and utilising a wider and more advanced array of skills. However, many suggest that this term is misleading, ambiguous and poorly understood by the service and the consumers of health care (Casey 1996, Castledine 1993, UKCC 1996c). It is argued that the characteristics of an NP embody a 'personal caseload, delegated prescribing powers and a higher order of decision-making in the case of discreet groups'. However, in the context of community nursing, these attributes are not unique to an NP as they relate to any nurse practising within this field. Indeed, to accept that there is a difference would be potentially divisive to the practice of nursing (UKCC 1993b).

Since the early 1970s, in the USA, reductions in the number of medical trainees and those entering the primary care field, as well as inadequacies in service provision, led to the creation of a range of roles, namely paediatric nurse practitioners, physician assistant and the nurse practitioner (Bates 1970, Burke-Masters 1986, Mundinger 1994, Stilwell 1982, Weston 1975). In many instances these nurses believed that their work related to the ethos of nursing values and they integrated a holistic approach to their care. However, this was unlike the proliferation of NP posts which took place during the late 1980s in order to:

- improve service deficiencies and enhance existing provision
- reduce the inappropriate workload of doctors by the transferring of certain functional medical tasks to nurses, thus freeing physicians to deal with the more complex cases
- decrease the costs of employing medical personnel in routine areas of medical practice and to enable nurses to maximise their potential following appropriate training
- prepare nurses to perform a broad range of primary care interventions

- satisfy the personal curiosity of nurses to develop a more technical and medical approach to their practice (Castledine 1995a).

This is clearly not a suitable description of the role and functions of the SNP and ANP in the community.

The UKCC's (1996c) interim report on the nature of advanced practice suggests that the work of the NP does not equate with advanced practice but loosely corresponds to the existing definition of specialist practitioner. The NP concept has also come under criticism in that the individuals are not fulfilling Council criteria in terms of the basis of their practice and their role preparation; many are now substituting the work of doctors (Mathieson 1996). Castledine (1995b) questions whether there is a potential for role conflict when balancing medical and nursing expectations.

In the view of Castledine (1995a), an NP should be described as 'A registered nurse who has been specially prepared to carry out and integrate a more medical model of care into his/her practice with the purpose of improving health assessment, management and delivery of services at the first level of access'.

However, there are several aspects to be considered within this definition which require further examination. Firstly, what is the nature of the specific preparation required and who determines this, bearing in mind that it relates to medical functions? Within the purchaser/provider system in nurse education, educators will need to ensure that nurse practitioners have access to the most appropriate curriculum which enables them to adapt and to be responsive to changing health patterns. However, with the changing nature of fundholding, general practitioners have an increasing control over the educational input of their employees, namely nurses. As Damant et al (1994) observe, 'if the GP takes the responsibility for the education of "his nurse", then there is the realistic possibility that she could become his assistant'. It may also be reasoned that as a result, the nursing component may be diluted, particularly if the training and preparation is dominated by a medical paradigm of a cure.

Again, the issue in question is whether undertaking roles, tasks and skills historically performed by medical practitioners necessarily means the adoption of a medical model of care; some believe it will and have predicted this may occur (Manley 1996,

Smith 1995). A viewpoint commonly expressed is that nurse practitioners, through the adoption of a medical model of care, are displacing nursing core values. An alternative to this is that perhaps community nurses with the appropriate preparation should undertake these aspects of care and dovetail them into a nursing model underpinned by a philosophy based on education, caring, counselling and comfort (Castledine 1993).

In undertaking these roles, community nurses are able to play a part in improving health assessment and delivery of services (Castledine 1993). The term 'improving health assessment' may be the crucial point within this definition. If improvements occur in terms of care and treatment to clients, then is this not the delivered product? Indeed, the nurse practitioner in the primary care setting has been found to be a highly effective health care provider (Mundinger 1994). Conversely, the product may not be the be-all and end-all. If community nurses are to claim to be specialist or advanced practitioners then a wider focus needs to be adopted within their practice. Community nursing is not solely concerned with an undertaking of medically orientated tasks, it actively promotes the delivery of a service that aims to meet the holistic needs of the community.

Misconceptions of specialist and advanced nursing practice roles

Whilst there are guidelines about the functions of specialist and advanced practice, there remain misconceptions over role expectations and responsibilities of these levels of practice which often reflect a lack of understanding and confusion throughout the profession.

At present, debates surrounding the nature of specialist and advanced nursing practice continue to attract much professional discourse and analysis (Albarran & Whittle 1997, Luft 1997, Murray & Thomas 1996). Many of the issues, however, remain unresolved as does consensus over the essence of these levels of practice (Murray & Thomas 1997, UKCC 1996c). As such, Salussolia (1997) suggests that caution should be exercised in responding to internal and external demands when no agreement has been reached by the profession. A GP or practice manager is unlikely to provide financial support to a nurse to progress to any of these levels if it is neither clear nor immediately recognisable what specialist and advanced community nursing practice embodies. As such, it is worth considering whether the profession is acting irresponsibly in publicly advocating such an enterprise without substantive clarity over definitions.

Interpreting the current situation is partly complicated because the number of self-styled specialists or nurse practitioner posts continues to expand. Often these nurses have either variable or no formal structured training (Briggs 1997, O'Hanlon & Gibbon 1996, Read et al 1992). Typically, these roles reflect the particular inclinations of employers (Stafford 1991) or have been introduced to fulfil a specific service need that has been identified as a result of a reduction of junior doctors' hours (Bowey & Caballero 1996). Similarly, within the practice surgeries, nurses are performing supervised minor operations or leading minor injury clinics to relieve the workload of GPs (Marsh & Dawes 1995). Castledine (1995b) adds that owing to manpower pressures, trust managers have begun to experiment with nurses' traditional roles by altering or redefining their work to meet services previously performed by house officers. Consequently, this lack of systematic coherence with regard to the development of professional roles has resulted in further confusion and collective mistrust in nursing. The introduction of criteria for registration of a recordable qualification which becomes official in 1998 (UKCC 1994a) will, it is hoped, ensure that the number of freelance specialists is regulated and will ensure public confidence.

Acceptance by the profession has also been hampered by the number of titles which abound. Since the early 1970s, advanced practice in the UK has been associated with a range of titles such as the clinical nurse consultant, clinical nurse specialist and specialist nurse practitioner (RCN 1975, 1988). The CNS role has been well-established in the USA where it is associated with a master's degree preparation in specific areas of nursing and linked with the ideals of advanced nursing practice. Other terms common in the USA include nurse specialist, nurse practitioner and advanced practice nurse which describe individuals with diverse skills, educational preparation and levels of autonomy for which additional licensing and certification is required. In the UK, PREPP (UKCC 1994a) referred to primary, specialist and advanced as distinct levels of practice. However, there has been a departure from the label of advanced nurse practitioner as it has not been viewed as helpful in describing this role, whereas the title of 'Nurse Consultant' has been deemed as more appropriate (UKCC 1996c). This plethora of terms is a source of confusion which means that nurses can never be sure whether they are discussing similar concepts and ideas, so adding to the degree of uncertainty (Albarran & Whittle 1997). This problem has been exacerbated as various terms are used interchangeably and because nursing publications are drawing from American literature (as is this case in this chapter) to inform the debates here (Salussolia 1997). As such, the message and ideology behind specialist and advanced practice inevitably remains obscured and misunderstood.

Scepticism towards the development of specialists within clinical practice has been equally reinforced by opinions of the past which, in turn, have prejudiced contemporary attitudes, resulting in a degree of opposition. For example, Dulfer (1981) was amongst those who resented the employment of specialist nurses in community nursing. It was claimed that they would fragment the delivery of care and it was feared that the introduction of Macmillan and other specialist roles would not only devalue the work of district nurses but deskill many. It was equally presumed that the practice of specialists would acquire a 'mystical' status and that the care of generalist practitioners would be of a lower order. Moreover, Chapman (1983) along the same vein of concern warned that the continued division of nursing practice into specialist roles would have an adverse impact on the provision of holistic care to patients. Chapman (1983) also proposed that as nurses accumulated their specialist skills and knowledge, they would be jealously guarded and employed amongst other things to strengthen their power and status.

The evidence, however, suggests that specialists in the community have selective 'hands-on' practice; thus they are neither infringing nor assuming the practice of district nurses (Haste & MacDonald 1992). This research has also emphasised that specialist nurses were viewed in a positive way by district nurses because of their resource role, counselling skills and teaching. In addition, the introduction of specialists led to improvements in the knowledge base of district nurses, patient care and communication between hospital and community. This was evident in another study which examined the patterns of community nursing for patients with HIV/AIDS (Layzell &

McCarthy 1993). The findings revealed that both patients and nurses benefit from the expertise and knowledge of specialists. Indeed, various studies have singled out the advice offered to patients and to community nurses as valuable, suggesting that they developed their knowledge and expertise as a result of discussions with specialist nurses (Graves & Nash 1991, Griffiths & Luker 1994, Haste & MacDonald 1992).

While district nurses have perceived that with the introduction of CNSs they would assume a minor position and their role would be eroded, this has not been supported in the literature (Haste & MacDonald 1992). Instead, many have sought to adopt some of the functions of specialist nurses but have been hampered by heavy caseloads and time constraints. Managers in contrast prefer to retain a generalist skill-mix rather than managing a group of independent practitioners, and feel that district nurses should be facilitated in acquiring the skills of the specialist (Haste & MacDonald 1992).

Perhaps another crucial issue emanating from these studies is that many specialists in the community are under-used and misused (Haste & MacDonald 1992). Arguably, because these roles have not been fully understood, their potential has not been realised and in some instances they have been perceived as a threat to the power base. For example, in one survey conducted in North America, it was noted that community health agencies have been unclear as to the benefits of masters-prepared CNSs. These nurses were thus employed either as administrators or educationalists and, as such, underscoring the 'multifaceted role' at the organisation's disposal (Mason et al 1992). To ensure effective utilisation of specialist and advanced practitioners in the community, nurses must be proactive in articulating their contributions to local and national health targets, in terms of providing skilled and cost-effective interventions which promote the well-being of the population.

Arguably, criticism of the maturity of the advanced nursing practice concept could be attributed to the dispute between the generalists and specialists. According to White (1985) this conflict has revolved around issues of professionalism, autonomy and accountability. For example, the generalist lobby has maintained that nursing is a practical occupation which does not depend on an academic base and that a first level registration is adequate preparation. Clearly, by denouncing the rationale for developing nursing expertise in a specific field of practice or need for life-long study, generalists and managerialists have attempted to regulate the profession. Equally, it may be reasoned that this explanation goes some way in disclosing why official acceptance of specialist and advanced practice has been slow to develop. More recently, the profession has witnessed the growth of more technical roles being performed by nurses, including surgeon's assistants in cardiac and laparoscopic gall bladder surgery (Bowey & Caballero 1996, Holmes 1994), and inserting central lines (Hamilton et al 1995). In other areas, at the instigation of medical consultants, nurses have been trained to provide the services associated with house officers (Dowling et al 1995, 1996, McDougall 1994). These innovations have been often described as advanced nursing roles; however, they do not fulfil the requirements as stipulated by the profession (UKCC 1994a, 1996c). The reasons include that the workload of these individuals remains non-nursing, based around prescribed protocols, and the nurses are clinically accountable to a consultant or a GP. In addition, in these posts the individuals are neither broadening nor pushing forward the horizons of nursing practice or patient care. Similarly, this applies to many nurse-led clinics which are utilising the skills of practitioners as a cost-effective substitute for a physician's time and thus reducing health care costs (Bowey & Caballero 1996, Mackie 1996, Marsh & Dawes 1995). There are, however, exceptions of nurse-led clinics running parallel to medical care where practitioners are able to make decisions without direct medical supervision and patients are reportedly highly satisfied with the care provided (Hill 1997).

This momentum of expanding similar roles in the primary care sector has also been evident. The rationale for this commitment has been endorsed by a range of bodies whose aim appears to ensure that national health targets are realised. To achieve this requires an adaptable and flexible workforce that is able to respond to changing health patterns; provide immediate access to meet the needs of the population; accommodate the reduction in junior doctors' hours and produce cost savings (DoH 1986a, 1994a, Healy 1996, NHSE 1996c).

The effect of NHS community reforms has also increased workloads for nurses and GPs because patients with higher-dependency needs are being discharged earlier into the community. This has led to a need for the updating and acquiring of additional skills. Consequently, many nurses have undertaken new extended roles or developed clinical roles within the community in order to achieve general practice contracts and/or to provide a range of other services. The claims advanced by reformers is to offer nurses opportunities for shaping the provision of primary and community health care in the next millennium, as well as enhancing job satisfaction and equity with GPs. Arguably, the sub-text of these documents is a recognition that nurses can deliver an efficient and effective alternative to health care provision in an era of increasing financial restraints.

However, while maximising the use of resources and skills is important for the Health Service, such roles rarely encompass the core values of nursing. Manley (1996) and Smith (1995) thus argue that the adoption of medical roles/tasks under the semblance of nursing titles serves only to expand practice by the medicalisation of nursing and this may jeopardise the core beliefs implicit within the current framework. It may also be reasoned that this unconditional acceptance of a medical approach may also stifle further professional initiatives. Indeed, the obvious distinction between nursing at specialist and advanced levels, and many of the roles cited above, is that these nurses are unsupervised by physicians but are proactive in terms of responding to both the individual consumer and organisation's needs by continuously developing and redefining the boundaries of clinical practice, education and research.

Misconceptions of specialist and advanced practitioners are also linked with extended roles. A study by Fox (1995) reported that senior nurse executives within trusts defined advanced practice as the ordering of chest X-rays, venepuncture and cannulation as central components of this level of nursing. Similarly, McGee et al (1996) conducted a national survey and identified that many individuals held the title of specialist or advanced nurse practitioner. However, under the area of clinical practice, similar work activities as those described by Fox (1995) were evident, including the verification of expected deaths, drug prescribing, suturing, treating minor injuries and managing nurse-led units. It thus appears that those in the position to appoint staff conceive the accumulation of certificates in extended roles as equating with a higher and sophisticated level of practice.

It would appear that the confusion and arguably acceptance within the profession has been constrained by this upsurge in nursing titles which continue to be used interchangeably, and by the diversity of roles which all claim to be either specialist or advanced nursing roles. The situation is untenable. Potential stakeholders may question any commitment to investing in a clinical career framework when there is disparity in the preparation and expertise of specialists and advanced practitioners. Clearly, for the sake of patients and the profession, the regulation and accreditation of practice and academic study must be immediate and broad enough to encompass the range of professional developments occurring within nursing.

Issues regarding educational preparation for specialist and advanced nursing practice

Debates in this area usually relate either to the academic level, whether the programmes are practice focused, relevant, or to funding issues. With regard to the expected level of education (UKCC 1994a), this raises a number of practical issues. For example, Dyson (1992) has suggested that the growth in post-registration courses and the emphasis on higher education has altered nurses' perceptions of the value of their registration and clinical practice. This situation has been compounded, as now most programmes of learning carry academic credit at either diploma, degree or higher levels. So, rather than elevate clinical expertise, a preoccupation with specialist or advanced practice may adversely lead to over-concern with academic accreditation. This has been reinforced by the relationship between clinical progression and academic achievement. In addition to this, with senior staff absent from the clinical environment because they are pursuing further studies, the development, clinical supervision and training of junior nurses and learners is threatened, which may have negative effects on standards of care owing to factors such as poor skill-mix and mentorship support.

Another area of major discussion relates to the education of ANP. The Council did not indicate the type of preparation or qualification necessary for this level of work. However, it acknowledged that advanced level practice requires additional knowledge and skills which are likely to emerge from studying at master's degree level or higher (UKCC 1994a). This is certainly a requisite in North America (Frick & Pollock 1993, Pridham 1990) and a growing view supported by many in this country

(Boore 1996, Castledine 1983, 1996b, Davis 1993, Gibbon & Luker 1995). The rationale is that at the advanced level, higher cognitive levels and knowledge are required, which go beyond the narrow focus of specialist knowledge. Arguably, a higher degree prepares the individual with a deeper and broader research base which enables the nurse not only to analyse and synthesise various clinical situations, but to instigate and develop research that enhances the delivery and quality of care.

At present, the programmes to develop advanced nursing practice emphasise both a clinical focus and the enhancement of patient care. However, of those who have reported the progress of their cohorts, it is interesting to note the range of participants attending these courses. For instance, in a sample of three intakes comprising 45 students following an ANP programme, 24% of the cohort were teachers with a commitment to practice (Brown 1995). In Northern Ireland, Boore (1996) similarly reports that the majority of students undertaking an MSc in ANP (part of Doctor of Nursing Science programme) held positions in education (15 out of 24). Moreover, financial support within a cash-constrained health service is also unlikely to be forthcoming. Interestingly, of the seven practitioners who were enrolled in Boore's (1996) programme, only one was receiving financial assistance and few had minimal support for personal study. On the basis of this, it is likely that the number of clinicians qualifying for this level may remain relatively small; thus opportunities for expanding the boundaries of nursing practice may be limited. The provision of funds for clinical staff to become specialist or advanced practitioners and whether nurse educators should undertake master's degrees in ANP are issues which merit further debate.

With regard to clinical staff, O'Hanlon & Gibbon (1996) have suggested that one of the difficulties for accrediting SPs is that nurses are undertaking generalist degrees which are not directly relevant. Similarly, those with post-graduate qualifications such as Master in Education or Business Administration cannot assume the role of advanced level practice, as the orientation of their curricula will be very different from that found in dedicated programmes. By appointing nurses with educational or administrative master's degrees, Arena & Page (1992) suggest that employers will have set up the role to fail; additionally such strategy will create and promote the impostor phenomenon. This in turn will convey the wrong signals to potential nurses wishing to pursue a clinical career.

The relationship between practice and education has also been a source of professional debate within academic settings. It appears that professors of nursing perceive these two domains purely in academic terms (Davis & Burnard 1992). Moreover, if university professors do not conceive professional practice as equal to theoretical study, then certain cultural values will be conveyed to the students.

Additionally, it would appear that there are also differences of opinion between educationalists with regard to the educational preparation for ANP. As can be observed from the listening exercise that the UKCC (1996) undertook, some advocated that the eduction for ANP should be based on a list of 'occupational competencies gained from a structured period of study' which would involve demonstration of specific knowledge and skills. In contrast, others proposed that 'pathways to advanced practice needed to be fuelled by many different experiences, structured reflection and individual tailored study' (UKCC 1996). In addition, the second group stressed that the knowledge base should be eclectic and process orientated. Rolfe (1998) supports this model, arguing that the most appropriate approach is one by which the educationalist facilitates the expert practitioner in exploring their own practice to produce knowledge from that practice and to disseminate to others. Rolfe (1998) is clear that at this level, educationalist and clinician are working in partnership both as experts in their own right. In particular, rather than developing any kind of practical skills, Rolfe argues that (1998, p. 274) advanced practice courses should emphasise 'the interface between theory and doing, with how knowledge is translated into practice and with how knowledge is generated and extracted *from* practice'. What seems to be advanced both by the UKCC (1996) and Rolfe (1998) is that courses cannot prepare individuals for the role. However, curriculums should be framed around the individual's needs and the assessment guided by critical evaluation of his/her own progress, project reports, and by the use of learning contracts and portfolios. Accordingly, by encouraging the advanced nurse practitioner to critically evaluate and reflect on their practice, educationalists can concentrate on assessing the quality of the critical evaluation. Since educators cannot be ANPs due to a lack of clinical credibility, their authority to assess the expertise of advanced level clinicians must be questionable. However, the approach advocated by Rolfe (1998) does legitimise the role of educators in respect to the preparation of ANPs, in that their key function is concerned with facilitating and enabling an individual to develop high-level cognitive skills rather than being passively engaged with the transmission of knowledge.

Finally, because there is a lack of accord about what constitutes specialist and advanced practice, it must be questionable whether existing programmes share commonalities and whether they educate nurses to perform at these levels. Thus, until a clear definition emerges, the content and structure of educational curricula will reflect individual interpretations, rather than a national and international approach. This is clearly an urgent professional agenda since others such as GPs may decide what is adequate preparation for nurses to assume certain functional levels, with many also believing that they are ideal practice supervisors and teachers (Marsh & Dawes 1995). Likewise, if SNP and ANP models are designed by educationalists, they may not be viewed as relevant by those for whom they are intended; it may be questioned whether the programmes should be driven by clinicians.

Debates around the nature of professional autonomy of specialist and advanced nursing practice

A recent viewpoint suggests that the levels of nursing autonomy and independence have increased as a result of professional development, although whether this change has been determined by external forces or internally orchestrated is a growing issue of discussion (Mitchinson 1996). With reference to ANP, most advocates have indicated that at this level nurses should be able to act autonomously and independently in decision-making (Gibbon & Luker 1995, Pearson 1983, Sparancino 1992). Equally, the Council has stated that the preparation of SNPs will enable them 'to exercise high levels of judgement and discretion in clinical care', implying that this is a new expectation. However, within the community, independent practice has been well recognised. Nurses in these settings typically work unsupervised, maintain their own caseloads for which they are accountable, are able to diagnose, manage patients' illnesses and prescribe as well as refer patients to other relevant services or agencies (Andrews 1988, Burke-Masters 1986, Trnobranski 1994).

Perhaps the greatest area of contention is whether practitioners' work will become blurred with the adoption of extended and expanded roles (which are integral within specialist community nursing practice – UKCC 1994a), as well as the idea that nurses will have full autonomy over practice. Realistically, the level of independence in decision-making or for instigating a treatment is likely to be confined for two reasons. Firstly, as nurses become the employees of GPs, most of the work devolved to them which traditionally was performed by physicians will operate within tight protocols and policies. Secondly, as GPs become business oriented, their priorities will be directed to efficiency and effectiveness and not with professional nursing initiatives (Mitchinson 1996). As such, centralised control over decision-making may be the dominant approach that guides practice.

One recent study has also questioned the authenticity of clinical autonomy experienced by community psychiatry nurses (CPNs) (Morrall 1997). The data in this research were generated through a combination of qualitative methods on a sample of 10 nurses. The findings revealed that in practice decision-making was chiefly characterised by an ability to determine their own case-mix and caseloads. However, the CPNs were not able to regulate or influence inappropriate referrals, either from psychiatrists or GPs. In other instances they employed covert strategies to avoid work being directed to them. Morrall (1997) thus suggests that the autonomy gained by CPNs was by 'default' and 'it is not ... legitimate and socially sanctioned'. The level of independent practice resulted because the nature of their work is unsupervised and unobserved, as well as difficult to monitor. Similarly, in a phenomenological study of seven CNSs, the respondents, describing the realities of their post, stated that they often felt isolated, unsupported and disempowered in their role (Bousfield 1997). Typical of the sense of disempowerment theme was a lack of freedom to exercise their professional autonomy, being unable to function independently, and lack of support from peers, managers and other disciplines (Bousfield 1997). Thus, despite being recognised as clinical leaders, knowledgeable and competent, autonomy was not automatically conferred on these CNSs. It also seems evident that despite progress within nursing, institutional, interprofessional, legal and intraprofessional regulators appear to dominate and sanction the degree of autonomy exercised by nurses regardless of their status within the health service bureaucracy. Additionally, without direct authority the advanced practitioner may be ineffective. This is particularly apparent when the individual is in a staff position (Harrell & McCulloch 1987).

Hixon (1996) suggests that organisations/employers must provide SPs and ANPs with the potential for autonomy and accountability in order to realise their wide contribution. For example, primary health care teams can demonstrate support for innovation by encouraging the growth of such roles from within the group that in turn will contribute to the vision of the team (Poulton & West 1993). Without such arrangements, it is unlikely that improvements in nursing services or quality of care outcomes will accrue and neither will the successful integration of such nurses into the practice setting – a view that was shared by Bousfield's (1997) respondents. It is also suggested that freedom to practice within the scope of one's role to a maximum potential does not exclude consultation and collaboration with other health professionals; indeed, this is a fundamental requisite for successful integration. Ultimately though, the effectiveness of SPs/ANPs will remain largely dependent on external forces as these tend to demarcate the margins of nursing activity (Hixon 1996, Mitchinson 1996). The reviewing of employment contracts, levels of autonomy for professional judgements and independent practice may be one way forward. Mitchinson (1996) and Gibbon & Luker (1995) also suggest that educating nurses at advanced levels to function independently may also assure the public and the organisation that nurses act within the scope of their defined practice.

Integrational dilemmas for advanced practice roles

A number of problems have been identified in connection with appointments to advanced practice roles which it may be reasoned also apply to specialist practitioners. Because of the novelty, many of the issues have not been addressed even though they are well documented in the literature (Table 1.1). Moreover, as neither role belongs to the traditional image of nursing, they

Table 1.1   Documentation of problems associated with appointments to advanced practice roles

Problems experienced	Authors
Role ambiguity	Harrell & McCulloch 1986, Nash 1993
Professional isolation	Bousfield 1997
Role conflict	Bousfield 1997, Hamric & Taylor 1989
Line accountability	Harrell & McCulloch 1986, Haste & MacDonald 1992
Stress/lack of support	Bousfield 1997, Hamric & Taylor 1989, Harrell & McCulloch 1986, Nash 1993
Pressure to prove worth	Hamric & Taylor 1989, Harrell & McCulloch 1986, Nash 1993

challenge the orthodoxy of their role; not surprisingly they may be viewed with hostility, resentment and suspicion by nurse clinicians, managers and medical staff. Likewise, these individuals can be perceived as outsiders and a threat to the stability of a practice or primary health care team.

This is often compounded by a poor grasp of what the role functions of these practitioners entail, and the fact that there is an inconsistent agreement over the responsibilities and goals associated with ANPs in particular.

As a consequence, managers have difficulties in utilising and managing specialist and advanced practitioners skills. The problems confronted by nurses currently in these roles need to be debated if those who are being prepared are to be integrated successfully.

Lack of support seems to be a major problem experienced by newly appointed specialists and advanced practitioners. Manifestations of this have included inadequate endorsement of authority, visible approval or official recognition from either nurse managers or peers. As a result, many have reported feelings of frustration and demotivation (Bousfield 1997, Hamric & Taylor 1989, Harrell & McCulloch 1986). Feelings of isolation are also described as arising because of individuals not being linked to a unit, the nature of the job and as a result of not being given direction. In this country, Cole (1991) speculated that only about 10% of nurses would reach the standard of ANP and by implication the amount of peer support would be minimal for these individuals. Arguably, the need for regular appraisals, feedback and supervision should be compulsory to enable the professional development of the nurse. A further source of stress has been related to the job descriptions as these tend to be broad and therefore allow for individual interpretation (Nash 1993). Ensuring that there is congruence between the individual's development and the organisation's expectations is an important activity which must take place and be formalised into a written action plan.

Conflicts may also arise because there is a requirement that, at these levels, nurses monitor and improve quality and standards through the supervision of staff and research implementation (UKCC 1994a). In doing so, evaluative judgements will be made about practice issues, which may result in negative behaviours that exclude or resist innovation being directed at the SNP/ANP (Bousfield 1997, Harrell & McCulloch 1986). Rather than being viewed as advisors and leaders, those in such innovative posts may be disapproved of and viewed negatively. Pressures to succeed can create role conflict for many, as the expectations of colleagues, managers and other disciplines can be both diverse and demanding. Menard (1987) also noted that CNSs did not expect success in their endeavours until their second or third year; this may be a source of friction and may be a difficult aspect to live with.

Evaluating personal effectiveness is perhaps the most sensitive and pertinent issue. However, as noted above, measurable outcomes may not be immediate and may not, if evident, satisfy all stakeholders. Nash (1993) suggests that because of a lack of clarity within role expectations, there may be a reluctance to make a commitment by setting measurable targets following appointment. For some there may be a sense of inadequacy or discouragement by the immensity of the role. In addition, the limited evidence on the effectiveness of such roles may place a burden on individuals in the justifying of their post and worth. However, learning to cope during the early stages can be through various mechanisms, including networking, focusing attentions on a small project and identifying a mentor figure.

Collectively, the problems highlighted in Table 1.1 can lead to 'burn-out' syndrome (Bousfield 1997) with many resigning from these clinical roles as a result of the negative experiences encountered in attempting to manage and balance the demands of these multifaceted roles (Arena & Page 1992). The costs of inadequate integration of specialist and advanced posts into the clinical environment are substantial, for which Bousfield (1997) and Page &

Arena (1991) have made recommendations. Institutional and managerial endorsement and support, they suggest, are vital in legitimising the future development of such roles, as well as encouraging others to progress. At a more practical level, official recognition can be demonstrated by participation in committees, working parties and the introduction to key personnel. Orientation and scheduled meetings in the early stages can increase confidence and promote networking. Moreover this, in combination with assisting those at advanced practice level to set short-term realistic goals and priorities that contribute to patient care and the organisation's objectives, will enable a more productive use of time, build effective working relationships and greater self-image and esteem (Bousfield 1997, Hamric & Taylor 1989). More research on the experiences of SNPs, ANPs and employers would be of value in further enlightening how integration of these key roles into clinical practice can be expedited with minimal human and resource costs and be of benefit to patient care. Woods (1997) suggests that the phenomenon of ANP is a complex subject and advocates using case study design as this methodology may shed additional light on some of these issues. It would also be appropriate for the Council to outline how they intend to communicate their recommendations for practice and education following registration to the wider health care disciplines and trusts, so that they can accept and understand the rationale and vision of nursing.

CONCLUSION

The ideology of a clinical career structure seems to be embedded in a need to strengthen the profile of clinical practice, to develop the quality of patient care and push forward the boundaries of nursing practice, education and research. Many of the examples cited have illustrated how SNP and ANP, through their unique contribution, have ensured the smooth and safe transition of children from hospital to the community setting, as well as enabled families to cope, through advice tailored to their needs. Other examples have demonstrated the effectiveness of this calibre of nurse in reducing the incidence of complications, promoting recovery, symptom management, and reducing the readmission rates of chronically ill patients. These improvements have been both cost-effective and related to government targets with many resulting in policy changes at the instigation of these advanced-level nurses. It is thus unquestionable that the clinical structure is here to stay as it offers much to the consumers of nursing services, the organisation and profession.

Despite this, it is self-evident that there are many areas of debate that need to be brought into the open and resolved before wholesale acceptance and promotion of both specialist and advanced nursing practice is declared. The current analysis seems to provide few answers to enable the profession to respond to internal and external demands. This is partly due to the lack of consensus over role expectations, titles, associated educational preparation/standards, level of autonomy and strategies for integrating nurses into a clinical career structure within a hierarchical and bureaucratic system of health care. A unified commitment that draws expertise from all nursing disciplines must continue to enable the profession to reach a satisfactory conclusion.

In terms of predicting the future, there are suggestions that one way forward that will serve the needs of a changing society, which also takes into account professional issues and patterns of health care provision, is the development of an advanced practice and nurse practitioner roles (Busen & Engleman 1996, Gilliss 1996, Kitzman 1989). This has the advantage of enabling nurses to combine preventive care, decrease costs, maintain continuity and holistic nursing services, as well as maximising the contribution to patient care. The blending of both roles can allow the registration of practitioners, providing they fulfil the criteria for specialist nursing practice, who will be capable of providing a broader range of services within a nursing framework, and assume greater responsibility for patient and family over a time continuum. In addition, external recognition from GP fund-holders and government may be forthcoming, as the potential for achieving national and local targets may be more feasible. In this country such roles are seen as ideal for primary care since they advocate utilisation of sophisticated assessment and evaluative skills, and a direct clinical role, as well as promoting collaborative practice – although it is envisaged that such roles will penetrate the 'grey zone' between nursing and medicine even further (Gibbon & Luker 1995).

In respect of education, a European project in the form of an international masters' programme in ANP seems to have succeeded and has established strong links with various universities (Davis 1993). Whilst it is recognised that health care provision varies across Europe and that there are cultural differences, studying with nurses from different nationalities in higher education is one advantage, as is a potential for cultural exchanges. However, the temptation for British nurses to work within Europe may not materialise, as in many countries opportunities for career progression, wages and professional recognition of community nursing are poor. However, through collaborative endeavours this may change.

Other initiatives that are beginning to respond to the current challenges include a framework for an ANP/consultant nurse role which links functions to context and outcomes (Manley 1997). Transformational leadership was a central theme which facilitated the adoption of a culture which empowered staff to become leaders and develop their practice further. In contrast, Castledine (1997) has proposed a clinical career structure that may accommodate those with a bias towards medical models of practice, generalist or specialist nursing. This would bring greater coordination and reduce the number of titles, as well as overcome the existing confusion within and external to nursing. This is an imperative that the profession needs to address and for which the luxury of time and debate has expired.

SUMMARY

Since the publication of 'The Future of Professional Practice' (UKCC 1994), much has been written about the specialist and advanced nurse practitioners. The evidence would suggest that individuals prepared to these levels of practice make a difference to patient outcomes and are able to effectively respond to the challenges of contemporary health care. It would appear, however, that there are a number of key areas that have not been addressed. These are in regard to the diversity of existing titles, consensus over functions associated with specialist and advanced practitioners, standards for preparation to these levels and whether these individuals can legitimately exercise autonomy and clinical discretion. Other unresolved dilemmas centre on whether nurse practitioners satisfy the Council's criteria for specialist or advanced practice, and whether the profession and Health Service can effectively integrate these nurses into the clinical environment.

POSTSCRIPT

Since the completion of this chapter, the UKCC has decided, following extensive consultation, not to pursue setting standards for ANP for the time being. Instead, it has decided to address the wide issues surrounding specialist practice and to consider whether those with Clinical Nurse Specialist or Nurse Practitioner roles can be incorporated within a much more simple and coherent framework.

It has equally submitted that 'higher level practice' may be a more appropriate term to embrace the notion of specialist level practice and to reduce the existing confusion amongst consumers, the professions and employers (UKCC 1998a). However, it has been proposed that to ensure that the public are protected, the regulation of those practising at a higher level will be mandatory. In addition, for individuals to gain recognition of higher level practice they will be expected to complete a programme of education to a nationally approved standard; be registered with the UKCC and regularly offer notification of their intention to continue practising at this level; finally, practitioners will be assessed for clinical competency against specified criteria, including the submission of reflective accounts and other relevant supportive evidence (UKCC 1998b).

2

Evidence-based practice

Jenny Littlewood   Mary Saunders

For many nurses the current term evidence-based health care (EBHC) will mean the same as research-based practice. However, despite similarities the two are different and the first part of this chapter seeks to explore what is understood by EBHC and its relevance for nursing practice. The second section examines how practitioners may develop skills necessary for this approach and the third section gives details of resources that may be accessed in the search for evidence.

HISTORY

Evidence-based health care has been defined as the conscious and explicit use of current best evidence in making decisions about care of individual patients. The practice of evidence-based medicine (EBM) means integrating individual clinical experience with best-available external evidence from systematic reviews of research (Sackett 1997). Cochrane, the originator of this approach, had not only effectiveness and efficiency as central to the search for best practice but also equity (Cochrane 1972). Within equity, he suggested, would be contained the notions of quality and humanity, though he did not specifically explore equity within his own book. Much of the current work on EBM has been developed at McMaster University, Sackett being its most famous proponent both in Canada and in its development in this country. The emphasis of EBM concentrates on effectiveness and efficiency in the form of therapeutic outcomes, using the randomised control trial as the method of choice in delineating variables and explaining outcomes. It is this emphasis that has led to controversy as much evaluation of nursing practice has not been based on this approach. Indeed it has been strongly argued that process approaches and quality issues are the essence of nursing care (Cowley & Casey 1995).

WHY THIS APPROACH?

The thrust for this approach has come from changes in financing the health service and some attempts to prioritise health care demands and patient needs. 'The New NHS' (DoH 1998a) has six important principles underlying the changes. The first two set the tone: that the National Health Service (NHS) is committed to fair access, high-quality, prompt and accessible service across the country; that it is committed to national standards being a local responsibility, local doctors and nurses will 'be in the driving seat' to shape the service. Recently, the focus of the health service has placed a strong emphasis on a research and development strategy focusing on clinical effectiveness, cost-effectiveness, value for money and quality assurance. Since the 1970s, various initiatives in the NHS have attempted to control costs of health care by focusing on efficiency manifested as an increase in productivity (the relationship between inputs and outputs, for example the number of bed days per operation) (Muir Gray 1997). However, efficiency is the relationship between inputs and outcomes (for example the number of extra bed days to obtain 1 extra year of life). Throughout the 1980s increased efficiency was still demanded but there was an emphasis on quality improvement with reference to work on costs involved and quality of life (QALYs) and disability (DALYs). Patient expectations were increased and clinical audit and other quality assurance mechanisms were introduced. In the 1990s the focus is on 'doing the right things right'. This period of intense change, incorporating the market principles of instability, insecurity, dehumanisation, fear, administrative chaos, lack of trust, different ethical stances from most health workers, have been discussed elsewhere (Littlewood 1995a). Evidence-based health care may be seen as adding stability to an otherwise chaotic world. 'The New NHS' (DoH 1998a) moves somewhat from market-led NHS to partnership and performance, quality being brought more clearly into underlying principles which incorporate the consumer perspective and need. Educational and clinical research will be increasingly valued, performance management oriented to quality and efficiency will be the hallmark. Purchasers and providers will have more opportunity to work together to plan local provision of health care. More importantly, the new NHS will extend the role of the expert nurse in acute and community care in the leadership and educational role which will cross organisational and professional boundaries, further emphasising the Government's commitment to continuity and integration of care. A quality organisation will ensure that evidence-based practice is in day-to-day use, with the infrastructure to support it.

The term EBM has been broadened to encompass health care in general and can be described as a movement initiated by a broad coalition of clinicians, researchers, educators, policy makers and others to accelerate and improve the application of evidence from sound clinical care research to clinical practice. It is essentially concerned with shifting organisational culture and individual behaviour so that a greater proportion of decisions in health care are based on research evidence. Assessment of the rigour and applicability of available research evidence and synthesis of research findings on a particular topic are regarded as cornerstones of evidence-based health care (Pickering 1997). However, a model developed for medicine is seen as inappropriate for nursing and other professions as it does not fully embody the principles of other disciplines. One of the key assumptions in evidence-based medicine is that the randomised controlled trial (RCT) is the best way to evaluate the effectiveness of interventions and a better basis for clinical decision-making than the clinical experience of the practitioner. Many nurses would refute this and cite Carper (1992) who identified empirical knowledge as only one way of many ways of knowing. Goding (1997), for example, discusses the use of tacit knowledge in health visiting practice and argues that practice guided by this is integral to the aesthetic experience of allowing the health visitor to see the whole problem rather than concentrating on the parts, combined with emphasis on the meaning rather than detail. This appears to be seen as a component of many specialist community nursing practices seeing clients outside of a hospital within the context of their own home, school or work.

THE GROWING NEED FOR EVIDENCE-BASED HEALTH CARE

The growing need for EBHC has come about because of the findings that current medical and nursing intervention may be as effective as the use of placebos; the idea of the rate of golden thirds (one-third get better, one-third stay the same and one-third die regardless of intervention); the existence of medical pluralism where cheaper forms of intervention may be as effective; situations where it may be patients' choice to reject the 'custom and practice' of past practitioner intervention if there is little evidence to support it.

However, considerable concern was raised by the Oregon experiment where the public were asked to decide the priorities for the health services. Cosmetic surgery was almost top of the priority and other more medically obvious priorities such as fractures were lower down. Further, a high proportion of people genetically at risk of developing cancer opted for radical surgery to prevent the possibility of its development.

Decisions in health care are made combining three factors: evidence, values, resources. Some of the factors influencing the need for EBM came from the need to rationalise resources in an increasingly ageing population. Some of the issues impacting on care are an ageing population, new technology and knowledge, patient expectations, easy access, high quality, redress and compensation for failures, professional expectations.

WHAT IS UNDERSTOOD BY EBHC?

The need for better assessment of effectiveness is not new. Normand (1996) suggested that the growth of work on effectiveness is more a response to changing understanding and attitudes rather than a change in the issues. Challenges to belief in the effectiveness of particular interventions and indeed questioning of the whole role of medicine and health care have opened up the debate. He states that evidence in nursing 'can be difficult to establish because of the complex nature of the objectives, that the interventions themselves are complex and there are many measurement difficulties'. He identified that it was risky to suggest that, because of the complexity, one should not try, as nursing has, like all other disciplines, to show that it is necessary and can defend a distinct and effective body of manpower.

Deighan & Boyd (1996) identified the strengths of EBHC:

- The practice of EBHC may help to overcome the political factors such as rationing schemes that are imposed on health boards, and may help providers make better use of limited resources by enabling them to evaluate and prioritise clinical effectiveness of treatments and services.
- EBHC has the potential for improving continuity and uniformity of care through common approaches and guidelines developed by practitioners.
- The use of individual clinical expertise as an important part of the prognosis of evidence-based health care can be reflected in more effective and efficient diagnosis and in more thoughtful identification and compassionate use of individual patient predicaments, rights and preferences in making clinical decisions about their care.
- The use of external clinical evidence could invalidate previously accepted diagnostic tests and treatments and possibly replace them with new and more powerful, more accurate and safer diagnostic mechanisms. Without current best evidence, practice is likely to become out of date rapidly to the detriment of patient care.
- EBHC helps to identify those clinical acts whose performance will meet the growing demand for increased clinical quality and will help with their appropriate purchasing and provision.
- As more clinical care is provided by health care teams, evidence-based health care provides a common language through which we can communicate multiprofessionally and rules of evidence by which we can agree on who will do what to whom.

Deighan & Boyd (1996) then list the weaknesses of EBHC:

- Other values might be included, not just those of effectiveness and efficiency, and equity of access and ethics beyond health economics may be sought.

- EBHC may be seen as a threat in exposing out-of-date practice.
- There is a lack of tools to evaluate the impact that the use of evidence is having upon clinical and managerial decision-making.
- Changing to EBHC may overburden workers already exhausted by change.
- Introducing EBHC clinical effectiveness and clinical guidelines will not necessarily reduce costs in the short term as the most effective treatment may not be the cheapest.
- The use of evidence will have to be incorporated into policy decisions.

They suggest that thinking about ways of measuring effectiveness might involve: the quality of the process; short- and long-term outcomes; providing approaches other than the RCT; measuring 'difficult to measure outcomes' (e.g. support or comfort); proof of efficacy.

Muir Gray (1997) identifies the following skills for practising evidence-based decision-making:

- the ability to define criteria such as effectiveness, safety and acceptability
- an ability to find articles on the effectiveness, safety and acceptability of a new test or treatment
- an ability to assess the quality of the evidence
- an ability to assess whether the results of research are generalisable to the whole population from which the sample was drawn
- an ability to assess whether the results of the research are applicable to the 'local population'.

IMPLICATIONS FOR HEALTH CARE PROFESSIONALS IN PRIMARY CARE

There are several 'levels' of evidence-based health care. First, there is the individual level, where practitioners aim to ensure that their practice is based on the best known evidence. Rosenberg & Donald (1995) have identified four steps that they feel can be translated across professional boundaries: formulation of a clear clinical question from the patient's problem; a thorough search of the literature for relevant clinical articles; evaluation (critical appraisal) of the evidence for its validity and usefulness; the implementation of useful findings in clinical practice.

However, White (1997) suggests that although at first glance these steps appear to be straightforward, difficulties may be encountered at each step. In community nursing formulating a clear question may be complex. It is usually easier to formulate questions about interventions that use health care technology than about those that use the therapeutic interpersonal skills of the nurse. In community nursing this could be illustrated by contrasting a nurse deciding on the best treatment for a wound where the clinical problem is relatively clear with a health visitor who identifies a mother with postnatal depression.

White (1997) identifies three areas to be addressed before the second step can be achieved: access to the literature; the person who is trying to answer the question must have literature-searching skills; research on the question being posed must be available in the literature – however, this does not take into account new fields where there may be a paucity of research.

Research shows that GPs have limited library resources (Sackett 1997). But there are guides to aid searches (Oxman et al 1994) though difficulties of access remain (McColl et al 1998, Millard 1997). It is likely that the situation is the same for community nurses. For some community nurses, access to libraries or databases is made more difficult by their employment status, e.g. occupational health nurses who may not have access to NHS library facilities, nurses who are not registered with universities may not have access to their library facilities and whilst schools of nursing libraries have now been integrated into universities, centralisation of facilities may cause increased travelling time. However, there are a number of different strategies becoming available that may assist in literature searching and these are discussed in the final section of this chapter.

The history of nursing research is relatively short but Mead (1996) highlighted the following areas where nursing research had developed significantly:

- *effective models of care* (significant impact on patient outcomes and cost-effectiveness)
- *patient teaching* (impact on shorter patient stay)
- *quality of nursing care* (a broad area encompassing direct patient care, patient safety, patient satisfaction, quality assurance)

- *reducing patient mortality* (research on direct patient care and research into skill-mix, the ratio of registered nurses is related to quality of care)
- *cost-effectiveness* (a relatively under-researched area).

The ICN (1996) identifies areas where nursing research makes a difference: answering needs; identifying effective models; patient teaching; quality of care – direct nursing, patient safety, patient satisfaction, quality assurance; reducing mortality; cost-effectiveness; improving the work environment.

White (1997, p. 177) highlights that: 'nursing is a young discipline and much exploratory and descriptive research needs to be carried out before the hypothesis testing stage is reached. A great deal of evidence, therefore may be neither the right type or sufficiently rigorous to place it high in the evidence hierarchy'.

The last sentence highlights one of the issues with EBHC. If the gold standard has been randomised controlled trials, other methods may appear to have less credibility. Broadening the scope of studies reviewed to include the 'grey literature' (reports or documentation that remains local) and the establishment of a centre for evidence-based nursing may have an impact on the range of credible methods.

The third step, evaluating the literature, requires nurses to have critical appraisal skills to evaluate the quality of the research. More recent nurse education has included appraisal skills as an integral part of pre-registration programmes. Current community specialist practitioner programmes are at degree level and will certainly include research methodology and processes and critical appraisal skills within the curriculum. The clinical leadership and management role of specialist practitioners means that there is a much greater awareness of clinical effectiveness, quality assurance and change management necessary for present-day community nurses. Consequently the skills necessary for practising evidence-based health care are more likely to be in place for the future. Some nurses are undertaking research projects as part of their degree and master's level studies, and there needs to be greater support from management and educationalists in identifying areas where evidence is sparse, as possible research topics, and in supporting students through to publication. However, the relative isolation of some community nurses and differing educational opportunities and peer support make this an area of concern.

The fourth step involves integrating sound research into practice and using this to inform clinical decision-making. At a wider level, findings can be disseminated to small groups or within the organisation and contribute to the development of clinical guidelines.

A fifth step should be evaluation of performance. Despite best intentions and the quality of the research evidence, performance still needs to be evaluated. RCTs are rigorously controlled and the application of findings may not sit comfortably within normal situations where many variables cannot be controlled. Although application of research-based evidence must take clinical judgement into consideration, evaluation and feedback to those developing guidelines is essential.

The ICN suggested that to improve the impact of research its relevance and rigour required greater attention. What was also required was appropriate dissemination by publication, presentations at conferences and so forth; evidence of its utilisation; then research into its utilisation; assuring potential for utilisation; and exploration of ways of using research in practice.

Mechanisms for encouraging EBHC

The discussion so far has focused on the individual adopting an evidence-based approach to practice. However, locally or nationally based guidelines are a widely advocated mechanism for encouraging EBHC. Many organisations support groups with a remit to produce guidelines on interventions or patient management issues. Conroy & Shannon (1995) identify the purpose of clinical guidelines as setting out the optimum management approach for a given condition, developed in the belief that they will improve health care outcome, health service efficiency and reduce levels of inappropriate practice. However, the success of guideline implementation depends on a number of factors, not least of which is whether the guidelines are easily available. However, practitioners still need to adopt a critical approach to guidelines and ask the following questions:

- How has the guideline been constricted and was the approach used in its construction systematic and sound?

- Do the guidelines draw on research evidence and clearly specify which of the elements are evidence-based and which are not?
- Is the evidence referenced? (Pickering 1997).

Practice nurses have been used to drawing up protocols for use in the practice management of certain chronic diseases. However, often these have been based on identifying roles and procedures rather than the best approach to effective practice. Many local guidelines draw on national guidelines such as those developed for asthma, hypertension and diabetes. However, the same questions must be applied to national guidelines and local factors taken into consideration when adapting them for local use. Box 2.1 identifies one format for the critical review of clinical guidelines.

Cluzeau et al (1995, 1997) have been at the forefront of developing an instrument for the purpose of critically appraising guidelines. There are a number of organisations that produce guidelines, for example the Royal College of General Practitioners, Scottish Intercollegiate Guidelines Network (SIGN), Clinical Standards Advisory Group, and a guidelines database is being set up by the Institute of Health Sciences, Oxford.

Clinical guideline implementation is fraught with difficulty. Despite the potential for improving practice there are a number of obstacles to be overcome. One common fear of practitioners is the potential reduction of clinical freedom in the managing of care and the stifling of innovation. However, the issue of clinical freedom can also mask inappropriate and inefficient practice. The rise of consumerism in the health services also means that patients should have the security of knowing that whatever nurse they see will provide them with a certain minimum standard of cost-effective care. Access to medical data on the Internet is likely to mean that patients have access to much more information, not only about their condition but also the most effective way of treating it.

Another issue in relation to the implementation of guidelines is that of ownership. Studies within general practice showed that participation in the development of guidelines encouraged implementation, as opposed to guideline implementation where the target general practitioners had no involvement in the development process (North of England Study of Standards and

Box 2.1 Questions (North Thames Research Appraisal Group)

1. Validity of the recommendations
1.1 Objective:
   a. Are the primary objectives of the guidelines clear?
   b. Are the health problem and desired outcome clearly stated?
   c. Is it clear in what setting the guidelines are to be used and which patients are to be targeted?
1.2 Evidence:
   a. Were all reasonable attempts made to identify and consider all available evidence?
   b. Was an explicit and sensible process used to identify, select and combine evidence? (Has the evidence been interpreted correctly, is it applicable to the population of interest?)
   c. How strong is the evidence?
1.3 Development:
   a. Who has produced the guideline? Have all key disciplines and interested parties, including patients, contributed to their development?
   b. Is there evidence of consultation or piloting of guidelines?
   c. Have the guidelines been subjected to a credible external review process?
   d. Have local circumstances been considered?

2. Use of the recommendations
2.1 Implementation:
   a. Are the guidelines clear, unambiguous and easy to read?
   b. Are clear recommendations made which are linked to recent available evidence?
   c. Are important and reasonable caveats identified?
   d. Are the guidelines to be used in the context of a clinical consultation process?
   e. Do the guidelines indicate how patient preferences are to be incorporated into decision-making?
   f. Do the guidelines state how and when they are to be reviewed?
   g. Do the guidelines offer ways to monitor the recommendations?
2.2 Dissemination:
   a. Is it clear how the guidelines are intended to be disseminated?
   b. Is the dissemination process one which is likely to be effective?

3. Value of the recommendations
3.1 Process of care:
   a. Is there evidence that the guidelines influence clinical practice?
3.2 Outcome of care:
   a. Is there evidence that the guidelines affect the outcome of care?
   b. From whose point of view are the outcomes valued?
   c. Is the outcome of value to my patients?
3.3 Cost of care:
   a. Have the benefits and harms of guideline implementation been considered?
   b. Have the costs of guideline dissemination and implementation been examined?

Performance in General Practice 1992). This must, however, be balanced against the cost of producing high-quality, authoritative guidelines, which can be a difficult and time-consuming process. The middle way is probably to encourage local modification of centrally developed guidelines to meet local needs. This participation may help to achieve the sense of ownership necessary for change.

Millard (1997) conducted a study which investigated how it was planned to implement guidelines from SIGN. Of the 11 guidelines published to March 1997, only 6 out of 11 community trusts had implemented, or were planning to implement, SIGN guidelines (three for prophylaxis of DVT and one each for diabetic retinopathy, immediate discharge and diabetes in children). It appears that local consensus directed the setting of priorities, with the priorities of the local health board being taken next into consideration. The study showed that there was a large demand for the sharing of local versions of guidelines and yet only 3 of the 46 trusts intended to disseminate local versions of guidelines to other trusts in the same area. There was a demand for the sharing of local versions and the reason for the low intended level of sharing needs further research, possibly to devise incentives to share.

A study by McColl et al (1997) to determine the attitude of general practitioners towards evidence-based medicine and their related educational needs showed that most respondents thought the best way to move from opinion-based to evidence-based medicine was to use guidelines or protocols developed by colleagues for use by others. The authors of this study are currently carrying out a similar one with practice nurses and it will be interesting to see if the findings are similar. Shortage of time and lack of access to facilities, cited by GPs, are likely to be similar experiences for community nurses and mechanisms for sharing both evidence-based summaries and guidelines may need to be considered. One such mechanism is a pilot study in Southampton where two GPs are paid to prepare summaries of evidence-based medicine for their practices, and it is hoped that this will make it easier for local doctors to have access to such evidence to influence implementation. Conroy & Shannon (1995) highlight a range of factors that affect the implementation of guidelines. These include:

- implementation strategy not included within the development of the guidelines

- identification of a 'performance gap', i.e. a sense of dissatisfaction with current practice and a realisation that something should be done
- recognition that there is no evidence to date of an ideal strategy or intervention and local conditions and personalities need to be taken into account.

However, any guideline implementation strategy should have an impact at four levels (Conroy & Shannon 1995):

- increasing knowledge – making clinicians aware of the guidelines
- changing attitudes – such that clinicians agree with and accept the recommendations as a better standard of care
- changing behaviour – such that clinicians change their clinical practice to conform to the guidelines
- changing outcome – by improving patient health and quality of care.

Such an implementation strategy has an application within nursing. However, there are other factors that also impact on implementation, and organisational powerlessness is one. Nurses have to be working in an environment where the organisational culture facilitates innovation and research. Many community nursing interventions have a multidisciplinary approach and focus on care rather than treatment. Guidelines need to take into consideration the interprofessional collaboration necessary for much of the successful care delivered in the community. Muir Gray (1997) highlights the importance of quality management in operationalising EBHC. He advocates that the key components in an evidence-based service are:

- organisations designed with the capability to generate and the flexibility to incorporate evidence
- individuals and teams who can find, appraise and use research evidence (see Fig. 2.1).

Another issue that needs to be considered in relation to EBHC is that of litigation. Tingle (1997) highlights that with the use of clinical guidelines there is inevitably a commensurate increase in the awareness of potential legal issues. He highlights the importance of accurate documentation, particularly in the exercise of clinical discretion. Explanations for the variance from the

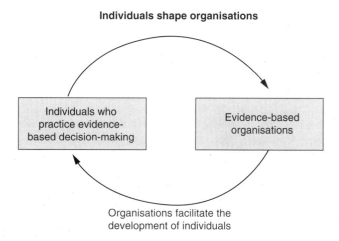

Figure 2.1 Key components of an evidence-based service.

guidelines must be fully documented and these trends should be subsequently analysed. Clinicians have a duty to consider the appropriateness of the guidelines to individual situations. However, he goes on to state that: 'Clinical guidelines are documents ... that represent channels of communication about patient care and properly drafted maintain an important potential to reduce health litigation and complaints (Tingle 1997, p. 640).

All guidelines should have a review date and be contemporary, evidence-based and reasonably achievable.

How are these applicable to nurses?

How is EBHC being operationalised within nursing?

The ICN definition of nursing research (ICN 1996) is: 'a systematic approach and a rigorous method with the purpose of generating new knowledge'.

Stevens (1997) suggested improving the integration between research and practice as a means of developing evidence-based health care. This was also an approach emphasised by Alsop (1997) in relation to professions allied to medicine, but particularly improving their skills for this approach. Kitson (1997) explored three implicit assumptions in the relationship between evidence-based medicine and clinical effectiveness, and demonstrated the essential pursuit of broadening methodologies to examine nursing practice.

As discussed earlier, evidence based on RCTs within nursing is relatively rare. Within community nursing one example evaluates the work of the district nurse and health visitor in relation to the elderly (Littlewood 1988); other examples are in relation to leg ulcers (Cullum 1994), hospital practice (Griffiths & Evans 1995), and venous ulcers (Layton et al 1994). In practice nursing guidelines for chronic disease management, where there is shared care between GPs and nurses, are in common usage and role exchange is being monitored (Richardson & Maynard 1995). Trusts are developing initiatives to produce evidence-based guidelines, and educational initiatives that offer units of accredited study for staff nurse grades are also developing. The educational packages have a theme of evidence-based practice in relation to clinical issues in the community but teach the participants the basic skills of literature searching and critical appraisal. Outcomes from the course are disseminated to others within local teams by seminars within working areas (Shuldham 1996).

Developing skills in critical appraisal

With a new development such as EBHC there is always a danger that it may become an academic exercise. Practitioners must feel that they have the necessary skills to participate effectively in the process. The next section highlights sources of information on EBHC that may be accessed by practitioners. However, many practitioners will want to examine their own practice and this section identifies the principle of critical appraisal.

The purpose of critical appraisal is to discover whether the methods and results of the research are sufficiently valid to produce useful information. Carter & Thomas (1997) provided an overview of this process for both quantitative and qualitative studies. They suggest that when faced with a large amount of literature, readers should first scan the titles, then look at the abstracts and, if it seems worthwhile, read the paper. It is useful to skim read the whole paper and then answer three questions:

- What is the message?
- Do I believe it?
- If true, how does it affect what I do at present?

If the answers are positive the paper should be critically appraised. There are many articles offering guidance on critical appraisal (Crombie 1996 – a pocket book providing checklists to use on different types of article, Fowkes & Fulton 1991). However, Carter & Thomas (1997) suggest the framework given in Box 2.2 for reviewing both methodologies.

Box 2.2 Framework for critical appraisal of quantitative and qualitative studies

Quantitative studies

Introduction:
What are the objectives of the study or the questions to be answered? Are they clearly stated? Is there a hypothesis? If not, why? Is the study ethical, has it been approved by an ethical committee? Literature review – is it adequate? Is it informative?

Method:
Design – is it appropriate to the objectives? Have the tools been piloted, e.g. questionnaires or interviews? Is there a control group or standard of comparison? What entry and exclusion criteria are used – are they valid? Does the timespan allow long enough for the outcome to occur?

Setting of the study – is it appropriate for the study and can the findings be related to your work?

Subjects – who makes up the sample, how big is it, was selection random, if not what attempts have been made to minimise bias? Were all the sample accounted for at the end?

Outcome measures – are there clear definitions of the criteria used, how were they developed, are they relevant to the objectives and reliable and reproducible?

What steps have been taken to minimise bias?

Qualitative studies

Abstract:
Is the qualitative approach the correct methodology? Although inductive in nature, the question should be clear by the time the research is written up.

Method:
Usually explained in greater detail. Detail should be given about the sample chosen, which should be sufficiently comprehensive to allow generalisability. Method of data analysis should be described and justified.

Box 2.2 (contd.)   Framework for critical appraisal of quantitative and qualitative studies

Quantitative studies

Results:
Are the findings clearly and objectively presented? Is sufficient detail given to allow readers to judge for themselves? Was the response rate adequate? What actions were taken with respect to non-responders or those lost to follow-up? Are the methods of data analysis appropriate for the nature of the data? Is the analysis performed and interpreted correctly? Are there sufficient data and analysis to decide if 'significant differences' are due to a lack of comparability between groups?

Discussion:
Have the initial objectives been reached, is the question answered or the hypothesis proved or disproved? Are the conclusions justified by the results? Are any results not explained? Are the results clinically significant and relevant to your colleagues or the profession generally? Consideration should be given to bias, confounding and chance.

Qualitative studies

Results:
Themes and concepts arising from the research should be clearly identified. What mechanisms have been used to validate the themes?

Results are likely to be much longer than in a quantitative paper – has enough of the original evidence been included to allow the reader to judge if the interpretation of the evidence is fair?

Discussion:
Should be based on the evidence presented and its analysis.

Systematic reviews and meta-analysis may provide important information. These are techniques for pooling research evidence on the effectiveness of a health care therapy or intervention. A systematic review is distinct from a descriptive literature review in that it is prepared using some kind of systematic approach to minimise biases and random errors and the components of the approach are described in detail in the methods section. Meta-analysis is a type of systematic review which involves the synthesis of research data from several studies to yield an overall summary statistic, although this method is not without its critics (Pickering 1997). Systematic reviews are published through the Cochrane Library (see below).

Many practitioners will already be involved in audit. If the audit cycle is completed, it should provide an excellent opportunity for evidence-based health care in practice. Evaluative research and audit are distinct but interrelated activities. Black (1992) identified that research involves establishing the value of health care where the results are generalisable, whereas audit involves assessing or monitoring the provision of health care to ensure that it is of as high a quality as research finding suggest can be expected and is essentially a local activity with the results being of value primarily at the specific time and place in question. The first stage of the audit cycle requires the identification of agreed standards and criteria and at this point the practitioner's knowledge of current best practice and guidelines available should inform this process. One of the key factors in successful audit is the implementation of change and, as previously discussed, this is a complex process in terms of individual behaviour and within organisational and professional cultures. Practitioners need to have an understanding of the principles of successful change management and there is much literature on this and, although not specific to evidence-based health care, it may offer useful approaches to follow. Integration of research findings into practice, however, has proved elusive (ENB 1995a, Foundation for Nursing Studies 1996, ICN 1996, McCleod Clark & Hockey 1989). However, evaluating what nurses do, its effectiveness in practice and education remains a cornerstone nationally and internationally (Hirschfeld 1998, Tierney 1998).

INFORMATION SOURCES ON EBHC

It has already been identified that many clinicians have limited time to search the literature for evidence and then critically appraise the material found. There are many new initiatives that have been or are in the process of being developed to help clinicians access relevant material. Below are a selection of resources.

Bandolier

This is a newsletter published by the NHSE Anglia and Oxford Research and Development Unit. It is designed to keep purchasers up to date with both local and national research on the effectiveness of health care interventions. There is free access to Bandolier on the Internet but publications may run several copies behind the printed version. For further information contact:

Pain Relief Unit
The Churchill Hospital
Oxford OX3 7LJ

Tel: 01865 226132
Fax: 01865 226978
Web site: http://www.jr2.ox.ac.uk/Bandolier/

CASP: Critical Appraisal Skills Programme

This is a UK project, started in Oxford, that aims to help health professionals develop skills in the critical appraisal of research evidence, in order to promote the delivery of evidence-based health care. Each region has, or is developing, its own CASP based on the Oxford model. Details of the national training programme are available from:

Oxford CASP Office
PO Box 777
Oxford OX3 7LF

Tel: 01865 226968
Fax: 01865 226959
Web site: http://www.ihs.ox.ac.uk/casp

Centre for Evidence Based Nursing

This is run from the Department of Health Studies at the University of York. Major current activities are: co-editing the journal *Evidence Based Nursing*; undertaking systematic reviews; undertaking primary research on nurses' use of information and decision-making; undertaking a systematic review of the clinical practice guidelines for nurses and PAMs. Further information is obtainable from:

Dr Nicky Cullum, Director
Centre for Evidence Based Nursing
Department of Health Studies
University of York

Innovation Centre
York Science Park
Heslington YO1 5DD
Tel: 01904 435222 or 01904 435137 (direct line)
Fax: 01904 435225

Centre for Reviews and Dissemination

The NHS Centre for Reviews and Dissemination (CRD) aims to identify and review the results of good-quality health research and to disseminate the findings to key decision-makers in the NHS and to consumers of health services. The review covers the effectiveness of care for particular conditions, the effectiveness of health care technologies and evidence on efficient methods of organising health care. It maintains databases of literature reviews and economic evaluations. Several databases are available through the CRD and librarians there will provide advice on searching for reviews of clinical effectiveness and economic evaluations and will conduct searches of their own databases free of charge. For further information contact:

NHC Centre for Reviews and Dissemination
University of York
York YO15DD
General enquiries: 01904 433648
Information service: 01904 433707
Web site: http://www.york.ac.uk/inst/crd

Cochrane Collaboration

The Cochrane collaboration is an international network of individuals who help to prepare, maintain and disseminate systematic overviews of the effects of health care interventions. The reviews are fed into the Cochrane Library. This is a computer database and is regarded as one of the key sources of information on high-quality trials research and systematic reviews. The Library contains:

- The Cochrane Systematic Review Database
- The Database of Abstracts of Reviews of Effectiveness (DARE) from the Centre for Reviews and Dissemination
- Abstracts of systematic reviews from ACP (American College of Physicians) Journal Club

- The Cochrane Clinical Trials Register (containing details of over 13 000 trials).

The database is available on CD ROM and available in many libraries serving nursing education.

Effective Health Care bulletins

These bulletins are based on a systematic review of literature on clinical effectiveness, cost-effectiveness and acceptability of health care interventions. They are produced by the CRD. Some of the published titles which may be of interest to community nurses include:

- Stroke rehabilitation
- The treatment of persistent glue ear
- Brief interventions and alcohol use
- Implementing clinical practice guidelines
- Treatment of pressure sores
- Preventing fall and subsequent injury in older people
- Preventing unintentional injuries in children and young people
- Preventing and reducing the adverse effects of unintended teenage pregnancies
- Obesity

Evidence Based Nursing (journal)

This is a new journal intended to help nurses by identifying and appraising high-quality, clinically relevant research and by publishing succinct, informative critical abstracts of each article together with commentaries from practising nurses who can place the new research in context. It is published quarterly by the RCN Publishing Group.

Guidelines Collaborators Directory

This directory is designed to share information and initiatives in collaborative work on guidelines related to nursing and to provide contact names in each of the contributing organisations. For further information contact:

Dynamic Quality Improvement Programme
Royal College of Nursing
Tel: 0171 872 0840

The list above is far from exhaustive. New resources are developing all the time and many disciplines are contributing to the growing literature on evidence-based health care. Apart from the resources listed, information may often be gained by contacting the regional offices of the NHSE who are likely to have their own developments or contacts with other organisations that may be of help. Organisations such as STaRNet in the South Thames Region have been set up to facilitate the development of EBHC and produce extensive resource packs for practitioners.

3

Advocacy and the mentally disordered offender

Nizam Mohammed

INTRODUCTION

To assist in understanding the role of the professional as an advocate in caring for the mentally disordered offender (MDO) it is important to examine the development of psychiatric care. Towards the end of the Dark Ages superstition was receding and witch hunting of the mentally disordered offender ceased; mental illness was explained as being due to superstition or being possessed by the devil. The mentally ill, however, were still being inhumanly neglected and allowed to roam; some perished. Those who survived long enough came before assizes and were committed to 'Bedlam', where many of them were permanently in chains, bedded in straw and went frequently naked. The inmates were exhibited by their keepers, and the lunatics at Bedlam were one of the sights of London, like 'bears at the Tower' (Clark 1958).

This general attitude gradually changed but took time. Pinel in Paris and Tuke at the Retreat of York ensured that there was a more positive attitude towards the mentally ill and saw these individuals as having rights. At the same time, several private 'mad houses' were established all over the UK, but gained a poor reputation due to the mentally ill being poorly treated. In these circumstances a select committee was set up by Parliament to investigate the care of the mentally ill (House of Commons Report 1763). As a result of this committee's findings, the first Act of Parliament, the Regulations of Mad Houses Act 1774, was passed to assist in caring for the mentally ill. It set up 'commissioners in lunacy' to supervise the running of institutions caring for the mentally ill (lunatics).

In 1835 with the reform of municipalities, power in the land was mainly vested in Justices of the Peace (JPs). Hunter & MacAlpine (1974) said 'in each county the JP met in Quarter Sessions, four times a year, to arrange affairs' and had the power to levy rates on the parishes 'for the maintenance and building of asylums'. They described these institutions as 'public institutions built for paupers and maintained by counties or boroughs; or hospital charities supported by voluntary contributions'.

The Lunacy Act

This Act of Parliament passed in 1828 indicated for the very first time where 'lunatics' should be cared for, that is, in institutions for the insane, the rationale being that during the preceding period 'lunatics had been poorly treated in Poor Law houses and houses of correction. During the period 1845–1860 the numbers of pauper lunatics rose from between 6500 to over 17 500, with no rights when kept in these institutions. However, the number of institutions continued to increase and the boom continued until the 19th century. At the same time, with the expansion in the economy, the number of potential recruits working within the institutions fell, owing to difficulty in attracting staff with the qualities necessary to care for the mentally ill.

Aldridge, writing in 1859, indicated that 'attendants had no training or preliminary instructions and had to learn their duties by what can be described as on-the-job training'. The attendants, however, considering all possibilities, did remarkably well in the performance of their duties.

The Commissioners of Lunacy (appointed since 1764 as a result of the 'Regulations of Madhouses Act'), when they undertook an examination of the role of the attendants, reported in 1858 that there must be some kind of training. They declared that 'under experienced and well trained professionals the bad habits of the patients had been removed.' In 1846, a handbook of duties was published by the Hanwell Institution (later known as St Bernard's Hospital, Southall), with others (Colney Hatch Asylum and Frien Hospital) soon following.

The Reverend Henry Hawkins, Chaplain of Colney Hatch Asylum, advocated a systematic training of attendants. He believed that the organisation for doctors, The Royal Medico-Psychological Association, should be responsible for the training. As this body was constituted in law with Royal Approval, it is believed that this must have set the scene for maintaining some rights of the individual, although this was not explicit. The first formal lectures were started in 1891 and successful candidates received the Royal Medico-Psychological Association's certificate. The first formal national training for any professions started about 1925. A search through the literature for this period indicates that patients' rights are either omitted or only briefly mentioned. Since their commencement, psychiatric nurse training and other professional training have undergone many changes and have been included in such reports as Platt, Salmon, Briggs and in the UKCC Project 2000: a new preparation for practice.

FORENSIC PSYCHIATRY AND FORENSIC PSYCHIATRIC CARE

Parker (1985) cites many examples of injustices in the creation of institutions caring for the mentally disordered offender (MDO) and the criminal justice system. 1810 saw the beginning of an argument between the Governors of Bethlem Hospital (Bethlem Royal and Maudsley) and the Under Secretary of State at the Home Office when he queried the possibility of setting aside part of a new hospital for a criminal lunatic asylum. Parker stated 'the new department should be under their absolute control and not be subject to visits from the country magistrates'. The lack of agreement is still seen today between clinicians and the 'C' Division of the Home Office, which has responsibility for the mentally disordered offender and, under the Mental Health Act 1983, has powers substantially to influence and even control clinical decisions (Mental Health Act 1983, Sections 41 and 49). This ongoing friction often results in the rights of the MDO not being recognised.

Parker, commenting on a select committee of the House of Lords appointed to enquire into the state of gaols, wrote 'witnesses agreed that it was undesirable to keep imprisoned people acquitted on the grounds of insanity or found to be insane on arraignment but there were often difficulties in transferring them to an asylum ... and due to the permissive character of the county Asylums Act 1808 many counties are without such provision' (Parker 1985).

Parker's quotation is extremely interesting when examining the rights of the MDO in the light of the Home Office/ Department of Health Circular 66/90 (Home Office/DoH 1992), which clearly states that no person detainable under the Mental Health Act 1983 should be detained in prison as such detention is a clear breach of the MDO's rights. This is because, when such individuals are detained in prisons, they are cared for by untrained professionals and are not given the care and treatment which is required.

Parker continued 'even when county asylums existed they were often reluctant to receive insane prisoners, knowing that the cost would fall on the parishes, whereas the expense of maintaining prisoners in gaols was met by the counties'. Similar problems continue to exist today because of the provider/purchaser split in the NHS, with both social services and the Home Office having responsibility. Hospitals rightly argue that if they are required to care for MDOs who would have otherwise gone to prison 'the money should go with the patient' and funds should be transferred accordingly. This does not, however, happen, and consequently there is still underfunding for MDOs.

The professional caring for the mentally disordered offender

A growing awareness of the links between mental disorder and clinical behaviour has led to increasing political, social, legal and professional pressure for the treatment of MDOs and to ensure that their rights are maintained. It is important to say, without pursuing any cause, that evolving legislation which offers 'defences' to certain defendants decrees that knowledge of an offender's 'mental disorder' at the time of committing an offence may permit a court to excuse the defendant of guilt and responsibility for his or her crime(s).

During the court process many expert witnesses, including psychologists and psychiatrists, give their opinions about the offender's mental state, diagnosis, prognosis and susceptibility to treatment. The court is then free to choose the options available to it in caring for the individual. Recommendations can be made to treat the individual in a special hospital such as Broadmoor, a medium secure unit or other such designated units rather than punish the individual under the criminal justice system. In the former institution, some rights are offered to the individuals under the jurisdiction of the Mental Health Act 1983. It must not be forgotten that the individual who is detained under the criminal justice system has all his or her human rights intact.

The Mental Health Act 1983 also allows for convicted prisoners to be transferred for psychiatric assessment and treatment to special hospitals, or other such environments, providing that the medicolegal justifications are met.

Burrow (1993) indicated that there is now a new and evolving role for professionals caring for the mentally disordered offender. This role involves the use of assessment skills to identify dangerousness, maintain control of the therapeutic environment and identify strategies aimed at targeting a client's health promotion and offending propensities.

Burrow (1991) stated that in some maximum security hospitals these intentions are achieved through a formidable battery of defensive procedures and technology. This policy works against the current policy in general psychiatry which has progressed from compulsory admission to voluntary admission, where open-door policies are fostered and where deinstitutionalisation of patients and closure of asylums is occuring, enhancing full integration of the mentally ill into society. A multidisciplinary approach to community care is replacing the medical model of care.

ADVOCACY

The word 'advocacy' has been bandied about both inside and outside the mental health world, but what does it mean? Why has the term suddenly caught on? Why not 'advice', 'welfare rights', 'litigation', 'counselling', 'enabling', or 'representing'? It may be because advocacy contains all these elements and a little extra.

The dictionary offers the definition of 'an advocate' as 'one who pleads for another: professional pleader, supporter' and advocacy is a function of these. This definition already offers several meanings, that is, one who pleads for another on a voluntary basis; one who is paid to undertake such a task or one who supports another, perhaps in presenting the other person's case.

The concept of advocacy as it is known today was first developed in the USA and Europe for individuals with learning disabilities (mental handicap), defining advocacy as 'one who pleads for another on a voluntary basis'.

Wolfensberger (1972) one of the key writers in this field offers the following definition of a citizen advocate: 'an unpaid competent citizen volunteer, with the support of an independent citizen agency, represents – as if they were his/her own – the interests of one or two impaired persons by means of one or several advocacy roles, some of which may last for life'. This concept appears to offer a new component in the formula, that of an 'independent citizen advocacy agency'. From this it can be assumed that this body will be funded, and paid advocacy becomes another part of the picture.

In Holland, where advocacy it is believed has made great impact in psychiatric services, all advocates are fully paid but are not employees of the service. However, paid employees have multiple roles and loyalties and this will obviously detract from Wolfensberger's definition of advocacy. In Holland, such advocates define their tasks as being 'to defend the interest of the patient as the patient himself defines them'. The outcome the patient prefers is the outcome the patient advocate tries to achieve (Legemaate 1985). The advocacy work in Holland was only able to flourish because of the groundwork undertaken by the 'patients council movement' and the 'clients union' who were determined and committed to self-determination and self-representation.

Clearly from this evolving scenario advocacy cannot be seen as one thing, but as many. However, its end remit is that of the realisation of one person's interest. The methods of achieving this maybe through a multitude of ways such as:

- lay or citizen advocacy – where skilled volunteers supported by an independent agency work with individuals on a long-term basis
- paid advocacy – where skilled workers are paid by an independent agency to work with individuals on a long-term basis

- self-advocacy – where, singularly or collectively, individuals work on their own behalf to realise their own interests.

Lay or citizen advocacy

Higgins (1993) describes lay or citizen advocacy as 'a relationship between two citizens one of whom is a service user with the other acting as an advocate'. It is anticipated that volunteers could fulfil this role with appropriate support and training. The role can be seen as totally independent of any organisational constraint and the advocate would be impartial.

The main thrust of lay or citizen advocacy has always tended to be with people with learning difficulties through such groups as Advocacy Alliance, launched in 1981 by five national voluntary organisations (MENCAP, One to One, The Spastics Society, MIND and the Leonard Cheshire Foundation) as a pilot project to introduce citizen advocacy into long-stay mental handicap hospitals. The Alliance's stated aim was 'to give residents a friend/advocate – someone who will stand up for their rights and interests as if it were their own'. This group has now spread throughout the UK although there is a higher concentration in the south. They have achieved many long-term relationships between people with learning difficulties and advocates. This has now spread into the psychiatric care sector with similar results.

Citizen advocacy has received legislative endorsements with the passing of the Disabled Persons (Services, Consultation, Representation) Act 1986 and Disabled Persons Act 1995. This stipulates that local authorities must permit disabled people to be represented at their request should services be requested. The person is allowed to represent the disabled person at all stages in the local council procedures when handling claims for services by the disabled person. Local authorities at the request of the individual must supply the representative with any information he or she may require, or make available for inspection any documents the user of the service is entitled to have or inspect. The only way in which this may be withheld is if the local authority believes that the examination of such documentation will be harmful to the disabled person, giving due regard to their expressed wish. However, there is no such right of access under the Mental Health Act (1983) for the mentally disordered offender.

Paid advocacy

Sometimes termed legal advocacy, this is a very specialised form of advocacy. Butler et al (1988) describe it as 'a process in which legally trained persons pursue and represent the rights and interest of people within existing legislation frameworks, or seek to extend the parameters of legislation to protect and/or promote the rights of the individual'. Gates (1994) cites Clarke (1985) who gave an excellent example of this type of advocacy. The case was of Smith, Stringfellow and Poyner versus Jackson, Blackburn County, which was concerned with establishing the eligibility of people with a learning disability to pursue and exercise their right to vote. In this case the electoral registration officer would not place the names of three people who resided at Calderstones Hospital (a large learning disability hospital) on the electoral register. The electoral officer's decision was based on the premise that these three persons were patients of an establishment that dealt with the reception and treatment of people with mental illness or mental defectiveness. He felt that these individuals were 'patients' at this hospital and therefore they could not be thought of as resident under the Representation of the People Act 1949. This decision was challenged and an advocate was sought for the men concerned, in order that their right might be properly represented. Following the court case, Judge Prestt QC presiding ruled that although these individuals resided within a hospital they were not receiving treatment for a mental disorder or mental illness. He also concluded that because they were not receiving treatment they could not be classed as patients in the context of the Representation of the People Act 1949, and were, therefore, entitled to have their names placed on the electoral register (Gates 1994, pp. 3–4).

This case shows that a thorough knowledge of the legal system is needed by those providing care to ensure that the rights of the individual are upheld. It is a good example of where this might be beneficial to the mentally disordered offender.

This form of advocacy, however, is perhaps the least available form of access as it must be paid for to ensure that somebody would be available to individuals experiencing difficulties, and most MDOs may be on benefits and may not be able to afford the costs. Also, with the removal of legal aid, access to such representation will prove more elusive to this client group. One way forward will be to have an independent body to ensure that the MDO is not disadvantaged in terms of having access to this form of advocacy.

Self-advocacy

Williams and Shoultz (1982) see this as individuals or groups speaking out or acting on issues on behalf of others who are affected in the same way as they are themselves. This form of advocacy has (perhaps mistakenly) tended to be linked with the move towards consumerism and client-centred planning and delivery of services, which has been the subject of vigorous debate in the mental health field during the late 1970s and early 1980s. It denotes a process of speaking for oneself.

At the World Health Congress in Brighton in July 1985, groups from the USA and Europe together with British users and mental health professionals produced radical demands in their declaration for 'Advocacy – Individual's Right to Self Determination'. Later that year British user groups campaigned at the MIND National Conference and won support, calling for the abolition of certain forms of psychiatric treatment, namely ECT, rejection of the concept of mental illness and the recognition of psychiatric medical treatment as a form of institutionalised violence. Other groups pressed for further legislative reforms in caring for the mentally ill.

More recently, professionals have been cooperating with user groups in planning and providing services. In the past such cooperation was seen as idealistic and impractical. However, the evidence shows that participation can mean sharing experiences and promoting empathy and solidarity whilst achieving user empowerment – not by putting users in an adversarial role but through cooperative work aimed at developing a better service. Users themselves are becoming increasingly aware of the responsibility entailed in participating in the planning process, and the work needed to balance individual perspectives, through involvement in user groups to whom they felt accountable. The English National Board for Nursing, Midwifery and Health Visiting have recommended that user groups be involved in the development of nursing curricula.

User groups and networks are now functioning in a number of cities, commenting on both hospital and community psychiatric services, all with the common aim of creating more awareness and control by users of the services they receive.

Nottingham Advocacy Group

The Nottingham Advocacy Group developed an advocacy service within Nottingham's psychiatric care system based on self-advocacy with initially three component parts: patients' councils, paid advocates and a citizen advocacy scheme, that is, uniting the three aspects of advocacy into a working unit.

The group was set up largely through the initiative of Nottingham MIND who drew together a number of individuals interested in or working on advocacy into a steering group to develop advocacy services in Nottingham. A legal advocacy project had already been in existence since January 1985, offering in-house advice and training for patients and staff at a local psychiatric hospital. This had been established by the Hyson Green Law Centre. An advice service was held on one morning and one afternoon every week, where a member of the Law Centre staff would be available to give advice on any aspect of legal and welfare rights. Although take-up of this service had been quite good (Mapperley Advice Project 1986), workers did not feel that it truly reflected the level of potential demand of people hospitalised. This finding was supported when a national meeting with other legal advocacy projects in hospitals showed similar results.

There were some structural reasons why more people were not using the service. For example when the project was first opened it was sited in an almost inaccessible office, little more than a broom cupboard right at one end of the hospital and on a corridor separating the day and night sections of a long-stay ward. Understandably, this was not an arrangement appreciated by either the ward staff or those involved in the project! Also, initially a large volunteer team was used to give advice and thus no-one became a familiar face about the hospital or was able to get to grips with the project. Although a great deal of negotiating and liaison had been done with the hospital hierarchy, the project had predictably failed to consult the most relevant group of all, the users themselves.

Experience of projects in the wider community concerned with the take-up and effective implementation of individual rights revealed that the most successful campaigns or projects are those that:

- cater for a particular community or group in that community
- are based, and have their roots, in that community
- create a level of expectation in the community that the consumers' demands should be, and can be, realised.

Although there are quite clearly marked differences between working in the wider community and within the institutions of psychiatric care, it is believed that some aspects of this model of take-up can be usefully transferred into both hospital and community settings.

A particular problem for users of psychiatric services is the power differential between consumers and providers. In hospitals, for example, services are either brought to the patient or the patient is brought to the services. Whilst there is a certain encouragement to change to fit in with notions of good health, there is little or no encouragement to alter the status quo of the active provider and passive receiver.

This situation is not too unlike that of many people in the community; moreover the problems of users of psychiatric services are compounded by the stigma of having a psychiatric label. We believe that to truly provide an effective advocacy service for users, the power differential must be tackled so that user expectations are increased.

The Nottingham Group promoted self-advocacy for users through a patients' council, an idea first developed in Holland. It involved users taking an active part in the power structure of the hospital. The council function rather like a tenants' associations and range from being mere tokens to genuine participants in the management of resources. However, there is evidence that they increase the accountability of services and create a climate in the hospital where participation in its operation is a partnership, albeit often unequal, between users and staff. In Nottingham both groups decided to work together through the umbrella of Nottingham Advocacy Group (NAG) to create a comprehensive advocacy service for the users. However, whilst access to a paid full-time advocate or a group committed to self-advocacy will enable many people to express their views, it must be acknowledged that this will not work for everyone. Some people will be too restricted by the long-term effects of institutionalisation, drugs, and/or their mental distress to use such services effectively, whilst for others, there may be barriers of language or differences in cultural background. In such cases it will be necessary for the interests of such people to be discussed in the context of a more intense, longer-term relationship. In these circumstances, it seemed appropriate that the model of citizen advocacy used in mental handicap could be usefully applied to this group and, thus, lay advocacy became the third part of the project. Now all we needed was for someone else to think it was a good idea and provide the funding.

Patients' councils

Since the inception of user's group involvement, there has been a move towards patients' councils as seen in the model developed by Mapperley Hospital Patients' Council (1989) (Fig. 3.1).

Hospital Council guidelines

1. There will be monthly meetings of the Hospital Council.
2. All wards are to have a spokesperson(s).

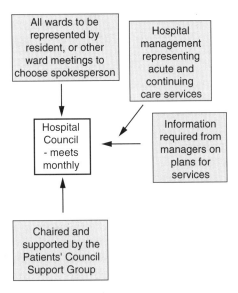

Figure 3.1 The Mapperley model.

3. All wards are to have a regular ward meeting: spokesperson(s) to be chosen for the Hospital Council.
4. Where possible, a resident (or residents) should represent the ward.
5. If a member of the ward team is chosen, it is recognised that this is a short-term arrangement.
6. With reference to point 5, the arrangement should be for a maximum of 6 months.
7. The aim is for the Council to consist only of residents within 9 months.
8. Staff can accompany residents if necessary.
9. The Hospital Council is to be chaired and facilitated by the Patients' Council Support Group.

Issues covered at Council meetings

These included:

* improving signposting in the hospital
* introducing more games and magazines to making the patients' lounge more homely
* discussion of complaints about menu choices not always being available, in some cases because of welfare benefit restrictions on self-catering wards (an issue later taken up in a DSS tribunal)
* possible funding for murals in corridors and wards
* plans to provide information to patients leaving acute wards
* complaint about waiting time before seeing a doctor on admission
* plans for hospital closure and community hospital replacements
* complaint about inadequate heating.

Attempts have been made in some areas to belittle this type of meeting because of the emphasis on catering, entertainments and other supposedly minor issues. However, it must be said that these issues are of great importance to people living in hospital, and they are always combined with matters of a policy nature, such as information on medication or plans for new facilities.

Such issues have far-reaching implications for the Citizen's Charter introduced by the last Government (conservative) (DoH 1992a) as many hospitals are setting up users' charters. One such example is the Brighton Users' Charter (Box 3.1).

Box 3.1 Brighton Users' Charter (Charter Steering Group, 22.01.90, Brighton, Sussex)

1. Users should have health/social services appropriate to their needs, regardless of financial means or where they live.
2. Users should be treated with respect as intelligent and equal human beings and be treated at all times with respect for their personal dignity.
3. Users should have their cultural, religious, sexual and emotional needs accepted and respected.
4. Users should be consulted about decisions affecting their daily lives, especially those involving risk.
5. Users should have information and explanation relevant to their individual needs.
6. Users should have privacy for themselves, both in their affairs and belongings, including consultations in private; the right to receive visitors in private; and for personal information to be kept confidential.
7. Users should not be judged on their sexuality and where confusion over sexuality exists, it should be respected.
8. Users should have the same access to facilities and services in the community as any other citizen, including registration with the GP and dentist of their choice and be able to change without adverse consequences.
9. Users should have written information about health services, including hospitals, community and GP services.
10. Users should have the right to negotiate a change of psychiatrist, other professional or 'keyworker' including male and female; and to have adequate time with their psychiatrist, other professional or 'keyworker'.
11. Users should have good and sufficient 'community care' when discharged from psychiatric hospitals so that people are generally satisfied and feel good about the quality of their lives.
12. Users have the right to both discuss and use alternative therapies, without fearing the loss of access to mainstream services.
13. Users should have access to a crisis service.
14. Users should be informed of their right to see their records which are held by Social Services and Health, in accordance with existing Statutory Policies.
15. Users should know whether they are able to accept or refuse treatment without affecting the standard of care given.
16. Users should be given an explanation of diagnoses in plain language, be able to say 'I don't understand' and ask for more information.
17. Users should know there is a recognised, active and practical complaints procedure.
18. There should be advocacy; self-advocacy and interpreting services; and users should be able to have the support of a relative or friend at any time if they wish.
19. Users should be able to feed their views back to a management structure that will listen and act upon them.
20. Users should not be destructively labelled by professionals.

Professionals as advocates

There is a belief that patients need advocates (Willard 1996). Willard says that 'the assumption that advocacy is required in healthcare implies that the process of becoming a patient results in a reduction of autonomy and that the patient's rights or interest may not be respected'. She contends that while some patients will lose autonomy because of the nature of their illness (for example conditions that cause unconsciousness or severe mental incapacity), service providers and professionals must consider the extent to which an individual, normally considered to be capable of self-determination, should lose this in the health care setting (Willard 1996, p. 61).

The move towards advocacy in the health care environment was due to demands for consumer rights from the American public (Starr 1982). This movement in the UK started in the early 1970s and peaked in the mid-1980s; however, the introduction of the Patient's Charter (DoH 1991a) has heightened users' and professionals' awareness. The United Kingdom Central Council for Nursing, Midwifery and Health Visiting (UKCC) states that advocacy should form an integral part of the nurse's duty to patients. McIver (1993), however, tries to differentiate between the work of the hospital representative such as the nurse, who is a professional carer, and that of an independent advocate. Professional independent advocates would work alongside patients who were using the services, seeking to empower them to self-advocate (Holmes 1991). The contrast, says Mallik (1997), is that hospital patient representatives are seen as functioning only within the establishment, being responsive to individual's problems and remaining strongly oriented towards consumer issues, and do not consider all the issues. She continues: 'the significance of the above development is in examining how nurses' perceptions of their particular advocacy function articulate with those undertaken by patient representatives'. Evidence exists that there is hostility between patients' representatives and professionals because of role boundaries (McIver 1993, 1994). Mallik cites Pullen (1995) who claims that advocacy can be best achieved by a specialist nurse practitioner. Pullen (1995) refers to this particular specialist carrying his/her own caseload of clients who will need advocacy. However, can a professional be a true advocate according to agreed definitions when caring for the MDO?

Public and patient interest

Crucial to illuminating the exceptional predicament of the forensic professional is the statutory, and other, documentation of recent years which helped generate significant changes in health care perceptions. The most pertinent is the UKCC Code of Professional Conduct which prescribes the professional behaviour of care. In its introductory statements, registered professionals are asked to: '(a) safeguard and promote the interests of individual patients and clients [and] (b) serve the interests of society' (UKCC 1992a).

In a similar vein the Department of Health and Special Hospital Services Authority produced the national objectives of the country's special hospitals in 1989. This body administers 1700 mentally disordered patients and other patients who are a serious management problem to other institutions. Its announced commitment is to: 'ensure the continuing safety of the public ... [and] the provision of appropriate treatment for patients' (DoH et al 1989).

The 1983 Mental Health Act makes about a dozen references to the medical–legal considerations for detaining a patient in order to protect both the patient and other persons simultaneously. For example, a person displaying signs of mental disorder in a public place may be conveyed to a place of safety by a police officer for the individual's interests and the protection of other persons (Section 136).

Bailey & MacCulloch (1992), highlighting 112 patients discharged directly into the community from Park Lane Hospital, revealed that 41 (36.6%) were convicted of post-discharge offences and 19 (17%) of serious offences. To add to these officially sanctioned discharges, there are the fatal repercussions of individual escapees into the surrounding population. A few infamous incidents such as the abduction, injuring or killing of children, members of the public and police officers form part of the risk-taking scenario which are the repercussions on the community if the forensic professional is not sufficiently vigilant.

This highlights the dilemma the professional encounters when attempting to assume the role of an advocate (Fig. 3.2).

The multifaceted role of professionals acts as a barrier to their becoming advocates. Mallik (1997) cites many authors who argue that nurses, as professional carers, are in a position to espouse the

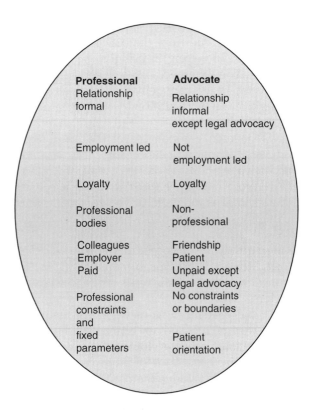

Figure 3.2 The multidimensional role of the professional and possible areas of conflict with that of an advocate.

advocacy role. Kalisch (1975) uses the word 'key', Kosik (1972) 'best', Gadow (1983) and Albarran (1992) 'ideal'. Mallik says 'authors are not only referring to the nurse's functional position within the healthcare team but also to the quality of contracted time with patients.' She continued: 'At a political and functional level, nurses are well placed in the division of healthcare labour and can act as natural mediators because of their location within the healthcare team'.

Bishop & Scudder (1990) posit the view that occupying the middle ground is a very positive asset for nurses, and they can have legitimate authority to foster team decision-making. Linking this mediating position directly to advocacy, Jezewski (1993), following Tripp-Rumer & Brink (1985), proposes a model of 'cultural broker' similar to Littlewood's theory of nursing (1991) and taking her cue from the discipline of anthropology, she outlines 'culture brokering' as bridging, linking or mediating between groups. The difference between the cultural system of the patient and the health care delivery system as a cultural system needs clarification or resolution by the mediator or the 'culture broker', i.e. the nurse.

Mallik says that at an emotional level, the position also allows nurses to develop a unique relationship with the patient. It is argued that such a relationship will encourage the nurse to act as the patient's advocate (Cooper 1988). It could be construed that nurses have a moral mandate to advocate, arising intrinsically from their unique knowledge of the patient. Even if this point is sustainable, the assumption is that such unique relationships actually and naturally always occur in practice.

In contrast, Morse (1991) is much more specific in placing the advocacy function within specific types of relationships. From her research, Morse maintains that there is a continuum of relationships, and patient advocacy occurs only when the relationship is 'therapeutic' and/or 'connected'. In her exposition of events that will hinder the development of relationships, Morse includes, among others, the issue of multiple caregivers and the lack of time. In a similar study, Ramos (1992) states that even in balanced relationships, the nurse was still in control. Nurses' actions were based on their own values, wishes and knowledge. Decisions were made unilaterally by the nurse if the patient was indecisive, if there was little time for discussion, or if nurses felt their professional knowledge was central to the decision-making.

THE FORENSIC SYSTEM

The term 'forensic' has its root in Latin meaning a forum or market place at which legal disputes would have been settled during the Roman era. Today's equivalent is the court of law which in terms of the mentally disordered offender is either a magistrates' court or the High Court.

The forensic process can be described as the successive stages in the forensic management of clinical behaviour. This commences with police detention and investigation of a crime, and goes on to include apprehension of the alleged perpetrator, examination of evidence, determination of a verdict in court, completion of a prison sentence in a custodial environment and, finally, preparation for release into the community. In relation to health care, the forensic process mirrors these details but include variations which enable the management of the mentally disordered offender to be more health related.

In the first instance it will evaluate whether, in committing a crime, defendants were able to make sound judgements about their actions, were able to control their behaviour and could differentiate between right and wrong in relation to these actions. In short, the court, with the help of expert witnesses such as the forensic psychiatrist, attempts to elicit whether there is an abnormality of mind. If this is found to be the case, the forensic health care process may continue with allocation of the client to an available and suitable facility. Treatment strategies for psychiatric illness and any other dysfunction which contributes to the offending behaviour will then be provided, followed by rehabilitation, community supervision and discharge.

Mentally disordered offenders' rights

Within the context of the Mental Health Act 1983, patients who are committed should, throughout their stay in hospital, be given as much information as possible about their care and treatment. Furthermore, information must be provided in such a manner that it is easily understood by the patient. It must be given at a suitable time to facilitate understanding, so that the patient is able to understand the nature of the information. Should the patient request information, this must be given in an honest and comprehensive manner. Information should be given periodically and checks must be made to ensure that patients continue to understand the information given to them. Under Part IV of the Mental Health Act every Section contains detailed information which should be given. These are the patient's legal rights, but if the patient fails to understand can the professional act as his or her advocate?

The professional within the forensic system

Examination of various curricula has shown that the role of the forensic professional does not lend itself to being an advocate. Lynch (1993) suggests that the subjects covered do not truly prepare the professional as an advocate.

Box 3.2 gives an overview of a curriculum which a nurse may follow undertaking a course in forensic nursing. No such curriculum exist for other professionals.

Box 3.2 Sample curriculum core course in forensic nursing

Course title: Introduction to forensic nursing
Credit: 3 semester hours – 3 contact hours, 6 laboratory hours

Course description
The application of academic and professional development of the forensic clinical nurse specialist (CNS) in advanced nursing practice in a clinical or community-based institution. The forensic nurse will fulfil the required 96-hour internship in field and laboratory experience – as well as required classroom contact instruction – under the preceptorship of a forensic, trauma, emergency, or other appropriate CNS; a medical examiner; or a forensic scientist. The course will include an incisive exploration of the principles and philosophies of clinical forensic nursing and the role of the forensic nurse in the scientific investigation of trauma. The role of the forensic nurse in biomedical investigation and community mental health as a nurse coroner or medical examiner's investigator/associate will be addressed.

Topics covered
1.   Role of the forensic clinical nurse specialist.
2.   Role of the sexual assault nurse examiner.
3.   Role of the nurse coroner/death investigator.
4.   Role of the forensic psychiatric nurse.
5.   Role of the medicolegal nurse consultant.
6.   Role of the forensic geriatric nurse specialist.
7.   Role of the forensic correctional nurse specialist.
8.   Role of the nurse in forensic research and education in medicolegal practice.
9.   Structure and function of institutions of legal medicine.
10. Forensic psychopathology.
11. Signs and legal aspects of death, certification of death.
12. Notification of death, victim management of survivors.
13. Legal/ethical aspects of nursing practice, bioethics.
14. Victimology/traumatology.
15. Sexual and domestic violence, forensic gynaecology.
16. Medicolegal documentation/rules of evidence.
17. Implication of bite mark evidence.
18. Recognition of patterns of injury, nursing management of gunshot wounds.
19. Nursing responsibilities in clinical forensic cases, protocol development.

Three other courses in forensic nursing are required to complete master's degree or postgraduate certificate in forensic nursing: Investigation of injury and death; Criminalistics/forensic science technique; and Courtroom procedure/expert witness.

Pullen (1995) has indicated that the role of advocate can be fulfilled by a specialist practitioner. However she did not give an outline of a curriculum for the education of such a person or substantiate her claim for this specialist practitioner. Walsh (1995) supports Pullen's claims saying advocacy is representing 'the interest of a patient as if she were representing her own interest'. This he claims to be appropriate on the basis of the qualification of 'closeness to their patient'. Such intimacy and proximity implicit in the nurse–patient relationship puts the practitioner in the ideal position to:

- know the patient's needs
- act as a buffer between the patient and other agencies
- protect the patient from all would-be wrongdoers.

In parts this may appear to be so, but is it a function of nursing or advocacy as defined?

Further exploration of the various health care professional curricula shows the multiplicity of functions as previously discussed and not that of an advocate.

Care role

From the stance of care, one might speak of an inclusive forensic care speciality which has evolved out of general psychiatric competencies and has adapted specialist care skills but is progressing towards a more discrete forensic focus. It is, perhaps, a measure of this that the current English National Board care course focusing on this area is entitled 'Care Within Controlled Environment' rather than 'Forensic Care.' Nevertheless, the Reed committee endorsed expansion of the forensic care provision and encouraged the academic ascendancy of forensic care (DoH & Home Office 1991).

A forensic focus requires the existence of a range of phenomena which are sufficiently exclusive to confer a specialist status on the care role. The case for forensic care is as follows:

1. The client category consists overwhelmingly of offenders with psychiatric personality disorder or offending behaviour related to psychiatric morbidity.
2. Care strategies are largely incorporated within institutional control and custody of patients.

3. The configuration of patient pathology, criminal activity, therapeutic interventions and competencies, court/legal issues, and custodial care creates the need for a formidable and accelerating knowledge base.
4. The advocacy role is different from that in other care specialities, embracing both the destigmatisation and decriminalisation of the patient group.
5. Clients' potential for future dangerousness requires the formulation of risk-assessment strategies.

This stance again does not include that of the role of an advocate.

Therapeutic detention

Care has often involved, historically, the pursuit of health and the detention of patients to effect the treatment programme. With the massive state institutional intervention of the 18th and 19th centuries, vast numbers of the 'mentally deficient' and 'pauper lunatics' were incarcerated within elaborate asylums. There was no polite invitation to these populations. Once formally certified, patients were enclosed by perimeter walls, bars to their windows, locked ward doors, padded cells, and seclusion rooms. Interpersonal management could be facilitated by the forceful restraint of patients – either to effect a specific treatment such as 'electroconvulsive therapy' or to handle 'refractory' behaviour – as well as the use of mechanical restraints such as 'strait-jackets' to immobilise a disturbed individual. As these institutions evolved, their regimes still included other invasive strategies such as the 'systematic searching' of the suicidal resident. McPhail (1940) describes how this would require care staff to search the patient's cap lining, shirt, drawers, flannel, outer garments, pockets, socks, boots, slippers, trousers, jacket-cuff, bedding for injurious implements, and then to bind and label the articles so that other patients could not access them.

Care is no stranger to the task of combining treatment goals with those of detention. Historically, the evidence suggests that the traditional involuntary hospitalisation of psychiatric patients was seen to be self-evidently moral and legitimate so that generations of psychiatric professionals were reared on a staple diet of unquestioning patient-detention.

In this context, a perception that the custodial management of mentally disordered offenders remains a legitimate service to society has militated against a thorough appraisal of the role conflict and the ethical dilemmas associated with the contemporary forensic care role.

Response to role conflict

It cannot be assumed that professionals working in this area even attempt to come to terms with this role conflict. Certainly, they are qualified as professionals to focus on psychiatric pathology and mental health care, but there is no formal education in restrictive custody demanded for their professional registration. Neither are they specifically educated or skilled in the management of offending behaviours. Yet, their professional purpose is to somehow organise strategies which coordinate these divergent dimensions.

Of greater significance is the likelihood that many care staff working in forensic settings find the conflict of interests quite untenable. This is most likely because, as individuals, they are oriented towards either more emphatically therapeutic interventions or uncompromising custodial considerations. In turn, their stance on these issues will derive from the diffuse social and political values they hold as members of a broader culture. Care staff will reflect every shade of opinion on the management of this client group. Some may actively despise the residents for whom they are responsible and take every opportunity to impede their progress.

Others may be periodically or irreversibly disturbed by the biographical detail in patients' histories or the stress from daily vigilance, occasions of violence and other deviancies. Many will believe that because of the infamous nature of their deeds certain types of offender, ill or not, will not benefit from treatment. At the extremes, views may range over a desire for retribution via capital and corporal punishment to terminal incarceration and irreversible surgery, to an aspiration that every possible resource should be committed to reconciling the client and society.

Phillips (1983) revealed the attitudes of Canadian forensic professionals on some of these matters. Asked about the status of residents: 17% of the respondents viewed them as criminals rather than patients; 30% believed that the care facilities should be located within the prison system itself; 25% felt that unlimited access to lawyers, social workers and probation officers was not warranted; and as few as 61% felt that forensic professionals required a specialist, post-basic certification.

Treatment strategies

Throughout the patient's period of therapeutic detention, care staff, along with other disciplines, develop a profile of each individual. This includes: an understanding of the circumstances in which individuals committed the acts for which they were apprehended; how they construed their behaviour then and now; the part that provocation or unpredictability played; whether denial of the incident is a factor; and to what extent any remorse is presented. Information that indicates biographical issues, such as morbid jealousy, lack of self-control, and difficulty in managing stress and violent fantasies, is gathered alongside material relating to poor compliance with treatment, impaired insight into mental state and limited social skills.

Most crucially, the professional tries to estimate the risk of future dangerousness in the patient. This may extend into work in the community in terms of accompanying patients on planned trips to monitor their progress in more normal conditions, as far as this is possible. The preventive role includes identifying risk factors for each individual rather than systematically predicting future dangerousness.

The full gamut of general psychiatric care skills, such as coun-selling, is utilised. Furthermore, specialist intervention with any of the major treatment models may be used. For example, sex offenders may receive medication for their sexual arousal or experience a behavioural programme targeting dysfunctional sexual behaviour; there may be individual or group analysis of sex-related meanings and events in the context of the past; or a therapeutic milieu may be created in which both staff and patients develop solutions to problems perceived to have arisen out of social and environmental influences.

This emphasis on the offence behaviour, e.g. sex offences, arson attacks and physical violence, alongside psychiatric illness, constitutes the exclusive focus of the forensic health care model. However, it is not unreasonable to expect considerable attention to be channelled into the management of challenging behaviours such as verbal and physical aggression, absconding, offensive weapon-making, manipulative behaviour and deliberate self-harm, since such activities are prevalent among this patient group.

Thus, the care role has to be incorporated within the legal and physical boundaries of custodial detention, even though the patients are being treated in hospitals. As Burrow (1991) pointed out, herein lies the essential paradox of the forensic treatment process and the care role, because of the incompatibilities of therapeutic custody. The therapy vs custody debate is about whether it is possible to provide individualised, patient-centred health-promoting care while confining patients, often for many years and sometimes without a clear treatment programme, to ensure the protection of the general public.

Forensic institutions lie on a custodial continuum from maximum through medium to minimal security. In order to operate secure custody, professionals can engage in an extensive repertoire of control. They require a continuous perimeter and locked internal doors, key straps, belts and keys for securing premises, two-way radios while physically escorting patients, regular accounting for patient numbers, maintenance of environmental and client safety checks, monitoring of relatives, gifts, mail and telephone calls, and three-person teams to carry out control and restraint techniques of violence management. Such measures are by no means wholly standardised, and they vary according to the security profile and policy of individual units. Notwithstanding this, control of the environment and its degree of restrictiveness can be greatly influenced by care staff.

Considering the notion of the varying role of the forensic professional and that of treatment, where should the MDO be housed when treatment is the option? Should it be in a psychiatric hospital, prison, or a specialised place capable of providing the right environment and taking account of what was recommended by Bloom-Cooper (1992), and how should their rights be safeguarded?

Special hospitals

In Britain at least, the criminal lunatic asylums have been superseded by special hospitals. These were constituted under the

Mental Health Act 1959 and their remit was elaborated under the National Health Service Act 1977 whereby the Secretary of State was obliged to 'provide and maintain establishments for persons subject to detention under the Mental Health Act 1959 who in his opinion require treatment under conditions of special security on account of their dangerous, violent or criminal propensities'.

In these particular institutions it is fair to say that the care role has followed the archetypal model of asylum care. However, they have endeavoured – despite serious periodic criticism and a considerable disadvantage over younger institutions – to adapt their traditional regimens to one that reflects a more contemporary type of health care. Special hospital professionals have become increasingly active in helping to instigate therapeutic changes despite the disadvantage of their heritage and a significant residuum of staff reaction.

Medium-secure units

Medium-secure units have been commissioned within regional health authority boundaries as a result of the recommendations of the Butler report (Home Office & DHSS 1975), which determined provision for the mentally abnormal offender, and the Glancy report (DHSS 1974a), which reviewed the security facilities of the NHS psychiatric hospitals. As largely purpose-built units, they were directed to become a focus for the development of forensic psychiatric services, to care for offenders and non-offenders, and to include separate facilities for the mentally impaired and a national unit for adolescents. They are geared for up to 2 years' residence, have a high staff complement, a clear therapeutic intent, and are purposefully located near populated areas to facilitate community access.

The operational criteria of medium security are based on the fact that residents would not represent a grave and immediate danger to the public (which, in effect, largely constitutes the admission criteria for special hospitals). They are also intended to provide a pivotal link point for liaison with other NHS hospitals, special hospitals, the prison medical service, probation and social services, and GP services, as well as the courts themselves. The care role extends well beyond the physical boundaries of the units, with regular community contact.

Prisons

Forensic mental health care in this country also extends to the prison services hospital wings and related specialist units (Carlisle 1990, Cooke 1989, Dulfer 1992, Evershed 1991, Gray 1974, McCarthy 1983, Saunders-Wilson 1992). The incidence of psychiatric illness among the prison population reveals the need for forensic care skills in these settings. Gunn et al (1991) investigating the male prisoners of 25 prisons, found that 652 (37%) had psychiatric disorders while only 52 (3%) required transfer to hospital for treatment.

However, the effectiveness of care for prison inmates is compromised by a number of factors. The environment is not conducive to mental health because of the limited range of diversional, recreational and occupational resources. Individual care cannot be attempted because of the limited number of staff available and the care is shared between hospital officers with 6 months' health care training, other registered professionals, and ordinary discipline officers.

The inadequacy of the present system of care can be gauged from an example of a young man with learning difficulties who admitted his sexual offence to his cell mate who promptly beat him, shaved his hair with a blunt razor and forced him to drink his own urine during one night when a total of eight officers were monitoring 850 inmates (Pitt 1993). To add to the difficulties, patients may refuse the medication they are offered since they are not formally detained under the Mental Health Act 1983 as they would be if they had been transferred to a hospital facility. The mental state of inmates may deteriorate rapidly so that staff have to confine them to solitary cells because they are perceived to be unmanageable.

The forensic care role is not confined to secure institutions; because of prior contact with clients as inpatients, the community forensic professional is better able to detect signs of dangerousness arising out of their relationships, social circumstances and mental state. Furthermore, as part of a psychiatric assessment panel, community professionals aim to identify people with a mental disorder before they are propelled into the judicial process. Most significantly, at the pre-court stage they can recommend the diversion of such individuals into the health care system in order that they might receive treatment.

Promoting patients' interest

There are many concerns over the safety of people with mental health problems especially those living in the community. The high-profile incidents of cases like the death of Jonathan Zito (Shepherd 1995), Georgina Robinson (Bloom-Cooper et al 1995) poses many problems for those caring for the mentally disordered offender and effective advocacy. Media attention has focused on the problems the mentally ill pose both to themselves and others, making it harder to promote positive perceptions of such individuals.

Glasman (1991) identified how the rights of the mentally ill could be safeguarded by introducing advocates in hospital services. Nottingham was the first city in Britain to have established a Patient's Council. It evolved as a result of the World Mental Health Conference in Brighton in 1985. Delegates from Holland where such councils were commissioned and advocacy was the face for individuals with mental health problems.

In what is called a process of 'diversion', Hillis (1989) describes how potential patients are transferred from police or magistrate court cells into hospital facilities to provide an opportunity of assessing the therapeutic potential. Often, this results in the discontinuation of legal proceedings against the individual so that he or she might be accommodated for immediate treatment. What are the rights of the individual in this situation is not made clear.

The clients' interests are also being sought when remanded or convicted prisoners are transferred for treatment as a result of displaying psychiatric symptoms while in prison, but not their rights. As part of ward-based clinical teams, the contribution of care staff could be a key element in the assessment of a prison inmate. Provided that a suitable hospital unit can be found with an appropriate level of security, a prisoner will then formally become a temporary patient for the duration of his or her treatment before returning to complete the prison sentence.

While this represents an admirable disposal of the mentally disordered inmate, in principle, it does have its accompanying difficulties. Describing their own experience at Rampton Hospital, Cordall & Phipps (1982) reveal their concern about the increasing introduction of inmates on their wards. This policy introduced a group with a distinctive, dominant status over other patients and provided them with an opportunity to manipulate younger patients. The increased admission rate of West Indians caused racial attacks among patients; imported more self-mutilatory behaviour; and increased the impetus toward more stringent security measures. Throughout their work and experience no mention was made of the patients' rights.

The most alarming feature for care staff is that a 'prison culture' is perceived to be imported into a hospital situation which identifies care staff as 'screws' thereby proliferating distrust for any genuine therapeutic endeavour and increasing the potential for a concerted 'hostage-taking', use of a weapon, or other violent encounter. What made this more likely in the Rampton scenario was that prisoners had enjoyed more privileges in prison than the necessary restrictions enforced in an admission ward in a maximum security hospital. It may change this scenario if professionals are able to start thinking about the rights of individuals and inform those individuals accordingly. Then the inmates may at last see that someone is interested in them as individuals and may alter their perceptions.

An increasing amount of forensic care literature relating to strategies directed toward the improvement of patient care and circumstances has appeared in the last few years. There has been a mixture of case studies, comment and research from secure units, special hospitals and the prison service, variously highlighting concern for professionals caring for mentally disordered offenders in conditions of security.

This work shows a concerted interest by forensic professionals on behalf of their residents, in initiating their own intervention strategies or adapting those from more conventional settings to their own therapeutic arena. These range from direct therapy initiatives to limiting dysfunction, enhancing skills, improving health, and increasing the patients' quality of life, representation and civil rights. This could be perceived as advocacy being contemplated.

Special status

What is special about forensic patients is that their health status is combined with a criminal or other deviant status. Accordingly, treatment can equally be 'special in that mental health interventions can be variously combined with any number of other targets relating to deviant or offensive behaviours (Brett 1987, Burnard & Morrison 1992, Burrow 1992, Carton 1991, Gudjonsson & Tibbles 1983). Specific individuals might receive treatment for their psychopathic personality, self-mutilatory actions, and sexual offending.

'A Strategy for Nursing' (DoH 1989) enumerates a number of targets for practice. Among these, it stipulates that consumers' wishes should always be included in health-delivery decisions. Similar mission statements are made in the Code of Practice, Mental Health Act 1989, the Reed Report (DoH & Home Office 1992), the Citizen's Charter (DoH 1992a), and the RCN's evidence to the Mental Health Care Review (RCN 1993b), all advocating for the patient a prime place in determining or contributing to an understanding of personal need, all bringing advocacy to the forefront.

So important an issue had this become even before the publication of the foregoing documents that in Broadmoor, the Health Advisory Service, an independent watchdog, vehemently criticised its failure: 'Little opportunity exists [to] afford the patient a prominent role in determining his or her treatment while in the hospital' (RCN 1993b). Likewise, the more recent Ashworth inquiry details the 'culture of denigration and devaluing of patients' needs' (DoH, Special Hospitals Services Authority 1992).

Clearly, when these criticisms were made, these institutions were out of step with mainstream thinking on the issue of patients' rights.

VOLUNTARY ORGANISATIONS AS ADVOCATES

One of the functions of voluntary organisations should be to speak out on behalf of their client groups and, where appropriate, represent them before statutory bodies with which they might be in conflict. Since the end of the 1960s the voluntary sector has been more active in this area of work. The success of Shelter, the housing charity, and the development of the National Council for Civil Liberties encouraged other bodies to take up issues that were appropriate to their expertise. The trouble is that there is a tendency to interpret the word 'political' wrongly. The political process is the pursuit of change or the maintenance of existing conditions through public argument and democratic choice. Such activity has nothing whatsoever to do with party political allegiances. It is surely right that if a voluntary organisation comes across abuses, whether these be personal or institutional, it should attempt to remedy such abuses. However, to obtain a remedy means campaigning, writing to the appropriate minister or local government councillor so that the abuse may be immediately remedied, providing evidence for members of the Government about policy plans. Social progress is not brought about simply as a result of individual or collective virtue but as a consequence of public campaigning. There is no reason at all why voluntary organisations should not play a full role in this area. The only restriction should be to ensure that such organisations do not become party political and, therefore, partisan rather than rational.

In 1974/75 MIND's Council of Management decided that the organisation should become more involved in the issues surrounding the rights of patients and so Tony Smythe, who had been General Secretary of the National Council for Civil Liberties, was appointed as MIND's Director, and subsequently Larry Gostin was taken on as Legal and Welfare Rights Officer. Over the last 7 years, MIND has developed a considerable reputation as a body willing to take up unpopular causes and represent those who find it difficult to pursue their own cases. Much work has been done on the 1959 Mental Health Act, and campaigning for changes in the law has culminated in the present Mental Health (Amendment) Bill at present completing its progress through the House of Commons. MIND has concentrated a great deal of attention on psychiatric hospitals and on the issue of consent to treatment. An individual's right to participate in decision-making, if he or she is competent to do so, has been the basic belief which has governed their responses to all issues.

Such a role has inevitably led them into conflicts from time to time with the psychiatric profession. That is inevitable and nothing to be overly worried about. If they concentrated attention on the quality and quantity of services provided by local authorities they would no doubt come into conflict with local authority leaders. But not all the advocacy with which they have been involved has been controversial. MIND has taken the lead in launching and supporting an Advocacy Alliance which will help to provide individual advocates for patients in hospitals. This is currently being done in some hospitals with the full agreement and cooperation of the hospital authorities. One of the aspects which we need to consider in the hospital sector is that a vast amount of the complaints we receive in our legal department about treatment or ill-treatment within hospitals comes not from the patients themselves, but from members of staff who clearly have no great confidence in their own complaints procedures.

RE-EVALUATION

The politicisation of the patient role has caused all branches of care to re-evaluate their service to patients. Concepts such as client-empowerment, individualisation of care, unconditional regard for clients and patients' rights, have altered the balance of power between health staff and their clients. However, with current professional documentation, recognition of the carer's responsibility to the interests of the patients could be made.

The circumstances of forensic professionals highlight the invidious role conflict in which professionals may find themselves in trying to fulfil both criteria. The Code of Professional Conduct (UKCC 1992a) is a well-meaning broad outline of professional guidance. If professionalism is to have any integrity, individual practitioners must have a clear, and unambiguous, philosophy about their parochial occupational purpose.

For forensic practitioners there is no acceptable argument for professionals 'conscientiously objecting' to working therapeutically with the mentally abnormal offender and similarly placed persons. It is equally unacceptable to perceive therapeutic custody as a vicarious, or even benign, form of punishment.

CONCLUSION

Professionals are not professionally empowered to sit in judgement of a client's criminal activity. The legal system will already have determined the client's culpability in relation to his or her behaviour or offence. Indeed, this raises the question as to whether professionals have the right to 'judge' any antisocial behaviour except from the stance of intervention to improve a patient's health status.

In the light of forensic patient histories and propensities, serving patients' interests cannot be aspired to without anticipating the possible repercussions on the interests of others. Further to embroil the argument, I feel that society's interests should not preclude the pursuit of those of the client. Also each individual must come to terms with, and examine, the attitudes he or she holds as a citizen towards offenders, criminal behaviour and other social deviations. It is asking a lot of professionals not to apply differentiating criteria to the mentally disordered clients vis-à-vis other psychiatric clients. But, when all is said and done, these folk are also members of society and also have a stake in the community. It is the responsibility of forensic professionals themselves to marshal these competing role tensions and present their case. Forensic professional managers, educators and leading clinicians cannot wait for such tensions to resolve themselves. They should be committed to confronting them and committing clinical and developmental time to reconciling their staff to the issues in order to enable them to invest in those clients the appropriate knowledge, skill and attitudes of health management. The custodial repertoire which accompanies this is indubitably a compromising factor, unless it is wholeheartedly embraced as a necessary parameter facilitating the health management of the mentally abnormal offender.

To provide experiential and reflective opportunities is to help resolve the conflict of interests, to assist personal development, and to produce a philosophy of care which generates a healthier, richer service in the interest of clients, staff and general public. Without this, it is tantamount to encouraging a debilitated service.

Patients' rehabilitation into the public arena is particularly difficult in the light of the historical folklore of the criminal lunatic and the current public and political antipathy towards offenders generally.

Therefore, one might say that the forensic psychiatric professional is a critical, clinical team member who manages the mentally disordered offender and others posing serious management difficulties within, where necessary, a secure environment. He or she may contribute towards the assessment and selection of appropriate patients for treatment, as well as undertaking their supervision within the community. Health-promoting rehabilitative interventions focus on any psychological, social and behavioural dysfunction within the professional remit and include the targeting of psychiatric and offending disturbance.

However, as the legal health care interface of forensic care gathers momentum it will become inexorably ensnared in more professional conflicts and dilemmas. For example, in addition to professional opinion the political climate demands that decision-making about the client group takes into account the social sensitivities of the media, the general public and politicians themselves. It is not inconceivable, and indeed is highly probable, that the future evaluation of the service (including the care role) will involve assurances that discharged patients will not reoffend. This will demand a rigorous and hopeless quest for the elimination of future dangerousness.

What forensic professionals may more realistically provide is a highly informed, ethical, skills-based practice which takes seriously the notion of therapeutic custody until the client's individual risk to the public has been conscientiously minimised. This is usefully facilitated by the range of institutional options within which forensic professionals can operate.

At first sight, the diversity of special hospital, secure unit, prison service and community roles may seem to indicate a widely divergent and diffuse alliance. However, provided that individual client needs are targeted, it is this very diversity which permits mentally disordered offenders to be treated and tested in varying environments to give both them and their therapists a better chance of success.

4

Addiction nursing: community-oriented approach

G. Hussein Rassool

INTRODUCTION

The use of psychoactive substances has been part of the social fabric of many societies and continues to be so to the present day. In many countries, the use and misuse of alcohol, tobacco smoking and the use of illicit and prescribed psychoactive substances constitute a serious public health and socioeconomic problem. The harms (physical, social, psychological, economic) caused by substance misuse not only affect the individual user but also the family or significant others and the community. These include: higher risks of premature death; risk of acquiring blood-borne viruses such as hepatitis B and C and HIV; overdose; respiratory failure; obstetric complications; suicide; and mental health problems. The World Health Organization (1987, 1993) targeted addiction as one of the major health problems to be solved by the year 2000. In Europe, Target 17 in the policy document 'Health for All' (HFA) of the World Health Organization (1993) states that 'by the year 2000, the health-damaging consumption of dependence-producing substances such as alcohol, tobacco and psychoactive drugs should have been significantly reduced in all member states'. Addiction nurses have an excellent track record in developing innovative health care initiatives and community-oriented programmes for their clients and many of the key developments in recent years have been nurse led. These include mobile methadone clinics, outreach work with drug-using prostitutes, and satellite clinics for homeless drinkers (Rassool & Gafoor 1997a).

The changes in health care needs and the widespread misuse of psychoactive substances in the general population demand a workforce that is skilled in nursing interventions and capable of providing effective preventive strategies and consultation, and specialist care to substance misusers and their families. Members of the primary health care team, which includes community psychiatric nurses, health visitors, practice nurses, district nurses, family planning nurses and school nurses, are increasingly coming into contact with clients with health-related problems in various settings. Besides, management of substance misusers is everyone's business rather than the responsibility and domain of a single health professional group. Many individuals who have substance-misuse problems do not use specialist drug or alcohol services but may be in contact directly or indirectly with the primary health care team and social care agencies. Members of the primary health care team and community workers are in an ideal position to identify, intervene and manage individuals with substance misuse problems, as substance misusers are more likely to use primary health care services (Grant & Hodgson 1991).

Substance use and misuse is unique in that it impinges on all aspects of the five key areas of 'The Health of the Nation' strategy (DoH 1992b): coronary heart disease and stroke, prevention of accidents, cancers, mental health problems, and HIV/AIDS and sexual health. Alcohol misuse, drug use and tobacco smoking are important contributing and risk factors in all the five key areas. In addition, the aim of the British Government's strategy, as set out in the White Paper 'Tackling Drugs Together' (1995), is 'to take effective action by vigorous law enforcement, accessible treatment and a new emphasis on education and prevention'. Substance misuse education for all health and social care professionals is therefore needed (ACMD 1990, Rassool & McKeown

1996, Rassool 1996, 1997b). Other relevant policy documents such as 'Working in Partnership' (DoH 1994b), 'Drugs and AIDS' (ACMD 1988, 1989) 'Report of an Independent Review of Drug Treatment Services in England' (DoH 1996a) have helped to activate the development of responses to meet the needs of the substance misuser.

This chapter will examine the prevalence and patterns of substance misuse in the context of recent policy initiatives. It will examine some of the parameters of addiction nursing with regard to issues related to nursing roles, nursing diagnosis and nursing models. In addition, it will also explore the development of community-oriented services in relation to the shared care model in the addiction field. Aspects of addiction such as public health, addiction prevention, screening and intervention strategies focusing on brief intervention will be presented. Implications for community nurses in relation to education and training are briefly examined.

PREVALENCE AND PATTERNS OF SUBSTANCE MISUSE

In the UK since the 1960s there has been an increase in the 'health-damaging' consumption of recreational, prescribed and illicit psychoactive substances across all strata of society, and substance misuse is now regarded as a major public health problem (Rassool & Gafoor 1997a). It is estimated that 6% of the UK population, around 3 million people, take at least one illegal drug in any one year (Tackling Drugs Together 1995). In England, it has been shown that over 90% of the population enjoy the occasional drink, one-third of adults smoke tobacco, hypnosedatives use and misuse is estimated to be in the thousands, and although prevalence figures for illicit drug use are patchy, owing to its covert nature, at least 6% of the population are believed to take an illicit psychoactive substance (Tackling Drugs Together 1995). The Department of Health Statistical Bulletin (1994) showed that of those clients presenting for treatment in 1993, by primary drug type (drug of choice), heroin was the primary drug in 54% of cases; in 18% it was amphetamines; and in 11% cocaine.

There is growing concern about the widespread increase of substance misuse among young people (Institute for the Study of Drug Dependence 1995). A study of 7722 pupils aged 15 and 16 conducted across the UK reveals that more than 40% of the sample had tried illicit drugs, mainly cannabis, with one-third reporting smoking in the previous 30 days (Miller & Plant 1996). There is also an upward trend in the number of young people experimenting and the use of amphetamines and psychedelic drugs (Parker et al 1995). Recent trends in the use and misuse of psychoactive substances suggest that there is increasing use among young females and the emergence of multiple-substance use as the norm in experimental users (HAS 1996). The phenomenon of polydrug use (the use and misuse of a multitude of psychoactive substances) seems to be the norm among established drug misusers rather than the exception. There is evidence to suggest that polydrug use is also common in young people experimenting with drugs, as the range of psychoactive substances now taken includes amphetamines, cocaine, LSD and ecstasy (DoH 1996a). There are other high-risk groups that are associated with alcohol and drug misuse and these groups include the elderly and the homeless.

There is evidence to suggest that there has been a significant increase in the incidence of alcohol misuse over the past two decades and to trends of problem-drinking in some professional groups, cultures, socioeconomic groups and geographical areas (Godfrey 1992, OPCS 1995). In the UK, each year the use of alcohol is associated with the premature deaths of between 8700 and 33 000 people (Godfrey & Maynard 1992). Psychiatric admissions associated with alcohol misuse total 17 000 annually and, with increasing emphasis on outpatient management, the true number of psychiatric clients is probably much higher (Paton 1994). Alcohol accounts for 25% of all deaths in road traffic accidents; 40% of all deaths from falls; 15% of all deaths from drowning and 65% of all deaths from cirrhosis. Alcohol misuse is a key factor in 20% of child abuse cases and in 30% of cases of marital conflict (Alcohol Concern 1995). In young people, alcohol drinking starts as early as 13 years of age (Alcohol Concern 1996).

Smoking is a major cause of both morbidity and mortality in the UK population (Callum et al 1992) and recent figures showed that the mortality rate is increasing; there may be approximately 120 000 deaths per year with about half of these occurring before or during middle age. According to West (1997) half of all lifelong smokers die as a result of smoking.

Benzodiazepines are the most commonly prescribed psychotropic drugs in the UK. The growing awareness of the risks of benzodiazepines and the rational use in prescribing among general practitioners resulted, in 1988, in a fall of 23 million prescriptions (Institute for the Study of Drug Dependence 1995). Recently there have been concerns over the injecting of benzodiazepines, particularly temazepam, and a link with increased HIV risk-taking behaviour (Darke et al 1993, Gafoor 1997a, Klee et al 1990). In Scotland and other parts of the UK, benzodiazepines use has been associated with a number of drug-related deaths and medical complications caused by injecting the contents of temazepam capsules or 'jellies' (Hammersley et al 1995, Ruben & Morrison 1992). HIV infection, which causes AIDS, is perhaps the greatest new public health challenge this century and is a greater threat to public and individual health than drug misuse (ACMD 1988, DoH 1992b).

Pattern of substance misuse

The levels of involvement range from the boundaries of the non-user to dependent or problem drug users/problem drinkers. Individuals vary in their pattern of drug or alcohol use and this is also reflected in their choice of psychoactive substance(s). Patterns of substance misuse include experimental use, recreational use and dependent use (Box 4.1). It is worth pointing out that an individual does not need to pass through all the stages of a drug-using career before shifting to abstinence or drug-free state. That is, moving from experimental to recreational to dependent use of psychoactive substances is not inevitable; there are exit routes at each level in the pattern of substance use and misuse.

It is stated that clear distinctions between experimental, recreational and dependent use are difficult to define, suggesting that it may be more valuable to identify whether the use of a psychoactive substance is problematic (ANSA 1997a). This is seen by the Advisory Council on the Misuse of Drugs' report on 'Treatment and Rehabilitation' (ACMD 1982) as a much clearer definition of a problem drug user: 'any person who experiences social, psychological, physical or legal problems related to intoxication and/or regular excessive consumption and/or dependence as a consequence of his own use of drugs or other chemical substances'.

Box 4.1   Characteristics of different patterns of substance misuse

Experimental use
- Refers to substance use in the very early stages of contact.
- Does not conform to any pattern or established pattern of use.
- Choice of substance is often indiscriminate and may depend on factors such as reputation, subculture, fashion and availability.
- It may be a group or individual activity.

Recreational use
- Recreational users may use psychoactive substance(s) frequently but not on a daily basis.
- Their prime motivation is mainly for pleasurable effects and relaxation.
- Choice of psychoactive substance is discriminatory, influenced by experience of experimentation, personal taste, expectations, availability and psychosocial and cultural factors.

Dependent use
- Users are characterised by physical, and/or psychological dependence.
- Use of drug is more important and frequent but less controlled, and situational factors such as time, company and settings are secondary.
- The chaotic behaviour pattern of users displaces rather than complements social activities.

This definition was widened to include any form of drug misuse which involves, or may lead to, sharing of injecting equipment (ACMD 1988). This holistic definition focuses on the needs and problems of the individual in acknowledging that the problem drug user has social, psychological, physical and legal needs, and is relevant to problem-drinkers. This definition could be expanded to incorporate the spiritual needs of the problem drug user or problem drinker. Some characteristics which may suggest potential or actual substance misusers are shown in Table 4.1.

DEVELOPMENT OF COMMUNITY-ORIENTED SERVICES

In the UK, health and social care policies implemented by the Government coupled with the changing health care needs of the population have provided added impetus in the care and management of a significant proportion of the population with substance use and misuse. Moreover, there has also been a growing

Table 4.1 Characteristics which may suggest potential drug and alcohol misuse

	Drug	Alcohol
How the patient presents for help	• With a specific request for drugs of misuse • Outside normal GP surgery • Repeated attempts for repeat/lost prescriptions • As a temporary resident	• Alcohol misusers are frequent attenders; however, alcohol use may be disguised by other physical or psychological problems
Signs and symptoms	• Injection marks, scars and pigmentation over injection sites • Pupils markedly constricted or dilated • Unexplained constipation or diarrhoea	• Smell of drink at interview • Withdrawal symptoms • Obesity, gastrointestinal symptoms, hypertension • Unexplained injury, bruising, memory blackouts • Anxiety and depression
Behaviour during consultation	• Unaccountable drowsiness, elated or restless • Loss of interest in appearance	• Inappropriate behaviour in the surgery • Emotionally labile • Aggressive
Social behaviour	• Family disruption • Frequent changes of GP • History of offences to obtain money	• Family disruption • Frequent changes of GP • History of offences to obtain money

Source: ANSA (1997b)

societal and professional recognition of the need for the prevention, treatment and rehabilitation of substance misusers. The attitude of 'laissez faire' or 'living with drugs' has been replaced by an interventionist approach in the 'war against drug misuse'. Community-oriented services for substance misusers emerged from this sociocultural and political paradigm shift.

In support for the development of community initiatives for problem drinkers, the Kessel report (Kessel 1978) suggested that general practitioners (GPs) were ideally placed to provide treatment and care for clients with drinking problems and gave impetus to the development of community-based services in the 1980s. In the 1970s the Government support for the first National Health Service (NHS) Alcohol Treatment Unit (ATU) in Great Britain, which had been established in 1955 at Warlingham Park Hospital (Glatt 1955), laid the foundation for the provision of a specialised treatment system for alcoholics in a variety of settings (Rassool 1997a). More recently, further development of alcohol recovery units such as Greenbank House (Checinski, personal communication, 1997) are dealing with a range of alcohol-related problems and those with dual diagnosis (substance misuse and mental health problems).

Kilpatrick (1993, unpublished work) has pointed out that drug and alcohol services have developed separately and at different times, and services for drugs tended to appear from the 1970s, later than the development of services for alcohol. Recently, alcohol has been put on the agenda, and GPs are required to offer health checks to their clients which include screening for alcohol consumption and offering help to the drinkers who are identified as being at risk (DoH 1989b). Furthermore, reports on the progress on the 'Health of the Nation' strategy (DoH 1995b) reiterate that health institutions should explore the incorporation of drinking history as part of the routine hospital admission procedure so that advice and minimal interventions can be implemented.

The Advisory Council of the Misuse of Drugs' report on 'Treatment and Rehabilitation' (ACMD 1982) highlighted the need for a comprehensive approach and multiprofessional response to substance misuse, calling for the active involvement of a wide range of both specialist and non-specialist service provision. This meant that health, social, probation and educational services and the voluntary sectors should coordinate their efforts and focus their services in meeting the needs of this client group. The first community drug team was established in 1983 and by 1991 more than half of the 192 district health authorities in England had such a team (Strang & Clement 1994). During the same period, the changing patterns of drug use and sudden increase in the number of young heroin users heralded the development of community drug teams, which were seen as a more effective service response to the problem drug-taker than the medically dominant drug dependency units (Rassool & Gafoor 1997a). Over the last decade, the growing demand for increased access to health care provision for substance misusers has resulted in some innovations in service provision such as development of community drug teams, alcohol liaison teams, day care programmes, street agencies, outreach work, needle exchange schemes and residential rehabilitation. Most of these innovations in service development have been nurse led. Addiction nurses have been at the forefront of these changes and many of the clinical developments and educational programmes for professionals have been nurse led, for example low threshold methadone programmes, satellite clinics for homeless substance misusers, outreach work with drug-using prostitutes, development of multiprofessional postgraduate educational programmes in addictive behaviour (Rassool & Gafoor 1997a).

ADDICTION NURSING IN PERSPECTIVES

Concept of addiction nursing

Historically, occupational labels such as alcohol nurse, drug dependency nurse, chemical substance nurse, specialist nurse in addiction and community psychiatric nurse (addiction) have been ascribed to those working with substance misusers. It was not until the mid-1980s that addiction nursing as a clinical speciality, within the broader framework of mental health nursing, began to put down its clinical and academic roots.

Addiction nursing may be defined as a specialist branch of mental health nursing concerned with the care and treatment interventions aimed at those individuals whose health problems are directly related to the use and misuse of psychoactive substances and to other addictive behaviours such as eating disorders and gambling (Rassool 1997a). Thus, the scope of professional practice in addiction nursing incorporates the activities of clinical practice (nursing, a range of psychosocial intervention strategies including complementary therapies), education, policy-making, research and all other pursuits through which nurse practitioners contribute to the care and work in the interests of their clients. It is argued that, although the concept of addiction nursing may be criticised on the grounds that it is too medically oriented and substance focused, other labels are too generic and lack the distinctive professional representation of addiction nursing (Rassool 1997a).

In the US, the concept of addiction nursing has been adopted by professional organisations and statutory bodies, producing two principal documents on addiction nursing addressing the rationale, scope, functions, roles and preparation for practice (ANA et al 1987, 1988). In the document entitled 'The Care of Clients with Addictions: Dimension of Nursing Practice' (ANA et al 1987) addictions nursing is defined as 'an area of speciality practice concerned with care related to dysfunctional patterns of human response that have one or more of these characteristics: loss of self-control capability, episodic or continuous maladaptive behaviour or abuse of some substance, and development of dependence patterns of a physical and/or psychological nature'. This definition denotes the concept of a specialist practitioner, and focus on both pharmacological and non-pharmacological addiction incorporates the diagnostic role for addiction nurses.

Nursing diagnosis

Nursing diagnosis originated in North America in the 1970s in an effort to combine the art, science and theoretical framework of nursing as distinct from other professional disciplines. The concept of nursing diagnosis within the framework of the systematic approach to care is accepted by the nursing professions and professional organisations in many American and European countries. However, in the UK, nursing diagnosis is not included as a component of the nursing process but the concept is slowly emerging in the nursing literature. It is stated that medical diagnosis describes the client's disease whereas a nursing diagnosis describes the client's current health responses. Recently, the North American Nursing Diagnosis Association (NANDA) had an unsuccessful attempt to have its taxonomy accepted for inclusion in the World Health Organization's 10th revision of the International Classification of Diseases (ICD 10) (Fitzpatrick et al 1989). This innovation would have made NANDA taxonomy the definitive classification of nursing.

Within the field of addiction nursing in the USA, 26 nursing diagnoses have been identified to guide nursing managers, researchers, educators and clinicians (ANA et al 1988). The 26 nursing diagnoses are grouped by four domains of human responses: biological, cognitive, psychosocial and spiritual. According to Murphy (1992), one of the strengths of addiction nursing as an emerging clinical speciality is that standards of practice and 26 selected nursing diagnoses have been identified by expert addiction nurses to guide clinicians, managers, educators and researchers. Murphy (1992) tested the 26 selected nursing diagnoses with a high-risk population of alcohol dependents, and her findings showed that diagnoses could be documented in 73% of the sample. This may indicate that there seems to be a consensus on the meaning and categories of nursing diagnoses. According to Lutzen & Tishleman (1996) nursing diagnosis is regarded as a strategy for advancing the professional status of nursing as well as a method of defining and organising nursing care. Other rationales for the adoption and implementation of nursing diagnoses include the shift away from medically-oriented nursing care plans to a more nursing focus; the provision of a common language to communicate clients' needs; and their use as a basis for monitoring the quality of care.

Nursing roles

Nurses have been the major component of the workforce, working as specialists in both alcohol and drug fields (ACMD 1990, Kennedy & Faugier 1989). Addiction nurses practise in both residential and community settings. With the massive expansion of community services for substance misusers such as the development of community drug/alcohol teams, drug alcohol liaison teams, day care programmes, street agencies, outreach work and needle exchange schemes, more nurses are entering and working in this developing field. This has heralded the potential development of addiction nursing as a community speciality. Neagle (1989) maintains that in order to provide services that are responsive to the changing health care needs of the population, nursing activities and nursing roles must adapt to changes and treatment trends. The role of nurses, midwives and health visitors, in relation to substance misuse, within the health care system is likely to change to meet the changing health needs of the population (Rassool 1996).

The roles of the nurse in relation to substance misuse have been highlighted in a recent document from the World Health Organization/International Council of Nurses (WHO/ICN 1991). These roles are: provider of care; educator/resource; counsellor/therapist; advocate; promoter of health; researcher;

supervisor/leader; and consultant. It has been identified that there is role differentiation between registered nurse practitioners and clinical nurse specialists working within residential or community-based settings (Rassool 1997a).

The roles of addiction nurses in the community are not as clear cut as those working in residential agencies. Owing to the nature of the work and the composition of many community teams, the blurring of roles among the disciplines is highly apparent. Much of the everyday work with drug users involves certain care skills (for example assessment, counselling and relapse prevention), and decisions regarding whether a client is seen by a nurse, medical practitioner or psychologist have, in the past, often depended upon which discipline was in charge of the allocation process and which staff member had a vacant slot (Gafoor 1997b). Both Rassool (1997a) and Gafoor (1997b) define a prescriptive role for the specialist nurse in substance misuse or addiction nursing: clinician; educator; consultant; manager; and researcher. The role of the addiction nurse as an advocate has also been suggested by Rassool (1997a). The skills utilised by addiction nurses include both nursing skills and psychosocial intervention skills and include assessment, counselling and motivational interviewing, relapse prevention, harm-minimisation, dealing with physical aspects of care, management, research, teaching and coaching. These skills need to be empirically validated so as to provide a more accurate representation of the role of the addiction nurse in the community setting.

Nursing models in addiction nursing

The implementation of nursing models has been slow to underpin the clinical practice of addiction nursing. The focus of the use of a nursing framework and/or model is to respond effectively in meeting the physical, psychosocial and spiritual needs of the clients. Hence, in addiction nursing, a limited number of models have been utilised as frameworks in the nursing care of addicted clients. Few nursing models have been adapted for use by addiction nurses in both residential and community settings (Rassool 1993) and these include Roy's (1980) Adaptation Model, Orem's (1985) Self-Care Model and Roper and colleagues' (1983) Activities of Daily Living. Anderson & Smereck developed the 'Light model' (Anderson & Smereck 1989) from a combination of

Martha Roger's theory of human–environmental energy fields and Aristotle's view of well-being to an optimal level. Although this model has not been fully empirically tested in the UK context, nevertheless, its main strength is to involve clients in their own recovery process and self-care within the framework of an informal contractual approach. Rassool (1997a) argue that no single nursing model, currently in use, is adequate to meet the diverse health needs of substance misusers, and the focus for clinicians and academics should be directed towards the adaptation and refinement of nursing models or the development of an integrated model of care applicable to the complexities and nature of substance misuse and addictive behaviour.

INTERPROFESSIONAL COLLABORATION AND SHARED CARE

The term 'interprofessional collaboration', as a practical construct has long been the trademark of many service-led drug and alcohol specialist agencies. This kind of working alliance has emerged as a result of the nature of the work, the problems associated with substance misuse and addictive behaviour and the blurring of roles. However, it is the cultural shift in the ideology of caring from institutional to community-oriented approach that has added new impetus and drive for more professional and clinical collaborative efforts amongst health, criminal justice and social care professionals. For addiction nurses, developing a shared care approach with other agencies helps to ensure that the client receives appropriate interventions which match the nature of the problem and prevent the silting up of the nurse's caseload (Gafoor 1997b).

Shared care has been defined in a recent Department of Health Circular (1995a) as:

The joint participation of specialists and GPs (and other agencies as appropriate) in the planned delivery of care for clients with a drug misuse problem, informed by an enhanced information exchange beyond routine discharge and referral letters. It may involve the day to day management by the GP of a patient's medical needs in relation to his other drug misuse. Such arrangements would make explicit which clinician was responsible for different aspects of the patient's treatment and care. They may include prescribing substitute drugs in appropriate circumstances.

According to Keating (1996), the concept of shared care between health services is not a new one as there has been, in the past, collaboration between the primary health care team and specialist services in dealing with substance misusers. The shared care model is advocated as the best way forward for substance misuse services (NHS Executive 1995).

The shared care concept was assessed in a randomised controlled trial (Drummond & Edwards 1990) and the findings show that after an initial detailed assessment and advice session by the specialist, the treatment provided by GPs (advice and counselling or brief intervention) is at least as effective as that provided by specialist clinics with respect to improvements in drinking behaviour and alcohol-related problems. The model of partnership between specialist and other members of the primary health care team based on the concept of shared care and interprofessional collaboration would appear to be the direction for community services to further strengthen its links. Key aspects of shared care are given in Box 4.2.

SCREENING, ASSESSMENT AND INTERVENTION APPROACHES IN SPECIALIST SERVICES

This section of the chapter focuses on screening, assessment and intervention strategies. It deals with different types of assessment and screening instruments that non-specialist community health care workers may incorporate within their particular assessment

---

Box 4.2   Core principles of shared care (ANSA 1997b)

- Clear roles and responsibilities of primary care team and specialist services, e.g. defining who is the lead care provider and responsible for the coordination of care.
- Agreement on patient records and confidentiality.
- Agreement on communication pathways between services involved.
- Agreement on cross-referral arrangements.
- Easy access to specialist services ('fast track'/urgent cases).
- Agreement on treatment policies.
- Agreed protocols (who will manage patient and when).
- Protocols for medical management (prescribing) for those requiring detoxification.
- Arrangements for urine analysis.
- Agreements with local pharmacists regarding dispensing arrangements.
- Consensus completion of Drug Misuse Database forms.

of their clients. The screening questionnaire and other screening tools are easy to use to identify the need for generic or specialist interventions. Brief or minimal intervention as an intervention strategy is also presented.

There are a host of physical, psychological and social problems related to substance misuse that are present covertly in almost every nursing encounter. Within the primary health care settings, there is ample opportunity for health care professionals to identify, recognise (screening and assessment) and intervene effectively (brief intervention, counselling, advice, health education). The following is a list of examples of occasions or situations when screening and assessment opportunities can be harnessed:

- new client registrations
- well woman clinics/family planning clinics
- well men clinics
- pre-birth checks
- under-5 and 16-year-old checks
- specialist clinics, e.g. asthma/diabetic/blood pressure/travel
- accessing primary care for other health-related problems.

Particular factors for those with problematic or dependent substance use (ANSA 1997b) include:

- The GP surgery/health centre is more accessible.
- Some clients are reluctant to attend specialist services e.g. fear of the label 'addict', stigma, etc.
- Some clients do not consider themselves as 'addicts' and do not wish to attend a specialist service.
- The specialist clinics may not have as flexible opening hours as the GP/surgery/health centre/clinic.
- Lack of knowledge about specialist services.

Screening

The purpose of screening and assessment is to determine the degree and patterns of substance use and misuse, the consequences of the sequelae, and the development of a plan for effective nursing care and health interventions. In addition, both screening and assessment serve to identify the appropriate professional help needed by the clients and significant others, and to monitor care, treatment and health gains. There are three types of assessment (ANSA 1997a,b,c): triage for emergencies;

screening; and initial/specialist assessment. Screening or taking a drug and alcohol history or simple health checks regarding the use of psychoactive substances should be incorporated within the health screening process. In triage the main objective is to identify and clarify the degree of emergency and health needs; the process lasts a few minutes and may include one-to-one telephone consultations. In emergency situations, a 'triage' assessment may be essential for those presenting within the primary health care settings with overdose, lost prescriptions, withdrawal seizures, delirium tremens, deliberate self-harm (ANSA 1997a) and those with dual diagnosis (substance misuse and mental health problems).

In primary health care settings, tools such as CAGE (Mayfield 1974) or the Short Michigan Alcoholism Screening Test (SMAST) (Selzer et al 1975) may be used as the next stage in the process of screening and assessment of problems. It is stated that in identifying the existence of problematic drug/alcohol use, a screening assessment may be an enabling process that can motivate problem drug users or dependent drug users to move from pre-contemplative to contemplative stage and action in changing their substance use behaviours (Prochaska & DiClemente 1986). The screening questionnaire in Box 4.3 may be incorporated within the assessment framework of any particular nursing speciality. The APPCP screening questionnaire was developed by the Addiction Prevention in Primary Care Programme (Ghodse et al 1994).

The outcome of screening would enable the nurse to determine the degree of intervention appropriate to this particular client. This is an opportunity for health care professionals to provide health information and advice, brief intervention or counselling depending on the health needs of the client. If substance misuse is identified as problematic (polydrug and alcohol users, pregnant clients, child care issues, dual diagnosis, etc.), referral to the general practitioner or specialist drug and alcohol services is recommended. A specialist or full assessment may be required to assess the degree of substance use problems and health status of the clients in order to plan for the appropriate clinical care and interventions. Addiction nurses, as part of a multiprofessional team, usually administer this type of specialist assessment. A specialist assessment tool is the Substance Abuse Assessment Questionnaire (SAAQ) (Ghodse 1995) which incorporates the following assessments: medical and psychological, alcohol use,

---

Box 4.3   APPCP Screening Questionnaire

1. Do you smoke or have you ever smoked?   YES/NO
2. How much do you smoke? (per day or week)

   • All smokers should receive further assessment and advice.

3. Do you drink or have you ever drunk alcohol?   YES/NO
4. In an average week, how much alcohol do you drink?

   • If greater than 28 units (male) or 21 units (female), a more detailed
     assessment of the patient's drinking history is necessary.

5. Do you use any pills, medicines, drugs or tablets other
   than those prescribed for medical reasons?   YES/NO
   e.g. to help you:
   – relax, sleep, cope with stress   YES/NO
   – feel good   YES/NO
   – have fun or excitement   YES/NO
6. Do you ever need to use more of your medicines than   YES/NO
   prescribed?
7. Do you regularly use non-prescription medicines from   YES/NO
   the chemist?

Source: Addiction Prevention in Primary Care Programme, Centre for Addiction Studies,
Department of Addictive Behaviour, St George's Hospital Medical School, University of London.

drug use, forensic, psychosocial and family, profile of the
substance misuser and treatment programme.

Brief intervention

A number of World Health Organization initiatives suggest that
early intervention strategies in primary care such as the use of
screening and offering brief advice (brief intervention) are the
way forward (Babor et al 1986, Wallace et al 1988). The term brief
or minimal intervention generally refers to intervention strategies such as health education in raising awareness of the problem
and advice on changing behaviour to a more healthy lifestyle. It
is cost-effective and can reach a wider population within the
health care delivery systems (Bien et al 1993).

The number of sessions varies between 8 and 10, each session
lasting from 10–30 minutes. The content of these sessions consists
primarily of simple advice and exchange of information, which
has proved to be effective in influencing a change in drinking
behaviour (Watson 1992). Prochaska & DiClemente (1986) suggest that problem drinking is likely to decrease or be modified to

less harmful levels at a point of change, i.e. life events such as the birth of a child, marriage and/or crisis, e.g. accident or hospital admission. The following offers some practical advice on brief interventions regarding alcohol use (Cooper 1995, 1997):

• When drinking is not seen as a problem: health education and harm minimisation.

• If alcohol is acknowledged as a problem but help seeking is not yet being considered: offer verbal information and health education literature on substance use and misuse. Provide details of support, self-help groups and advisory alcohol services.

• High consumption of alcohol is not perceived as a problem and the individual does not request help: offer advice within the individual limitations, and contact details of helping specialist agencies. Liaise with other agencies if needed.

• The individual wants to cease consumption or modify drinking behaviour and may require clinically supervised withdrawal: make contact with substance misuse agencies or alcohol advisory service for further advice and guidance or referral.

Elements that have been included in brief or minimal intervention that have been shown to be effective are feedback, responsibility, advice, menu, empathy and self-efficacy (or the acronym FRAMES) (Miller & Sanchez 1993). A framework on brief or minimal intervention for alcohol misuse has been suggested by Anderson (1990). The intervention strategies are:

• Ask clients if alcohol consumption is affecting their health.
• Make a note of their drinking behaviour: weekly consumption, types of drinks, regular heavy drinking days, etc.
• Fill in a drink diary to record and monitor consumption for the previous week.
• Indicate the client's health status in comparison to the general population. Methods of delivery include diagram, histogram of pattern of consumption.
• Raise awareness of risks or negative effects.
• Mention the benefits of reduced or controlled drinking or abstinence.
• Give sound but friendly advice.
• Give client health education literature, a pamphlet on alcohol or self-help manual.
• Arrange a follow-up appointment within 2–4 weeks to review client's alcohol consumption or monitor behaviour change.

The level of intervention may vary depending on the level of skill and expertise of the community nurse providing such therapeutic responses. This type of intervention can easily be adapted within the therapeutic framework of any community discipline. However, brief intervention is likely to be effective with drinkers with moderate dependence rather than those with severe alcohol-related problems. Brief intervention may also be extended to the misuse of prescribed, over-the-counter, or illicit drugs. Jarvis et al (1996) stated that there is no reason why early and brief forms of intervention should not be extended to opiates or stimulants, especially in those settings which have embraced a harm minimisation approach to drug use.

PUBLIC HEALTH AND ADDICTION PREVENTION
Public health

Licit and illicit substance use and misuse remain the largest cause of preventable morbidity and mortality in the UK. Nurses and, in particular, community nurses are involved with parents and school children and are well suited to identify needs and to give a clear direction for effective education and prevention strategies (Rawaf 1996). In addition, the aim of the British Government's strategy, as set out in the White Paper 'Tackling Drugs Together' 1995, is 'to take effective action by vigorous law enforcement, accessible treatment and a new emphasis on education and prevention'. For the first time there is a comprehensive approach to substance use problems in the UK with the emphasis clearly on education and preventive programmes. In addition, consumer interest groups and parents are also providing the impetus to combat the complex challenges of substance misuse. The spread of HIV/AIDS, hepatitis and, more recently, tuberculosis, has also influenced health and social policies and unveiled new prevention initiatives and challenges towards substance misuse. The realisation that some substance misusers engaged in high-risk behaviours such as sharing injecting equipment or having unsafe sex and the danger of transmitting the HIV virus to the wider population provided new impetus for the broad application of a harm-minimisation approach in the substance misuse field.

Public health campaigns are there to maximise current awareness of the risks of tobacco smoking, drinking and driving, and the misuse of over-the-counter drugs, alcohol, and prescribed and illicit drugs. Multimedia campaigns, in their role as a pro-social influence, have been influential in enabling individuals to withdraw from benzodiazepines (Beattie 1991). It is argued, however, that local-level campaigns working with self-help groups, outreach workers and the local community can be more effective than high-profile national campaigns (Rodmell & Watt 1986). Generally, strategies that focus on specific areas of drug or alcohol health education directed at multiple target groups within the community may be the most effective prevention efforts.

Prevention and harm minimisation

The cultural shift in the attitude of policy makers and professional bodies and institutions has made prevention activities to be everybody's business. This proactive process, according to the National Institute on Drug Abuse (1980), utilises an interdisciplinary approach which is designed to empower people with the resources to constructively confront stressful life situations. At a societal level, the drive to minimise the use and misuse of psychoactive substances and its sequelae has been reflected along two main fronts, that is, the reduction of the supply of and demand for drugs. Strang & Farrell (1989) suggested that prevention programmes must be directed to encourage drug users to approach care services earlier in their drug-using career rather than wait for the complications to appear before coming forward for help.

Traditionally health education activities have been viewed as existing on three levels of prevention: (a) primary, (b) secondary and (c) tertiary. This three-stage public health model has been modified by the Advisory Council on the Misuse of Drugs (ACMD 1984) on the grounds that it was not sufficiently comprehensive to cover all the elements of prevention policies in the context of substance use and misuse. The ACMD's approach to prevention is based on meeting two basic criteria:

- reducing the risk of an individual engaging in substance misuse
- reducing the harm associated with substance misuse.

There is no single appropriate model of health education in the field of drug prevention and drug education. The model or

models used by addiction nurses and other health care professionals in preventive efforts would depend on the ideology and
professional practice of the 'health educator' (Rassool 1997b). In
addition, the health needs of the client, the context and setting,
the client–worker relationship and the level of preventive health
education will, undoubtedly, influence the choice of model(s). In
the addiction field, a combination of approaches is utilised to
complement other intervention strategies such as the harm-
minimisation approach.

The concept of harm minimisation or harm reduction may be
viewed as the programmes and policies which attempt to reduce
the harms associated with drug use (Strang 1993). The concept
of harm minimisation, therefore, goes beyond measures aimed
at changing drug users' behaviours and involves wider societal
changes such as legal sanctions, public attitudes and educational
policies regarding drug use (Rassool 1997b). Thus strategies and
approaches that aim to reduce the harms associated with drug
use may be more pragmatic and realistic for some individuals
depending on their health-related problems. However, although
harm minimisation is an important clinical principle, it must
take place within practice that is, lawful to the benefit of the
young people (HAS 1996) and those attending treatment
programmes.

The ACMD (1988) further recommended that services 'should
adopt a hierarchy of goals in dealing with drug users' which
should include:

- cessation of sharing injecting equipment
- the move from injectable to oral drug use
- decrease in drug use
- abstinence.

Other sub-goals were later added to the hierarchy such as:

- cleaning injecting equipment before sharing
- reducing the number of people with whom injecting
  equipment is shared
- switching from illicit to prescribed drugs.

The concept of harm minimisation has always been associated
with illicit drug use rather than prevention of alcohol misuse.
However, there is a trend towards harm minimisation in alcohol
problems prevention, with increased attention being given to

measures which focus on reducing the adverse consequences of drinking without necessarily reducing drinking per se (Plant et al 1997). Plant et al argued that they did not see any conflict with abstinence-oriented approaches to the prevention of alcohol problems as harm minimisation does not imply the approval of drinking, and that the eventual goal of intervention might not include abstention. According to Plant et al (1997) the term harm minimisation refers to the policies and programmes which attempt to reduce the harm associated with drinking, without the drinker necessarily giving up his or her use of alcohol.

Addiction prevention

The Addiction Prevention in Primary Care Programme began in September 1991 as a joint initiative by the Department of Addictive Behaviour, St George's Hospital Medical School, and Merton, Sutton and Wandsworth Family Health Authority. The concept of prevention in the primary care setting is not new but the establishment of the Addiction Prevention in Primary Care Programme (APC) with specialist interest in substance use and misuse is the first of its kind in the UK (Ghodse et al 1996). The programme embraces the concepts of early identification and intervention and reflects the transition from ward-based health care delivery to a community-oriented prevention programme (DoH 1992b, Ghodse et al 1994, McShane 1997). The main aim of the programme is to equip community-based health care professionals with the appropriate attitude, necessary skills, knowledge and confidence to enable them to respond effectively to clients at an early stage of problem or hazardous substance use/misuse.

The roles of the addiction prevention counsellor include one-to-one counselling and usually take a client-centred approach. In addition, the underpinning principles of patient treatment matching, a brief intervention and motivational interviewing, in the APC's experience increase the likelihood of a successful treatment outcome. They are also involved in establishing smoking cessation and/or other substance misuse clinics or programmes as appropriate.

SPECIALIST INTERVENTION STRATEGIES

A model of change that has been influential in the substance misuse field is the model of behavioural change (Prochaska & DiClemente 1983). Prochaska and DiClemente first described the model as a result of their study of smokers who were successful in quitting, and their findings suggest that change occurred in a series of steps. These include stages of pre-contemplation, contemplation, action, decision-making and maintenance (Prochaska et al 1992). The model also provides a framework to identify the individual's readiness, in terms of motivation and commitment, to change, thus enabling the choice of suitable intervention strategies to achieving change. For example tobacco smokers will be at different stages in this dynamic process at any one time. In the pre-contemplation stage, the individual smoker is not thinking about stopping and may not be aware of his addiction. In the contemplation stage, individuals are aware of their dependence on nicotine and may consider stopping. In the third, decision-making and preparation stage, the individual may decide to stop. The action stage involves the individual in quitting smoking. In the final stage, maintenance, the individual is involved in maintaining the desired change of being drug free and avoiding relapse.

The intervention strategies used in the care, management and treatment of substance misuse or addictive behaviours incorporate the pharmacological, psychosocial and behavioural treatments. With early identification or recognition of substance use and misuse, clients may sometimes stop smoking or become drug/alcohol free on their own, in other words, have 'spontaneous remission'. As with smokers, spontaneous remission also applies to individuals with alcohol or drug misuse or problems and, like smokers, it may involve several attempts at being drug or alcohol free (Sobell et al 1993). For a comprehensive examination of methods of treatment see Ghodse (1995) and Jarvis et al (1995); only a brief overview of specialist treatment of substance misusers is given below.

Self-help groups such as Alcoholics Anonymous (AA) and Narcotics Anonymous (NA) are part of the treatment packages for substance misusers. The bases of AA or NA programmes are self-help recovery or self-care through following the 'Twelve Steps' and group participation or therapy. Pharmacological treatments involve the clinical management of withdrawal and detoxification from alcohol or drugs. Benzodiazepines such as chlordiazepoxide (Librium) are the preferred drugs for detoxification from alcohol rather than Heminevrin (chlormethiazole). For relapse prevention, the most popular and widely used drugs are disulfiram (Antabuse) and calcium carbimide (Temposil). Naltrexone and acamprosate (Campral) have also been used in the treatment of alcohol dependence to reduce craving following detoxification (Omalley et al 1992, Volpicelli et al 1992). For treatment of drug addiction, for example opiate dependence, methadone is used in a detoxification and maintenance programme. Buprenorphine, a mixed opiate agonist–antagonist, and desipramine (an antidepressant) have been used in the treatment of cocaine users. For critical reviews of pharmacological therapies for substance dependence see Ghodse (1995) and Borg (1997). Psychological and behavioural interventions with substance misusers within specialist agencies (hospital, outpatient and community settings) include the use of motivational interviewing (Miller 1983), cue exposure (Drummond et al 1995), relapse prevention (Marlatt 1985), and individual and group psychotherapy and counselling. The following case vignettes highlight the specialist interventions for alcohol-related problems and polydrug use.

Case vignette 1

Colin is a 32-year-old man who is married with two teenage children. Although he is usually pleasant and cooperative, he becomes verbally argumentative and physically aggressive whilst intoxicated. During the last 5 years his alcohol consumption increased markedly and he has been drinking seven to eight pints of Super Strong Cider (8.5% volume of alcohol) daily. Hence, he consumes 28 units daily and 196 units weekly. Colin visited his GP complaining of insomnia, depression and marked mood swings. He also is having problems with his memory and concentration, and has experienced blackouts on a number of occasions. The GP referred Colin to the local community drug and alcohol team.

Specialist interventions

Colin was assessed to determine the extent and nature of his problem-drinking, identify current problems, complications and the past triggering factor resulting in his present condition. On assessment, Colin was found to meet the inclusion criteria for home detoxification and his partner agreed to support and help him. A plan of treatment for home detoxification was formulated involving both Colin and his partner, as the involvement of the carer is of paramount importance in this process. Both the role of medication in facilitating alcohol detoxification and the overcoming of withdrawal symptoms was explained to Colin. Medication such as chlordiazepoxide (Librium), prescribed by his general practitioner, was administered as directed on a reducing dosage for 10 days. Colin successfully completed his home detoxification and continues to receive ongoing support and counselling from the community addiction nurse. He attends AA twice a week. During the recovery phase, the addiction nurse was also able to discuss the effects of alcohol and the ways of preventing lapse and relapse.

Case vignette 2

Peter is 20 years old, single and unemployed. At the age of 13, his father was made redundant and the family moved from Ireland to live in a small market town in the south of England, where his father found work in a local factory. Stephen found it difficult to settle into his new environment and was teased for his strong accent. He frequently truanted from school before finally being expelled at the age of 14 for aggressive and violent behaviours. Over the next 5 years he smoked cannabis almost daily and took amphetamines, LSD and ecstasy tablets at weekend raves. He was also drinking up to 30 units of alcohol per week. Peter left home when he was 19 and rented a room in a large house which was also shared by a number of substance misusers. He quickly became immersed in the local drug subculture and acquired several convictions for shoplifting and burglary to fund his drug and alcohol problems. He was injecting up to 4 g of amphetamines and drinking up to a bottle of spirits daily. In addition he was also injecting temazepam capsules that were either bought illicitly or obtained from various doctors. Peter was referred to the local community drug and alcohol team by his probation officer following a conviction for shoplifting.

Specialist interventions

Peter presented in an anxious and agitated state constantly asking for something to calm him down and threatening to leave if he did not receive a prescription of some sort. He had injected amphetamines immediately prior to his appointment with a member of the community drug and alcohol team (CDAT), but denied using alcohol or temazepam. Peter agreed to complete the interview after being informed that a prescription could only be issued after a full assessment had been made to determine his medication and health needs. His physical condition was poor and he had lost nearly 12 kg in weight over the past couple of months; the injecting sites on both his arms appeared infected. Shortly after his assessment, Peter was prescribed dexamphetamine elixir and diazepam tablets by his GP on the condition that he avoided injecting and kept his appointments with the CDAT for the next few weeks. After a while, both his physical and mental state improved, and with the help of the social worker he managed to find new accommodation in a quiet part of town and away from his drug-using peers. In addition to counselling and harm-minimisation, Peter attended sessions of anxiety management and relapse prevention and he was gradually weaned off dexamphetamines over an 8-week period. He is currently reducing his diazepam prescription by 5 mg a week.

PROFESSIONAL DEVELOPMENT

In the UK, owing to the changes in registration and professional development (UKCC 1994a) coupled with current policy (DoH 1992b, 1995b) and educational initiatives (ENB 1996a), nurses, midwives and health visitors must engage in continuing education and professional development as a statutory requirement to maintain their professional competence. Substance use and misuse are a key component in continuing education.

The lack of adequate educational preparation of nurses, midwives and health visitors is reflected in several documents (ACMD 1982, 1988 1989, 1990, Advisory Committee on Alcoholism 1978, Alcohol Concern 1994, ENB 1995b, WHO 1993, WHO/ICN 1991). Evidently the substance misuse component in pre-registration, post-registration and specialist practitioner education programmes lags behind current awareness of substance misuse. In addition, few centres provide specialist courses in addiction studies (ENB 962 and 612), and they are arbitrarily distributed through the English health authorities. In its recommendations for nurses in relation to substance abuse, the

WHO/ICN (1991) document states that nurses should be educated at the basic training levels and that continuing education should be provided for those working in this field. Furthermore, it is stated that education and training must be an integral part of service planning for all areas of treatment, and include specialist and non-specialist personnel (WHO 1993).

The failure of current professional education and training at undergraduate and postgraduate levels in nursing and health sciences curricula has reinforced the legitimacy of regarding alcohol and drug problems as somebody else's business (Rassool 1993b). Several studies have shown that education and training on substance misuse and addictive behaviour can enhance positive attitude and increase confidence and skills in identifying and working with substance misusers (Hagemaster et al 1993, Kennedy & Faugier 1989, Rassool 1993a, 1994). The curriculum content of both pre-registration and continuing professional education programmes need to be modified to incorporate aspects of substance misuse. Rassool & Oyefeso (1993) and the English National Board (ENB 1996) have suggested the use of a vertical-integration approach for the integration of substance use and misuse within existing nursing and health sciences curricula. This approach focuses on teaching aspects of drug, alcohol and tobacco use and misuse alongside the content of nursing or health studies curricula. Guidelines for good practice in education and training of nurses, midwives and health visitors on substance use and misuse are outlined elsewhere (ENB 1996). These guidelines are for use by programme planners and provide indicative content for both pre-registration and continuing professional education programmes.

The effectiveness of a professional development programme can be more pronounced when it is part of a strategic plan to create an organisational learning culture. It is argued that the dual development and integration of a substance misuse curriculum at pre-registration and post-registration levels should be part of a parallel process of change (Rassool 1996). If education and training in substance misuse and addiction for all health care professionals are to become a reality, policy makers, professional associations, educationalists and clinicians need to capitalise on the current political climate and cultural shift to genuinely implement policy initiatives. Special grants should be provided for those implementing substance use and misuse education at undergraduate and postgraduate levels.

CONCLUSION

The community responses to the health and social care needs of substance misusers have, in the past, failed to provide adequate and accessible services. To some extent, substance misusers have been marginalised by professionals and by society at large. The implementation of the Community Care Act 1990 has brought some positive results in the form of assessment and care planning. Primary health care professionals because of their close involvement with clients are in a unique position to deliver effective public health interventions and management.

However, while health professionals can provide clinics for preventive activities, brief intervention and counselling (for example smoking cessation), there is a strong need for the prevention of smoking (or other drug misuse) to be supported at a national level to alter the context in which health care is defined (Littlewood 1995). In the UK, there should be a proactive preventive policy reflecting the changing nature and extent of substance misuse. In addition, an integrated preventive policy covering alcohol, tobacco smoking, prescribed and illegal drugs, service provision and health education measures should be the hallmark of future policy development (Rassool 1997b). Interpersonal collaboration and shared care need to be strengthened between the primary health care team and specialist alcohol and drug agencies. A 'healthy alliance' could be developed for the provision of interprofessional education and training in substance misuse, and in multiprofessional collaboration in clinical and evaluative research into the addictions. Above all, the way forward is for community nurses to become the prime movers towards the process and maintenance of change.

ACKNOWLEDGEMENTS

I wish to acknowledge my thanks to M. Gafoor, Chief Executive, Addiction Counselling Trust, Buckinghamshire, and S. Derage, Clinical Nurse Specialist, Surrey, for providing me with the case vignettes.

5

Palliative care

Edna Elias

INTRODUCTION

Cancer can affect anyone regardless of race, religion, culture or socioeconomic status.

There are over 200 different types of cancers each of which has its own characteristics, incidence, spread and survival rates, but all share one common characteristic: that there is uncontrolled division of malignant cells, generally from a single primary site (Taylor 1992).

The most recent estimate of the world burden of cancer was made by Parkin (1993). An estimated 7.62 million new cases of cancer occurred in the world in 1985 and, if the rate remain unchanged, the number will rise to an estimated minimum of 8.4 million new cases in 1990 and 10.3 million in the year 2000, despite the fact that in many countries it is difficult to collect reliable information on cause of death, let alone register new patients with cancer (Cancer Research Campaign 1995).

About one person in three in England and Wales will develop cancer at some stage in their lives; approximately one person in four will die as a result. In 1988 there were around 300 000 newly diagnosed cases registered within the UK. In 1992 nearly 165 000 people died from cancer (Austoker 1994). Cancer is a major cause of death and avoidable ill-health, accounting for about 25% of deaths (OPCS 1992). It is predominantly a disease affecting elderly people. The increasing number of elderly people in the population has contributed to an increase in the demand for inpatient services. This has resulted in changes in treatment practice and development of preventive measures and early detection (Hawket 1995). It has been stated that the treatment of cancer accounts for about 7% of all NHS expenditure, amounting to about £1000 million per year at 1986/87 prices (UKACR 1994).

Development in the planning of health care provisions, and growing emphasis on financial management, have given increased focus to the study of trends of cancer incidence and mortality and to the active promotion of cancer prevention. This was given a high priority in 1985 with the development of the Europe Against Cancer programme. This aims at reducing the number of deaths from cancer by 15% by the year 2000.

The UK 'Health of The Nation' strategy is also aimed at disease prevention and health promotion, with cancer forming one of the five target areas (DoH 1992b).

HISTORY OF PALLIATIVE CARE

The original hospices go back to the early fourth century to Fabiola, a Roman matron who opened her home for those in need after seeing earlier Syrian hospices setting out to fulfil the Christian 'ways of mercy', feeding the hungry and thirsty, visiting the sick and prisoners, clothing the naked and welcoming strangers. At the time the word 'hospice' meant both host and guest, and 'hospitium' both the place where hospitality was given and also the relationship that arose. That emphasis is still central to hospice care today.

Religious orders attempted to carry the burden of caring for the poor, sick and dying, and continued to do so throughout the middle ages. Most closed after the reformation and those left became alms houses for the poor or elderly, or resting places for travellers. By the 19th century the few still open provided an alternative such as the workhouse infirmaries which catered for the destitute (Twycross 1980).

The word 'hospice' to describe a place caring solely for dying patients was first used in 1842 when Mme Jeanne Garnier founded the Demeudu Calvaire at Lyons in France. The name was adopted by the Irish Sisters of Charity in 1879 when they began carrying out similar work in Dublin.

In 1885 at the Friendenshe House of Rest, later St Columba's Hospice, began the establishment of the hospice movement in Britain. This was followed by the Hostel of God (now Trinity Hospice) in 1891 staffed by the Sisters of St Margaret. This was the result of an appeal by the Hoare banking family for funds 'to fund a home for persons in an advanced stage of a mortal illness' – thus establishing a heavy reliance on charitable giving which continues in the hospice movement to this day (Saunders 1984). A few years later St Luke's House (later Hospital) for the Dying Poor was started by Dr Barrett and the West London Mission. Cardinal Vaughan's expressed concern for the plight of the sick in the slums of London brought the Sisters of Charity across from Ireland. They set up St Joseph's Hospice in Hackney to serve the community in the East End of London in 1905 (Taylor 1983).

In 1911 Douglas Macmillan, a 27-year-old civil servant, watched helplessly as his father died painfully from cancer. The shock of this sudden illness and the sight of such needless pain and suffering moved Douglas to found the National Society for Cancer Relief with his father's final birthday gift of £10 (Ogden 1994).

As early as the 1920s the need was recognised to provide special homes and home-care nurses. The Marie Curie Memorial Foundation, named after the scientist who devoted her life to research into radiation and its uses in cancer therapy, was founded in 1948 by Squadron Leader Bernard Robinson, together with a few like-minded friends, inspired by Winston Churchill's comment that casualties from cancer were far worse than those suffered in the Second World War, thus establishing national cancer nursing. The Marie Curie Foundation worked closely with the Queen's Institute of District Nursing and medical officers of health to investigate the present position of cancer patients being nursed at home, and make recommendations concerning the best methods of providing the necessary help. It recommended that the Marie Curie Foundation provide, as a matter of urgency, 'special' residential homes for the care of cancer patients – both for the seriously ill and for convalescent care – with skilled nursing care in a non-stressful and cheerful environment.

By the end of the decade the first such homes were up and running. Now there are eleven nationwide with special emphasis on rehabilitation, continuing care, pain relief and symptom control, while Marie Curie nurses work with district nurses to provide care for terminally ill patients in their own homes.

The Sue Ryder Foundation, another charity, was set up in 1953 keen to embrace cancer work, but is now an international foundation dedicated to the relief of suffering on a much wider scale, caring for patients with many different disabilities.

St Christopher's Hospice, unlike nearly all the modern hospices, grew into the local community rather than out of it (Saunders 1991). This was really so because, working as a district nurse in the area from the mid to late 1970s, it was difficult to get patients to agree to be admitted to St Christopher's because they felt it was the place where people went to die, and 'if you go in there you never come out'. Also, because of the name, many thought it was a religious place and that certainly was not for them.

It was at St Joseph's Hospice in the 1950s that Dr Cicely Saunders, as a medical officer, began to develop techniques of pain control which she had first observed as a medical student while working as a volunteer nurse in St Luke's Hospital. St Joseph's were giving their drugs 'as required' and were using injections rather than oral medication. She firmly established that it was possible to achieve better control of pain by giving analgesic drugs at regular intervals before the patient appeared to need them.

Although other forms of cancer treatments have subsequently been developed, it is the regular administration of pain-killing drugs, together with the detailed control of other symptoms, and the personalised care of patients and support for their relatives, which has become the hospice trademark (Lewis 1989). So when Cicely Saunders set up St Christopher's in Sydenham in 1967 as the first research and teaching hospice, it quickly became the acknowledged international pioneer in the field of hospice practice, earning her the unofficial title of Founder of the Modern Hospice Movement (du Boulay 1984). Under her direction, hospice work was extended to home care in 1969 and much further work was done to increase understanding of the biological mechanisms of pain control drugs, opening up a whole new area of specialist medicine, of which some innovative anaesthetists were part.

Alongside pain control came a realisation of how important it was to help not just the physical suffering of the patient, but also the emotional anguish of relatives. New York's system of family support (mainly by social workers) set up by the American Cancer Care Organization in the 1950s was visited by Dr Saunders in 1963. But the main plans for proper bereavement services in British hospices came from the work of the Tavistock Centre for Human Relations, CRUSE, a national organisation set up in 1959 to help the widowed and their children, and St Christopher's (Kubler-Ross 1970, Saunders 1988).

The hospice movement developed these ideas by training volunteers who were especially sensitive to the effects of death and dying on bereaved loved ones. This twin approach to pain control and bereavement counselling was quickly picked up by hospices, NHS hospitals and community alike. As a number of hospices grew, experiences were shared and lessons learnt. With the exception of a few in London, the hospices are mainly in the suburbs and tend not to meet the needs of all the community. Hospices should be creating equal access and delivering a culturally sensitive service to our multicultural society (National Council for Hospice and Specialist Palliative Care Services 1995).

CANCER BELIEFS

The word cancer elicits an immediate emotional response, a response that seems to have no relationship to rational thinking, depth of knowledge of the individual, or the individual's role in society (Burns 1982). It is not naming as such that is pejorative or damning but the name 'cancer'. As long as a particular disease is treated as an evil, invincible predator, not just a disease, most people with cancer will indeed be demoralised by learning what disease they have. The solution is hardly to stop telling cancer patients the truth, but to rectify the conception of the disease, to de-mythicise it (Sontag 1991). In some cases, cancer is conceived as invasion of the body by an external living 'entity' which then grows and eats up the body from within (Helman 1994).

Cancer equates with more than death; it is equated with a manner of living and dying in chronic and endless debility accompanied by loss of muscular power and control. It is equated with a withering away of life's essential elements, and is associated with foul smell, feelings of dirtiness, severe and relentless pain and eventual death after months or weeks of this suffering. It is also associated with fear of being a burden or abandoned. Many people consider cancer to be the leprosy of our time. The social stigma associated with it is devastating to both patient and family (Winder & Hlam 1978). Because of the shame associated with cancer, the diagnosis is sometimes communicated to other people in whispers. Those who die of it are often said in their obituaries to have died from 'extended illness' (Burns 1982).

Cancer is still the most feared of all diseases, people continue to think of cancer as a killer, and both patients and doctors use euphemisms to avoid the dreaded word. 'Rogue cells' or 'tumours' are said by doctors to be kinder words to say to patients than cancer. The big 'C' or being subject to 'a fate worse than death' are words cancer sufferers use to describe their illness, and family and friends will make statements such as 'you don't look – or smell – as though you have cancer!' or 'you look well' as if cancer is usually visible.

The worse thing I did was to tell my best friend about the cancer, now when she sees me she crosses the road and pretends that she did not see me coming.

I am coping better now with my breast cancer; 5 years ago when my sister had it she found it quite difficult to talk about it with her friends. 10 years ago my husband developed cancer of the oesophagus our friends shunned us when they heard. One even thought that it was contagious and told the other to stay away, now 10 years later he is still with me, the friends have come back and I was able to tell them that they could not have caught the cancer in the first place. The stigma that was associated with cancer is much less now.

Health beliefs and the Health Belief Model

A source of contemporary medical opinions about patients and their beliefs has been research work utilising the Health Belief Model. This work, quoted extensively by some medical educators, can also be considered to have reinforced some aspects of the medical type and to have diverted attention from the pressing issues relevant to how patients' beliefs could be utilised in consultations. Health Belief Model research has contributed to the idea that patients influenced by social groups with 'inaccurate' beliefs present a major threat to improved care and has provided the theoretical backbone of attempts to provide 'health education' (David et al 1985).

Indeed, according to a working party of British General Practitioners influenced by it, the main barriers to patients' participation in preventive health care 'appear to depend chiefly on their beliefs and knowledge about health and disease.' (Royal College of General Practitioners 1981). The same beliefs are also widely held to influence inappropriate visits to doctors and non-compliance with treatment. The Health Belief Model began principally as an attempt to organise and make theoretical sense of the diverse relationships between social and cultural groups and patients' utilisation of medical services or compliance with treatment. Proponents of the Health Belief Model have, undoubtedly, helped to indicate which aspects of patients' belief systems need to be changed if they are to be made consistent with biomedical thinking. Some beliefs may seem more or less psychologically attractive to patients because they enhance or threaten feelings of control or guilt (King 1982).

PLAYERS IN THE FIELD

Standard of care

The Expert Advisory Group set up to advise the Chief Medical Officer of England and Wales on the organisation of cancer services and to make proposals for advice to purchasers of cancer care said that: 'All patients should have access to a uniformly high quality of care in the community or hospital wherever they may live to ensure the maximum possible cure rate and best quality of life' (EAGC 1994).

Access to modern resources and expertise was poorly coordinated and poorly integrated and the service lacked the structure to facilitate comprehensive evaluation or the implementation of new development in a uniform fashion. Medical oncology could contribute towards the resolution of the problems facing the provision of cancer care (Association of Cancer Physicians 1994).

Documents from bodies such as the Department of Health ('The Patient's Charter' 1991), Royal College of Nursing (1991, 1993a), Joint Council for Clinical Oncology (1993), The Royal Marsden Hospitals NHS Trust (1994), Cancer Relief Macmillan Fund (1994) and EAGC (1994) reiterated similar themes over the years, that patients should be offered the most appropriate therapy in the light of current medical knowledge, taking into account the stage of the disease, their age and general health. The

EAGC (1994) also stressed the importance of a diagnosis being confirmed without delay. Delays are distressing for all concerned, and can be detrimental to long-term outcome. Consideration of the needs of the patient in relation to the quality of life was very important.

The standard of care is inextricably linked with the providers and deliverers of care. The SMAC (1984) report stated that the NHS could not be insulated from the economic realities. The resources allocated need adequately to reflect the very large number of patients affected and a sensible balance of provision between different aspect of specialised diagnostic and therapeutic services. It is recognised that the prevalence of cancer is likely to rise and will continue to do so for the foreseeable future. The Association of Cancer Physicians (1994) commented that the changing structure of the NHS, the increasing tendency towards specialisation and the awareness that resources are finite lends some urgency to developing a plan for the provision of cancer services across the nation.

It has been recommended that in a cancer unit (a designated unit within a district general hospital for the care of the commoner cancers), surgical management of cancer patients should be carried out by surgeons who specialise in a particular anatomical area (EAGC 1994). In the past, 30% of the work of surgeons was the management of cancer (SMAC 1984). They might be general surgeons or surgeons with an interest in certain types of cancer. The advantage of specialism is the accumulation of experience in complex procedures and high throughput of patients.

Radiotherapy and chemotherapy standards have also been covered in the SMAC (1984) and EAGC (1994) reports with specific reference to training and experience of specialist doctors and nurses in obtaining optimum results for patients.

Development of services

Services should always be developed to meet the needs of the local population. The EAGC (1994) report has given advice on the organisation of cancer services and has made proposals for advice to purchasers of cancer care. The structure recommended for cancer care is:

- Primary care is seen as the focus of care. Detailed discussions between primary care team, units and centres would be necessary to clarify patterns of referral and follow-up to ensure the best outcomes.

• Designated cancer units should be in district general hospitals with expert clinical teams and facilities to manage common cancers.

• Designated cancer centres should provide expertise in the management of all cancers. They would provide specialist diagnostic and therapeutic techniques including radiotherapy.

Community

The Tomlinson Report (1992), with its emphasis on primary and community care, offers great scope to develop community health services, which are particularly poorly resourced in London. The overall aim of Tomlinson is to create services that break down the barriers between primary, secondary and tertiary care, and to concentrate on providing high quality care tailored to individual patients' needs. Thus a flexible range of options needs to be developed between acute hospital-based care and the standard home-care arrangements currently provided by district nurses.

Most people, given the choice, would prefer to die in their own home, but instead of this, death from terminal cancer still happens more frequently in hospital or hospice (Townsend et al 1990). Townsend et al concluded that with a limited increase in community care 50% more patients with cancer could be supported to die at home, as they and their carers would prefer.

The practical aspects of nursing patients requiring palliative care until death within their own environment will differ subject to the availability of resources and the quality and expertise of professionals. There is little or no continuity in the availability of services throughout the UK. Tomlinson (1992) is intended to improve patient care in the community, by creating a new strategy between the social services, medical and nursing services.

Discharge planning

For care to be viewed as a continuum between hospital and home it requires planning. It has been argued that discharge planning should be considered at the time of admission to hospital (Turton & Barnett 1981). All too often hospital staff underestimate the effect that imminent discharge may have upon the patient and family. If patients are relatively self-caring, then discharge is viewed as a release from the confines of the sick role, which all too often is still imposed on patients; but if patients are less well, then there will be fears of how well they will cope without the additional support of the hospital in maintaining pain control, pressure area care and mobility.

Today, discharge planning is the responsibility of all the member of the multidisciplinary team from medical staff to pharmacist. The nurse tends to take on the role of coordinator of the process; some hospitals have specialist nurses with community expertise to coordinate discharge planning and community liaison. It is important to involve the patient, GP and the primary care team, i.e. the district nurses, social worker and the relatives.

The key to a successful discharge is communication. Information to the community care team regarding all aspects of a patient's care is vital if care is to be continued appropriately. 'Relevant, effective communication between hospital and community (nurses) is the only efficient way to ensure continuity of care for patients and their families' (Houlton 1988). The use of a discharge sheet serves as a guide to care and treatment received in hospital, and the patient's needs after discharge. The discharge sheet should be written in collaboration with the patient and his or her family, and if possible the community care team should be made aware of its contents before discharge. All too often the community care staff are unaware of the patient's needs until they perform a home visit, and the information on the discharge sheet may be inadequate to meet the needs of the health care professionals (Owen & Black 1996).

Communication, however, is a two-way process, and it is just as important that the primary health care team communicate effectively with hospital staff prior to admission. All too often an aspect of care has changed in between hospital admissions, and hospital staff are rarely made actively aware of this. Changes could include newer increased medication, different wound dressings or changed dietary needs. Patients and their families are not always aware of why changes have taken place. Hospital staff may therefore undo all the care that has been given in the community because of lack of information. This leads to feelings of frustration in the community staff, and confusion over appropriate care when the patient is discharged home once more.

Whilst written information and care plans may be shared between the hospital and the home, it should be remembered that 'elaborate and lengthy care plans have little or no place in the home. Simplicity and practicality are the nurse's guides upon which educational efforts are based' (Maloney & Preston 1992).

In 1966 the RCN Cancer Nursing Society published two reports: 'Guidelines for Good Practice in Cancer Nursing Education' (1996a); 'A structure for Cancer Nursing Services' (1996b). These set standards for cancer education which should in turn improve the standard of cancer care developed by nurses.

Specialist nurses and nursing in specialities

When providing cancer nursing services it is important to differentiate between a nurse working in a speciality and a specialist nurse. Nurses working in specialities provide everyday care to patients in wards and departments in cancer units and centres. These are practice-based positions with limited in-depth knowledge and experience. Although experienced in the care of cancer patients, they will need to draw on the expertise and support of specialist nurses.

Specialist nurses are registered nurses who have successfully completed higher and advanced level educational programmes. They possess in-depth and specific knowledge and skills (RCN Cancer Nurse Society 1996b).

The RCN has described specialist practice as: 'Involving a clinical and consultative role, teaching, management, research and the application of relevant nursing research. Only when a nurse is involved in all of these is he or she a specialist' (RCN 1988).

More recently the UKCC has described a specialist practitioner as someone: 'able to demonstrate a high level of clinical decision making, able to monitor and improve standards of care through clinical supervision of practice, clinical audit, the provision of skilled professional leadership and the development of practice through research, teaching and the support of professional colleagues' (UKCC 1994b).

The role of the nurse specialist working in the community

The dynamics in cancer and palliative nursing require specialists who can support, advise and act as clinical leaders. These specialist nurses have a major role in designing standards and packages of care in collaboration with the community nurses and primary health care team.

Whilst generic services have caseloads of patients with many diseases, the specialist nurses may be treatment focused (for example chemotherapy) or patient group focused (for example paediatrics). Specialist nurses deal constantly with specific patients with disease-related needs and are therefore able to advise, educate and support the primary health care team. This in turn enhances levels of knowledge, clinical practice and encourages collaborative working practice.

The success of home-based treatment is dependent on multi-disciplinary, flexible and collaborative working practices involving the specialist cancer team and those working in primary health care. An effective community service will require the services of the pharmacy, laboratory (including haematology and chemical pathology), social services, medical oncology and radiotherapy personnel (RCN Cancer Nurse in Society 1996b).

Breast care nurses

Since the 1970s there has been increased awareness of the problems that patients with breast cancer face, and in some instance, what might be done to help (Tait 1995).

In the late 1970s researchers in the UK identified some of the unmet needs for psychological and practical support of patients with breast cancer (Maguire et al 1982, Morris et al 1997). The first breast nurses were recruited in the mid-1970s in the hope that they might help alleviate some of these problems. Since then, the work of breast care nurses has been evaluated in particular settings. Though few nurses were involved in these projects and these studies have not been replicated, in each case the breast care nurse was shown to have made a significant contribution to patients' well-being. Consequently, it is now known and accepted that adequate psychological assessment of patients' needs, using a limited intervention strategy, information-giving, supportive counselling, practical help and referral to appropriate psychological agencies has improved patients' outcome. Other possible influential factors have been facilitation of informed choices and the nurse's personality (Cotton et al 1991, Maguire et al 1980, 1983, Watson et al 1988, Wilkinson et al 1988). Maguire et al (1982) found that the breast care nursing service was cost beneficial within the National Health Service.

Breast care nurses have increased in number over the years thanks to the influence of Breast Cancer Woman and their Families, the National Breast Screening Programme, Cancer Relief Macmillan Fund and the Royal College of Nursing.

In the interest of the cancer sufferer it is important for all the support services, whether they be statutory service or voluntary organisations, to work together to ensure a high standard of care. In some areas they provide:

- a home care team – who will provide specialist cancer care from a local hospital
- a palliative care team – who will provide care for terminally ill patients
- a pain control team – who are mainly based in hospitals and hospices, but go out into the community if their services are needed.

Macmillan nurses

Background. The first Macmillan nurse posts were set up by the Cancer Relief Macmillan Fund (CRMF) in the mid-1970s to provide care in their own homes for patients with advanced cancer, the area of greatest need at the time. Macmillan nurses and others have gradually spread awareness and knowledge of palliative care skills among other health care professionals, so the role of the Macmillan nurse in the community has evolved to reflect these developments, and CRMF has also been able to meet other needs, such as for patients in hospital and patients with particular kinds of cancers. There are now over 1600 Macmillan nurses, including 768 in community care, 285 in hospital support, 141 in breast care, 58 in hospital liaison, 36 in paediatric care, and 22 chemotherapy and 16 lymphoedema nurse specialists.

Macmillan community-based nurses. Macmillan community-based care nurses work in the community with people with cancer and their families, to provide help with pain and symptom control, emotional and psychological support and information for the patients and their family and friends. They work alongside district nurses, GPs and other health care professionals, complementing and enhancing the care that they provide and helping to coordinate services for people with cancer. Macmillan nurses are often able to lend specialist equipment for home care and to identify other sources of help for patients.

Macmillan hospital support nurses. Macmillan hospital support nurses work in NHS hospitals supporting patients with cancer form the time of diagnosis. They will work in most of the departments of the hospital, providing information, emotional and psychological support for the patient and the family and help with pain and symptom control. They support staff caring for patients and are involved in passing on palliative care skills to a wide range of hospital staff, doctors, nurses, paramedical and ancillary staff. There are over 200 Macmillan hospital support nurses currently in post.

Macmillan paediatric nurses. There are about 1200 new cases of paediatric cancers every year in the UK and about 400 children die from cancer. The rates of cure are very good, but treatment can take years, and both the child affected and the family need a lot of support and advice throughout the disease process, whatever the outcome. There are 22 Macmillan paediatric nurses, mostly based in regional specialist units. In addition to direct patient care, they are involved in supporting the local GP and district nursing and health visiting staff in caring for the child with cancer out of hospital. Children may spend periods in hospital where there are many facilities and both they and the families can be very worried by the prospect of going home; the Macmillan nurse will remain in touch, providing a source of expert advice to the family and carer and an essential continuity of care and link to the hospital. Within this number are included two specialist nurses working in paediatric neuro-oncology (Macmillan nurses 1998).

Marie Curie nurses

Marie Curie Cancer Care provides almost 5000 part-time nurses nationwide to look after cancer patients in their homes throughout the day or night when the pressure on relatives or carers become too great. Having a good night's sleep knowing that your loved one is being cared for can make the difference in keeping a family together in such a stressful time and helps the carer, who is usually the wife and mother, to continue in her role.

Marie Curie nurses work with local district nurses and half of their cost is paid by the community health care trust. Marie Curie Cancer Care provides specialised medical, nursing and day care in 11 Marie Curie hospice centres. They are involved in cancer research and strive to improve the quality of cancer care through the education of health care professionals.

District nurses

District nurses work closely with GPs as members of the primary health care team. The GP has overall responsibility for the care of the cancer patient in the community; the patient is referred to the district nurse for needs assessment and care. It is understood that they as a team will take care of the patient regardless of who the patient is. The district nurse visits the patient at home, assesses his or her needs, meets the family and discusses the care plan which involves them. It is important that patients and their families feel in control of the care they receive in their homes; the district nurse by working with the family enables them to do this.

Here is the story of one family. John was discharged home from hospital terminally ill after treatment for stomach cancer. He had three children, two boys and a girl of 9 and was referred to the district nurse for assessment and care. A week later he returned to the hospital for his check-up. His wife was with him when the consultant asked him, 'how was your daughter's birthday?' to which he replied, 'it was wonderful!' His wife was astonished, because it had not been their daughter's birthday, and asked for an explanation, to which John said, 'I wanted to come home. There are things I have to do for my family, I could not do in a hospital bed.' John's wife was worried and felt that she could not cope, but she had support from his seven brothers and sisters, his parents, the district nurse and GP. John died peacefully at home with his family in attendance.

ALTERNATIVE THERAPY OR COMPLEMENTARY THERAPY

This covers a wide range of help and services the cancer patient may wish to know about and to use. Some NHS hospitals are beginning to incorporate some of the less extreme treatments into the services they offer to cancer patients. It is important for nurses to be informed; then if patients ask, the information can be made available to them to enable them to make informed choices. After proper assessment, the patient may need referral for counselling to a dietitian, or for massage or relaxation therapy. Patients can also be referred to the National Homeopathic Hospital. Some patients because of their culture may wish to use home remedies or traditional medicines. It is important to encourage them not to use the home remedies as alternatives to hospital treatment, but as complementary to the treatment from the hospital.

CULTURAL NURSING CARE

The people of the world can be seen as a tapestry woven of many different strands. Those strands differ in size, shape, colour, intensity, age and place of origin. All strands are integral to the whole; yet each retains an individuality that enriches the beauty of the cloth. The tapestry symbolises the cultural diversity among people.

It is also important to understand and respect the health care 'culture' within which the nurse is practising. That culture, whether located within the hospital, home or community, is influenced by intersections of forces larger than the individual. For example, capitalism affects the financing of nursing care, especially in a market-driven system such as 'managed care'. Nursing care is also influenced by shared values about what constitutes ethical professional practice (Lipson et al 1996).

African and Afro-Caribbean patients tend to be labelled 'difficult' for not responding to questions, or questioning procedures, which it is their right to do.

Carefully explain planned procedure in very simple language, using diagrams and pictures to illustrate, since patients are unlikely to' ask for clarification or admit to not understanding. Consistent with their respect for authority, some patients will sign consent forms with little hesitation. Some patients are very sensitive about maintaining privacy; personal and private matters are kept strictly within family. They may be hesitant to disclose to nurses information about matters pertaining to sex or private body parts, even though the information is relevant to the diagnosis. Extra measures should be taken to minimise patients' exposure during examinations or treatments.

SERIOUS OR TERMINAL ILLNESS

Patients' significant other(s) should be the first ones notified. They will decide among themselves if and when the patient is to be told the prognosis. It is recommended that family members are present when the patient is being told the news. The presence of supportive others makes the occasion less traumatic for the patient, given the numerous myths and fears surrounding notions of death and dying in this culture.

Home vs hospital

Most families will care for chronically ill/dying relatives at home. This is done out of sense of family obligation and loyalty as well as respect for the dying relative. When death is imminent, close friends and family will want to gather at the bedside of the dying person to pray and witness the loved one's passing. Nurses, having made sure that the patient is comfortable, should leave the family to themselves (St Hill 1996).

COMMUNICATION

Communication in cancer care has been a focus of concern for many years (Fallowfield & Roberts 1992, Faulkner 1980, Maguire & Faulkner 1988, Maguire & Rutter 1976). More recently, research has been undertaken that concentrates not on the problems of communication between cancer patients, their families and health professionals, but more on whether the necessary skills of effective interaction can be taught and maintained over time (Faulkner & Maguire 1994). Much of the work undertaken has focused on effective interaction between the patient and doctor or nurse while the patient is in hospital. There are, however, particular issues in the community where the patient is away from the safety of the hospital and often attempting to maintain a normal life while struggling with the many problems raised by living with a diagnosis of cancer. Those who work with patients in the community need to consider the particular problems of interacting with individuals in their own homes, and also be aware of particular issues which may be raised for the patient (Faulkner 1996).

Communication between the health professionals involved in the care of cancer patients at home is very important if the patient is to get coherent care and know where to go to discuss concerns that may arise.

The lack of open communication clearly distresses cancer patients. A number of studies have shown that up to one in four patients will have significant problems and would benefit from help (Green 1985, Maguire 1985). Furthermore, up to 80% of psychological problems in cancer patients go unrecognised and therefore untreated (Bond 1982).

Staff sometimes assume that patients will always disclose any psychological problems they have and that there is no need for them to enquire. Some doctors and nurses are reluctant to enquire because they fear that patients will reveal strong emotions such as anger and expressions which they feel unable to handle.

Patient satisfaction research also continues to indicate that cancer patients are not satisfied with the information they receive regarding their treatment and nursing care (Anderson 1988, Karani & Wilshaw 1986, Maguire 1976). It would seem that most patients with cancer would prefer to know if they have a diagnosis of cancer (Cancer Relief Macmillan Fund 1988). It also seems clear that most patients appear to benefit from open, truthful communication with health professionals, as active seeking of information about the disease and its treatment has been identified as a coping mechanism (Weisman 1979) to help people gain control over the situation (Friedman 1980). Open communication also appears to reduce anxiety and depression in patients with cancer (Hames & Stirling 1987, Morris & Royle 1987).

There is as yet no evidence to suggest that open communication or information-giving has the detrimental effect of increasing anxiety or depression in those cancer patients who want to be fully informed about their disease. The key issue in giving information to patients, therefore, is not so much whether or not to tell, but to identify just how much information patients require, so tailoring it to individual needs (Wilkinson 1995).

Nurses in hospital and in the community are in the forefront of care during the period when patients may want to discuss their diagnosis or prognosis, and yet regardless of an emphasis on communication skills training over recent years the majority still appear to use the avoidance behaviours described by Quint more than 20 years ago (Wilkinson 1991). Why is this still happening?

Cancer information organisations have developed over the past 15 years. They perform a valuable service for cancer sufferers and their families. They produce a variety of information on all aspects of cancer, which is free to the general public, as well as a telephone help line.

ETHICAL ISSUES AND CANCER CARE

Caring for people who have cancer raises a host of ethical issues and moral questions. Perhaps one of the biggest dilemmas we have to face is when medical intervention fails to cure a cancer and the client asks the question: 'Nurse, am I going to die?' Such an enquiry asks for much more than a purely clinical response; if we are to show true understanding and empathy then we must search for the ethical insights to underpin our answer (Kendrick 1995).

You will have learnt many skills since joining the profession of nursing. When nurses recall their early days of training it becomes apparent that many rich and diverse experiences occur on the road to becoming a competent practitioner.

With training and experience comes responsibility. In a normal working day we will be expected to give patients information and obtain consent from them for procedures they are required to have. Telling the truth should be the central part of the relationship nurses have with their patients, but this is not always so, because most nurses feel bound by the story that is told by their superiors or the doctors, which sometimes is not the full truth but has been decided on as the best information that the patient can handle at the time. This creates a dilemma in obtaining informed consent. Patients may give permission for a procedure to be performed on them, but do they really have sufficient information to make a decision? As nurses, we also tend to say that we are the patient's advocate. In the true meaning of the word, very few of us during our daily work with patients can say we are truly their advocate.

Working in the community, health care workers are not exempt from ethical issues. In fact, they are often involved far more comprehensively and intimately with cancer patients and their families than hospital colleagues or other workers in other institutions, e.g. hospices, nursing homes or residential homes. This often means that patient and family will turn to them for ethical guidance, which in turn may create serious dilemmas for them when the hospital's advice and guidance is somewhat different. Good communication between professionals goes some way to alleviate this problem but in the real world this is not always achievable, not least because of time restraints (Crowther 1996).

The patient's and family members' viewpoint must be taken into consideration. Doctors and other health care workers have a different set of moral issues to contend with, starting with the communication of bad news to a patient and family. No one enjoys this and it is often done badly. Increased training in communication skills is improving the situation but it requires the scarce commodity – time – to achieve the best for patients and families. Many doctors have particular difficulty since they still feel that not being able to cure the patient is a sign of failure. Continued and further training at medical student level and during the pre-registration appointments may help in this area.

Each patient is an individual and some investigations and treatments are unpleasant and frightening for patients. With the patient's participation, a judgement must be made in each case of whether the benefits of doing the tests and having the treatment outweigh the disadvantages of not so doing.

Self-preservation is a normal attribute of all of us, and it applies to our feelings and coping with 'awkward questions' from patients and their relatives. May (1995) concluded that the effect of gate-keeping strategies is to manage patients' uncertainties through controlling access to information about what is currently known about their disorder and its effects. Because nursing staff may themselves be highly uncertain about this, the nurse represents herself as dependent on knowledge constructed and mobilised elsewhere (in the pathology laboratory, by the patient herself, or by the doctor).

Living wills

As nurses working in the community with cancer patients, it is important to build up a relationship with the patients and their families. Encouraging patients to make a will is important for them and for the family members who are left behind. It is normally said that it is important to 'put your house in order' which sometimes may avoid unpleasantness after the patient's death.

A living will is different. Living wills are documents in which people state their wishes in relation to medical treatment and intervention at the end of their lives. Should patients become unable to speak for themselves, their wishes have been clearly recorded and can be used to guide their care. Living wills often focus on aspects of intervention a person wishes to decline, such as a request not to be considered for cardiopulmonary resuscitation. A living will may also express a positive wish to receive all possible interventions to prolong life.

One of the major limitations of such a document is that it can reflect only a person's wishes at the moment it is signed and circumstances may change rapidly (Cowe 1996). The House of Lords Select Committee on Medical Ethics (1994) supported the development of advance directives on the basis that they enable expression of individual preference and stimulate discussion between doctors and patient.

Patients are no longer passive recipients of care but are increasingly recognised as active participants, despite some continuing to be labelled as 'difficult' when expressing their wishes. The teaching of some religions may run contrary to the underlying principles of living wills. For example, the Catholic Church emphasises that God alone should make decisions about life and death (Pope John Paul II 1994).

Living wills are in their infancy in the UK, but nurses have a duty to be aware of current health-care issues including some information on living wills. The Royal College of Nursing (1994) issued a statement on living wills, taking a generally positive view of the contribution of such documents to patient care, while emphasising that supporting the use of living wills does not alter their anti-euthanasia stance.

Euthanasia

The debate on euthanasia, which occupies the medical and legal press with increasing frequency, is complicated by the terminology used. Withdrawal of unproductive treatment of some commentators is passive euthanasia to others; some speak with approval of 'mercy killing' while others regard it pejoratively as active non-voluntary or involuntary euthanasia; it is difficult to make any national distinction between assisted suicide and active voluntary euthanasia (Mason & Mulligan 1996). Although most people would believe that medical, moral and legal distinctions exist between the broad categories of letting a person die by withdrawing treatment and suicide or euthanasia, there is still substantial disagreement as to what these distinctions are and which are most relevant (Cranford 1995).

Much of the opposition to any form of euthanasia stems from its popular association with terminal disease and old age. The picture changes, however, if we consider death due only to incurable and progressive neurological diseases and persistent vegetative state. They are similar because they affect a wide age group and both lack effective treatment.

BEREAVEMENT

Caring for loved ones through terminal illness can be rewarding or devastating; it can be an event in the family which brings them together or pushes them apart.

After the death of her husband Mary said: 'Thank you sister for making it possible for my family to share the most important part of our lives.' The children who lived away came home and helped their mother care for their father during the final 2 weeks of his life.

Grief is a normal process and the majority cope without needing any additional professional help. One of the key ways nurses can help bereaved families is by recognising those people who are at risk of having difficulty with their bereavement and referring them for appropriate help. Research has, however, identified that certain individuals are at 'high risk' with regards to their adjustment to a significant loss (Parkes 1990, Worden 1991).

Bereaved adults caring for young children often deny them the opportunity to understand what has happened to a parent or sibling who has died, in the mistaken belief that the children are best protected from the knowledge or cannot understand it (Black 1996). The nurse, seeing a patient alone, may find it difficult to extend care to other family members and sometimes this may fit in with the family style. However, the exclusion of other family members means that problem-solving is reduced and individuals are left to carry their own pain. Two workers together may find it easier to involve all the family. Living with cancer can make families feel as if they are on a roller coaster. Feeling out of control leads children to show symptoms of anxiety such as nightmares, bedwetting, tantrums and nervous habits. The constancy of support offered helps to create a degree of containment (Firth & Anderson 1994).

Children need to talk. They may have been excluded at home and are able to open up in a group. With all the best intentions, the families might not talk to children and think they are protecting them. The child may also believe he or she is protecting the parents by not asking questions (Cohen 1994). Kids Can Cope is a group intervention designed to help children and teenagers who currently have a parent diagnosed with cancer (Taylor-Brown et al 1993). In previous generations, children grew up with the inevitability of loss, and a sense of the rituals and customs surrounding it, in a way that placed death as an integral part of living. The decrease in infant mortality, combined with an increase in life-expectancy, and advances in medical science, have all contributed to a state of affairs in which death can intrude very little, in any real sense, in many children's lives (Pettle & Britten 1995).

Amy aged 14 describes her feelings of surviving cancer after her friend Beth died. 'Just before Christmas she did die and the news of her death affected me deeply. I feel very guilty that she has died and not me. I went to her funeral. I found it very hard to do. While I was there I felt that I had swapped places with Beth and I suddenly felt like it was me who was suffocating in the coffin and that Beth was standing where I was, singing her favourite hymn. It sounds very strange, but it was a very real experience. I also began to wonder who would have come to my funeral if it had been me. Whether Beth would have come or not, would she have cried as I was crying? I was frightened to face her family who might hate me for surviving when Beth did not. What bothered me most of all though, is that I never said goodbye' (Shindler 1992).

There are a variety of bereavement counselling services available today. It is important that nurses should visit patients during that period and refer them on when necessary.

RELIGION – SPIRITUAL CARE

The nurse's role is to respect patients' spiritual concerns and help them and their families explore and express issues related to spirituality. Spiritual care can be given by any member of the professional team and the goal is to minimise 'spiritual distress' and promote 'spiritual well-being.' A positive outcome will be deemed to have been achieved if the patient and/or the family state that their spiritual needs have been addressed and the spiritual needs of the patient have been documented (Bradshaw 1996). A belief in God, rather than a vague notion of a 'higher or supreme being' is still held in some way by the majority of patients. The danger is to consider that for most patients the label Anglican or Methodist, for example, is merely nominal and that the chaplain, religious services and practices would therefore be out of place. At the same time, there is a major focus on other religions (Andrews & McIntosh 1992).

Obviously, it is important that the nurse seeks to address the religious needs of all patients, but we need to remember that a relatively small number of patients in the UK belong to non-Christian religions (OPCS 1995). There also seems to be an assumption that people who are Sikh, Hindu, Buddhist, Muslim or Jewish take their religion seriously, unlike the rest of the population. The NHS 1992 guidelines state: 'The NHS should, where necessary, make every effort to provide for the spiritual needs of patients and staff,' and 'as far as reasonably possible, this provision should recognise the welfare needs of both Christians and non-Christians.' But it stresses it is 'for hospital management to decide what arrangements should be made' (NHS Management Executive 1992).

Spiritual pain may be recognised by the questions asked by the patient, and the feelings expressed – 'Why me?' 'What have I done to deserve this?' 'God doesn't care about me.' 'Why am I being punished?' 'It just isn't fair.' These questions and statements express self-doubt, isolation and a search for meaning, they are often indicators of spiritual pain (Elsdon 1995).

Spirituality is central to holistic health care, and interacts with physical, psychological and social aspects. In the dying person, as physical health recedes, the spiritual dimension may grow in importance, so the profile of spirituality in palliative care should be raised. Nurses are in an excellent position to assess the spiritual needs of a dying person, and to facilitate resolution of spiritual pain.

CONCLUSION

The prevalence of cancer, its diagnosis, treatment and final outcome, has been the subject of increasing public awareness and debate throughout the 20th century. In tandem with this has been a growing commitment to cancer prevention, screening and early detection as well as to cure and palliation, particularly within the developed world.

Palliative care is an essential and integral part of effective cancer care. It can be provided in a variety of settings – in the community, hospital, hospice and nursing home. It is, however, from hospices that much of the skill and motivation for change has emanated in supporting cancer patients and their families.

Palliative care is a multidisciplinary activity which crosses professional boundaries between health and social care. The needs of patients facing a life-threatening illness are multifaceted and may be shaped by a variety of personal, social and cultural factors. Palliative care principles can support people at different points of their illness and need not be confined to the terminal stages (Hawket 1995).

Nurses are in a unique position to play a major role in cancer care in the future. Documents from the UKCC (1994b) and the ENB (1995a) have shown that on preparing for specialist practice, the nurse requires expertise in clinical practice, education, research and management related to cancer care. Access to a wide range of resources, including a recognised cancer centre, contributes to the development of this level of expertise (RCN Cancer Nursing Society 1996a).

As we approach the 21st century, caring for people who are terminally ill should reflect the society we live in. There should be culturally sensitive care provision for people from black and minority ethnic groups dying from cancer. Services should aim to provide a caring environment which reflects individual choice.

SUMMARY

Cancer care has developed over the years, in hospital, hospice and community services. More than any other group, nurses have close daily contact with users of health care services; about 80% of direct care is delivered by nurses. Patients are individuals and have different needs. The care should be holistic and cater for the individual, physical, psychological, social and spiritual needs.

USEFUL ADDRESSES

Cancer BACUP
3 Bath Place
London EC2A 3JR
Tel: 0171 613 2121

Cancerlink
11–21 Northdown Street
London N1 9BN
Tel: 0800 123905

Cancer Research Campaign
Cambridge House
Cambridge Terrace
London NW1 4JL
Tel: 0171 224 1333

Women's National Cancer Control Campaign
Suna House
128–130 Curtain Street
London EC2A 3AR
Tel: 0171 729 2229

Breast Cancer Care
Kiln House
210 New Kings Road
London SW6 4ZN
Tel: 0500 245345

Macmillan Cancer Relief
Anchor House
15–19 Britten Street
London SW3 3TZ
Tel: 0845 6016101

Marie Curie Cancer Care
28 Belgrave Square
London SW1X 8QG
Tel: 0171 235 3325

Hospice Information Service
St Christopher's Hospice
51–59 Lawrie Park Road
London SE26 2DZ
Tel: 0181 778 9252

6

Intensive care nursing: supporting the community

Sotirios Plakas

Who but you?

Who cares for families threatened by critical illness
and injury?

Who radiates hope when others would rather surrender?

Who inspires confidence when others doubt?

Who comforts families, helping them bear the unbearable?

Who makes the impossible seem effortless?

Who is the cornerstone of acute health care?

You a critical care nurse.

(Leske 1991a)

ROLE OF THE SPECIALIST CRITICAL CARE NURSE

Nursing as a growing and dynamic discipline contains numerous and diverse speciality areas. The first intensive care units (ICUs) started in the 1950s as centres to provide care to polio victims. In the 1960s, recovery rooms were initiated for patients undergoing major surgery and coronary care units were established for patients with cardiac problems (Sole & Hartshorn 1997). Critical care nursing developed as a speciality in the 1970s and within a few years it had evolved to include areas of practice such as patients with renal, pulmonary, metabolic and neurological disorders. Critical care had an important impact on the profession, the image of nursing being one of the first areas to be affected (Dracup 1993). Nurses working in ICUs developed a knowledge and confidence that could not be seen in any other hospital setting. Patients and their families were grateful for their high competence and compassion. The best of the nursing profession has been embodied for the public in the critical care nurse. The relationship between medicine and nursing has also been affected by critical care nurses. In ICUs doctors must work collaboratively in mutual respect with nurses or otherwise patient care is compromised. The high level of knowledge of the body systems that nurses must have in order to respond quickly and intelligently to subtle alterations in a critically ill patient has contributed towards that appreciation (Dracup 1993). Intensive care is a highly interdisciplinary speciality; thus nurses need to communicate with all other member of the health team in meaningful ways. Nursing care in ICUs also goes beyond the patient to the family system. Nurses know that when caring for families they are performing the same critical function as if they were assessing the haemodynamic status of the patient or titrating drugs (Dracup 1993).

The American Association of Critical Care Nurses (AACN) defined critical care nursing in the following way: 'nursing is defined as the diagnosis and treatment of human responses to actual or potential health problems. Critical care nursing is the specialty within nursing that deals specifically with human responses to life threatening problems' (AACN 1984, cited in Hartshorn 1993).

Critical care nurses deal with the total human being and his or her responses to actual or potential health problems. This means that the critical care nurse is responsible for prevention of disease as well as the cure of the patient. The nursing care that is provided is intended to restore health, alleviate suffering and pain and preserve the rights and dignity of individuals (Clochesy et al 1993). It is inherent also that the focus of the critical care nurse involves the family of the patient and their response in addition to the response of the individual patient. Furthermore, human response can take the form of a physiological or a psychological phenomenon. Critical care nursing is specifically concerned with human responses to life-threatening problems; trauma or major surgery are some examples. Prevention can also be viewed as consistent with this definition. A critical care nurse could teach a patient about methods to lower blood cholesterol levels which may then prevent a life-threatening problem (Hartshorn 1993).

The AACN's 'Scope of Critical Care Nursing Practice' statement of 1996 (cited in Sole & Hartshorn 1997) provides a definition and description of the practice of the critical care nurse. This includes the critically ill patient and family, the critical care nurse and the critical care environment, with nurse–patient interactions central to its scope. At the centre of critical care practice are the critically ill patient and family who experience compromised health status, are physiologically unstable and cannot compensate, and are dependent on caregivers. The nurse provides leadership for the care of the patient and incorporates the values and preferences of patients and their families. A critically ill patient is one with life-threatening problems or at high risk of developing such problems. This kind of patient requires constant, intensive multidisciplinary assessment and intervention in order to restore stability, prevent complications and achieve and maintain optimal responses. In the process of care for this patient the critical care nurse is identified as the coordinator for the interventions directed at resolving life-threatening problems (Hartshorn 1993).

The critical care nurse is the professional who is responsible for ensuring that all critically ill patients receive optimal care. The nurse should practice in accordance with standards and within an ethical framework. Interactions of the nurse and the patient are of prime importance (Hartshorn 1993). Unique aspects of critical care practice include: focusing on the patient and family; receiving a multitude of data and prioritising information; providing research-based interventions; monitoring patients continuously to detect changes; collaborating frequently with members of the health care team; intervening proactively to prevent complications and exacerbation of illness and promoting wellness (Sole & Hartshorn 1997). The critical care nurse must demonstrate caring behaviours, make skilled clinical judgements, act on behalf of others, use teamwork and innovation, and work in collaboration with the other health care providers (Sole and Hartshorn 1997).

The critical care environment is viewed from three perspectives. The equipment and the supplies are the resources which contribute to the interactions between the nurse and the patient.

The institution or setting in which critically ill patients receive care is the second perspective of the environment. Here critical care management and administrative structure ensure effective care delivery through provision of resources, quality control systems and maintenance of standards of nursing care. The final perspective includes all of the factors that influence the provision of care to the patient and these include legal, regulatory, social, economic and political factors (Hartshorn 1993).

Critical illness is dramatic for both the patient and the family. In most cases the ICU hospitalisation comes without notice and there is no opportunity to consider the critical care experience. Psychological insult occurs over the major physiological one. This insult affects the family as well as the patient. The critical care nurse has the privilege to understand this phenomenon and initialise techniques that will help both patients and families cope with the situation. Interventions for psychological insults are as crucial for the well-being of patients and their families as are the physiological interventions (Hartshorn et al 1993).

The role of the critical care nurse includes identifying the family that is at risk for crisis, assessing the family in crisis, and choosing strategies to deal with either situation. The strategies that can be used are: health teaching and information giving; anticipatory guidance; development of a nurse–patient–family triad to maintain a unified family system. Providing effective, meaningful, open and honest communication is important. A caring concerned humanistic attitude towards families, using their names and eye contact, means that excellent care is being provided to the families. Using simple terminology in answering families' questions will do much in alleviating anxiety (Caine 1989).

It is very interesting to see the differences and similarities in nursing practice in different nursing settings. Schultz & Daly (1989) administered an interview schedule to 16 nurses with experience in ICU and non-ICU nursing. The focus of the questions was on the nursing care responsibilities, the technology of care, and the relationships with physicians. The perceptions of differences included: 'ICU nursing is more stressful'; 'Floor work is harder'; 'We have to work with sophisticated equipment here'; and 'It takes a better nurse to work here'. The results showed that clear differences existed between nursing in ICU and non-ICU settings. To the question 'How do you see the relationship of the practices of medicine and nursing?' most nurses replied that there is an overlap rather than the two being mutually exclusive. When requested to describe ICU and non-ICU nursing, the nurses found the first more technical, curative, knowledgeable, and the second more 'dependent'. To the question on similarities and differences of ICU and non-ICU nursing, the respondents replied that the use of the nursing process was essentially the same in both areas but the depth of knowledge and the responsibility for patients were greater in the ICU. ICU nursing requires more in-depth assessment of patients, is more demanding and specific, requires the use of more technology to accurately assess changes earlier, is held in higher esteem by physicians, requires more independence and provides more stress. Non-ICU nursing was found to require more physical labour but less intensity from the nurse, to provide more continuous care and demand more planning on the part of the nurse. Overall most of the respondents were found to have strong negative biases against nurses in other settings (Schultz & Daly 1989).

NEEDS OF FAMILIES

Over the last 15 years, nurses have become increasingly aware that the family context makes a significant difference in health outcomes for individuals (Murphy 1986). Nancy Molter, one of the first nurses to study the needs of the families of critically ill patients, when interviewed by Leske (1991b) expressed the reasons which led her to study this subject. She stated:

In 1973 I was working in the burn unit of a large hospital; at that time about half of our patients died. I was overwhelmed with the distress among the families and felt inadequate to meet their needs. I did not even know what their needs were, only what I imagined them to be. So I decided to study families, their needs, how important they were and which ones required the assistance of a nurse.

Nursing research on families has taken a big place among the research literature. VanGott et al (1991) studied the nursing research that was published in nursing journals from 1979 to 1988 and identified that 8.5% of all the research was concerning family member's needs. Since 1988 more studies on families' needs have been performed (Coutu-Wakulczyk & Chartier 1990, Davis-Martin 1994, Forrester et al 1990, Freichels 1991, Quinn et al 1996, Rukholm et al 1991, Warren 1993, Wilkinson 1995, Zazpe et al 1997).

Leske (1992) performed a quantitative literature review with the work of 27 nurse investigators in 15 states of the USA over a period of 10 years (1980–1989) to describe the importance of the needs of the family members of critically ill patients during the 24- to 72-hour timeframe after admission to the unit. Seven of these studies had been published; 20 were unpublished. In addition, she compared family member age, gender, relationship to the patient, prior ICU experience and medical diagnoses in relation to the perceived importance of the needs.

She found that the most important needs of the families were:

- needs for assurance such as 'honest answers, best possible care provision, knowing the prognosis, feeling hope'
- needs for proximity such as 'to be near and see the patient frequently'
- needs to have daily information, to know the treatment, progress, and procedures done for the patient.

Concerning the relative importance of these needs, it was found that there was no statistically significant differences as far as age of the family members was concerned. The female family members rated the needs for support, comfort, information and proximity as being significantly more important than did male family members, but there was no statistically significant difference in the category of assurance needs. No statistically significant differences were found either among spouses, parents and adult children concerning needs for support, information, proximity and assurance, while the need for comfort for the adult children of the patients was significantly less important. No significant differences were also found in needs for support, proximity and assurance between family members with previous ICU hospitalisation experience and those without, but the needs for comfort and information were perceived as more important for those with previous ICU experience. Finally, the family members of cardiac, trauma, medical and surgical patients, rated all but the comfort needs similarly. Comfort was rated more important for the surgical patients than for the other patients (Leske 1992b).

Warren (1993) conducted an exploratory descriptive study to identify the importance of the needs of the family members of the critically ill patients during the first 18–24 hours of admission. A convenience sample of 94 family members rated the Critical Care

Family Needs Inventory (CCFNI) but the results were not analysed by item but by needs category. Therefore the category 'assurance needs' which included 'to have questions answered honestly and be assured that the best care possible is given' scored the highest among all categories. Information, proximity, support and comfort were the categories following in order of importance. This analysis does not permit us to compare need statements with the previous results but the assurance needs were rated very high in all the previous studies.

Coutu-Wakulczyk & Chartier (1990) tested the CCFNI in Canada in the French language. In the surgical ICU of the university hospital in Sherbrooke, Canada, 207 family members were interviewed to provide the data on the CCFNI. The average length of stay in the ICU, the time of data collection, was less than 48 hours but no exact timeframe was given. 74.9% of the sample were female and the mean age of the sample was 45.4 years. Alpha coefficient reliability for this study was 0.91. They found that the most important needs were consistent with the previously mentioned results from studies that used the English language version of the CCFNI.

Rukholm et al (1991) performed another study using the CCFNI to investigate needs and determine the relationship of these needs with the cultural background of the population, especially between the French- and English-speaking populations in three hospitals of Sudbury, Ontario. The sample consisted of 155 family members, 107 English speaking and 48 French speaking. Both groups were considered similar in age; 72% of the English and 75% of the French group were females; all the French-speaking group were Roman Catholic in contrast to 43% of Roman Catholics in the English-speaking group. The 'English' group scored a mean of 115.69 on the whole CCFNI while the 'French' scored 118.58 giving higher importance to their needs. It was suggested that cultural background influenced the importance of the needs but certain limitations of the study decrease the value of these findings. The fact that, even though French speaking, most of the subjects felt more comfortable to complete the questionnaires in the English language, and the smaller number in the 'French' group are certain methodological inconsistencies of the study. However, the findings of this study have implications that cultural differences influence the perceived importance of the needs of families.

Davis-Martin (1994) conducted a study to identify the needs of the families of long-term critical care patients. Researching 26 family members of patients who had been in an ICU for more than 2 weeks and using Molter's Critical Care Family Needs Inventory, this researcher found that needs remained constant over time and continued in a crisis mode regardless of the length of time of being in an ICU. The need for information remained the top need for the families. Quinn et al (1996) conducted another similar study to identify the needs of the families, how satisfied they were and who satisfied their needs. In 24 units in the Republic of Ireland and a total sample of 255 family members, they found that assurance and information were considered to be the more important needs. Only 10 out of 30 needs were found to have been met satisfactorily for the families, while nurses were identified by both the relatives and themselves as the most appropriate people to fulfil the needs of families.

Hammond (1995) conducted a descriptive study of the positive and negative attitudes of ICU nurses and patients' families towards their involvement in the physical care of the patient, to identify areas of care that would be appropriate for the families to undertake and to determine the benefits of lay participation in care.

It was found that both nurses and relatives agreed that involvement in care of the patient by the family would make them feel that they were helping their loved one directly, and would make them feel closer to the patient. Both agreed that all aspects of care should be explained to the families wishing to participate in physical care.

Wilkinson (1995) conducted a small qualitative study with six participants using unstructured interviews to establish the needs of the relatives of patients in a general ICU. Relatives were interviewed after the first 72 hours of patient admission, which should have been an emergency one. The findings highlight that relatives experience shock at the ICU admission, and they need to be near the patient, to receive social support, to be in a positive environment, to feel hope and receive information.

Zazpe et al (1997) conducted another descriptive study in Spain, this time with 85 relatives of patients, to identify their needs and whether they were met satisfactorily. Using a modification of the CCFNI they studied the families when at least 48 hours had passed after the admission of the patient. They found that at least

94% of the needs expressed by the family members were met. Needs for information and confidence were among the more important.

THE ROLE OF THE CRITICAL CARE NURSE IN SUPPORTING FAMILIES
Why bother with families?

The critical care nurse is the person from the health care team who has been most often cited as having the responsibility for meeting the needs of the families of critically ill patients (Daley 1984, McIvor & Thompson 1988, Millar 1987, Molter 1979, Rodgers 1983). Hickey & Lewandowski (1988) have stated some factors that affect critical care nurses' attitudes toward families. They are: the amount of available time for the nurse to deal with the families; the nurse's stress levels; the nurse's knowledge about the psychosocial aspects of dealing with families in crisis; and the role security of the nurse. Hickey & Lewandowski (1988) investigated the views of 226 critical care nurses on family visiting and the role of patients' families in the unit, how nurses themselves view their role with the families, and the factors that influence nurses' involvement with families of critically ill patients. The results indicated that critical care nurses, although considering the effects of the families on patients' fatigue and unit confusion, generally believed that frequent visiting by families was beneficial for the patients and important to their recovery. As far as the nurses' role with families was concerned, one-third of the sample did not believe that they had the knowledge to meet the psychosocial and emotional needs of families. Another important finding was that 77% of the sample believed that it is emotionally exhausting to become involved with families in need of support; however, they agreed to become involved with the families, no matter the costs to themselves.

There are specific interventions the critical care nurse can use while working with the family. Boettcher & Schiller (1990) described the use of a multidisciplinary group meeting to support the families of critically ill trauma patients. Families were able to attend any group without making prior arrangements; they could do so as often as they wished and were not required to attend a set number of sessions. The goals of the groups were:

- to help meet the emotional needs of families of trauma victims
- to orient families to the hospital and ICU environment
- to explain medical terminology and information
- to promote mutual support among families in crisis
- to provide a forum for discussion and to answer questions pertaining to other generic issues that arose.

The group met in a room next to the unit as families did not want to go far from their patients. From the evaluation of this programme, 100% of the respondents said that the programme met some of the emotional needs of the families, 87% answered that they were better oriented to the unit since attending the trauma support group, and 75% said they had been more supportive of each other and of other families since the group began.

Cray (1989) described how the implementation of a family intervention programme was evaluated. In a 12-bed medical intensive care unit (MICU) in a major university medical centre an 'MICU visitors teaching booklet' was given to all families with 'information regarding policies of the unit equipment, disease processes common to the critically ill, medical and nursing treatment, local hotels, churches and common feelings and concerns of dealing with an acute illness of a loved one.'

The families were assessed about living situation, marital status, level of education, previous experience with illness, the patient's significant others and the family's perception or expectations of the present situation. A strategy of telephone communication and personal visiting from nurses was also implemented. In fact, twice a week, a significant family member was called at home and, at least three times a week, families were visited by a nurse in the waiting room to develop a trusting relationship with the family and to keep them up to date.

Educational classes were offered to the family members once or twice a week and later, because of a good response, three or four times a week. These included 15-minute sessions on MICU procedures and equipment, respiratory failure, kidney failure and stages of awareness. Families being selected for the evaluation were provided with a pamphlet explaining the goals and activities of the programme. Also when the patient was transferred to the intermediate care unit, information about the new environment was given to the family but no specific programme or pamphlet was used. The ICU nurse also visited on the ward to see the patient. All interventions were evaluated after 14 weeks of their implementation. The classes were evaluated after their end and were highly favoured. 76 participants were asked to rate the following statements on a Likert scale of 1 (disagree) to 5 (strongly agree): the programme was helpful in understanding the patients illness; it would have benefit for other families; information was easy to understand; questions were answered. The vast majority of the 76 participants answered 'strongly agree' with the statements; no participant had received similar classes before. Additional comments also showed that this intervention was a beneficial and excellent idea.

The evaluation of the entire programme was also positive. Here the families were selected to participate and were followed up after the discharge of their relative to the intermediate care unit or for 2 weeks after the death, if their relative had died. Criteria for selection were that patients should be in a critical condition, having 'no resuscitation' orders, or be withdrawn from life-support systems and as selected by the nursing and medical staff.

14 families, from which only one member was required to evaluate the programme on behalf of the whole family, were selected to evaluate the programme using an instrument with seven questions on a Likert scale of 1–5 (1 = not helpful, 5 = very helpful). With almost no exception, all answered that all the aspects of the programme were very helpful to them. In their comments, statements were made that the programme was very helpful because they had information and they felt that somebody cared for them.

Chavez & Faber (1987) conducted a pre-test–post-test experimental study to measure the stress levels of the families as reported by the subjects and as derived from measures of their blood pressure and heart rate. The intervention in this study was *an education orientation programme and a visit to the loved one.* During this programme they had an orientation in the unit, to the equipment and to the patient's levels of comfort and mentation, and individual concerns were discussed. A hand-out with the unit policy was given. This lasted approximately 10 minutes.

In the intensive or coronary care unit of a large veterans administration medical centre a convenience sample of 40 spouses and offspring who visited their patients was randomly assigned to two groups. The instrument used was the Subjective Stress Scale (SSS) by Kerle & Bialek (cited by Chavez & Faber 1987) which consists of 25 descriptor words incorporated into two forms, each consisting of 15 words. These words range from *'great'* to *'terrified'* in form A and from *'wonderful'* to *'scared stiff'* in form B. Respondents were required to make a single response on how they felt and scale values were calculated for each word. Chavez & Faber (1987) highlight the wide applicability of this instrument and its previous use but no tests of reliability and content validity are offered. The control group had their blood pressure and heart rate recorded and then they were asked to complete the SSS. Then they visited their loved one for 5 minutes according to the visiting policy and the same data were collected again. The experimental group, in contrast, had only their blood pressure and heart rate recorded initially. Then they attended the education orientation programme. After the programme, blood pressure, heart rate and the SSS were recorded. Then the family member was escorted to the bed area by a nurse and left in privacy with the patient. After the visit, the same data were collected again. No information is given about the duration of this visit. No statistically significant difference was found in the control group between pre-visiting and post-visiting scores. In the experimental group the only statistically significant difference was in the heart rate which was decreased after the programme and further decreased after the visit ($p = 0.016$). The other scores had no statistically significant differences. Demographic data between the two groups was considered similar.

Sabo et al (1989) evaluated how family support group sessions benefited families and more accurately investigated the relationship between these sessions and the family's appraisal of stress, of social support and feelings of hope. Although the description of the family support session is not provided in the original article, generally the authors describe these groups as having a facilitator or group leader to provide the participants with information, to foster hope and share and ventilate common concerns. The criteria for the participants were to be a relative or significant other to a patient hospitalised for more than 24 hours and 16 years old or more, and being able to speak and write English.

In a 900-bed university-affiliated hospital with a 16-bed medical ICU, 18-bed cardiological ICU and 20-bed surgical ICU, a two groups (control and experimental) comparative design study was performed. A convenience sample of 67 subjects, 36 in the control and 31 in the experimental group, was used but no information is given about whether or not the allocation to the groups was random. The demographics of the participants were considered similar. 83% were females in the control group and 64% were females in the treatment group. 61% were older than 46 years in the control group and 67% in the experimental group.

The control group completed over a 3-week period an instrument of 27 statements that express feelings of stress, social support and hope, on a five-point Likert scale. Three open-ended questions were provided for information about the participants' perceptions of stress, assessment of hope in their situation and how the staff could be more helpful. The instrument was developed by the investigators. A panel of experts established content validity. No reliability tests were performed. The treatment group completed the study over a period of 8 months. Part two of the questionnaire was administered additionally to this group. Its purpose was to identify the benefits of attending the support group sessions. Three fixed alternative questions were used to identify the influence of the group sessions on their perceptions of stress, social support and hope. Three open-ended questions asked them to describe the most and least beneficial aspects of the group sessions and if they would recommend the groups to other families.

The analysis of the data using mean scores showed no significant difference between the stress scores of the two groups. However, for the open-ended question 'What is the most stressful aspect of being here?' 15 categories of aspects were identified from the control group and 8 only from the experimental group. To the question of whether the support group influenced the feelings of stress, 23% felt no change, 52% felt somewhat decreased stress levels and only 9% felt strongly decreased feelings of stress. No significant difference between the social support mean scores was identified: 51% responded that the most beneficial thing that the staff could do was to give information; 71% felt that they received increased feelings of support in attending the group sessions. Neither was there a significant difference identified between the hope mean scores: 45% felt an increased sense of hope after attending the sessions and 32% felt no change; the rest did not answer the question. To the question about what was the

most beneficial aspect of the session, 33% responded 'they listen …
a chance to express feelings', 23% responded 'someone trying to
help us understand what is happening … give us information' and
23% responded ' being aware that they are here … feel cared about'.
77%, however, would recommend the sessions for the future.

Freismuth (1986) conducted a quasi-experimental study to
find if there is any difference to the degree the family members'
needs are met when the visiting policy in an ICU is open in comparison with when the visiting policy is strict. In a 15-bed
medical–surgical ICU, 24 control group subjects and 20 experimental group subjects were interviewed within 48–72 hours of
the patient's admission. On a 30-item needs questionnaire developed by the investigator, participants were asked to rate the
extent to which each need was met. Characteristics of the participants and reliability and content validity of the instrument are
not provided. Analysing the data using a t-test showed a statistically significant difference ($p < 0.05$) in favour of the experimental group. Needs such as to be with the patient more often, to be
allowed to visit at any time, to have someone tell the visitor what
he or she is able to do at the bedside and to know what treatment
the patient is receiving were the needs for which the statistically
significant difference was identified.

Henneman et al (1992) conducted a comparative study with
one way between subjects design to evaluate the effectiveness of
two methods of meeting the information needs of families of
critically ill patients – an open visiting policy and a family information booklet. The booklet, entitled '*Where Caring is Critical*',
was professionally designed to convey a caring attitude of the
staff towards the family. It included information on the purpose
of the medical ICU, what the family could expect to see in the
unit, the various personnel involved in patient care and their
roles, and finally the family's role. In a 12-bed medical ICU of a
west coast university medical centre, 147 members of families of
patients admitted to the unit were the convenience sample used
for this study. The criteria of relevance for the participants were
to be family members or significant others, 18 years of age and
older and English speaking. The requirement for the Group 3
participants was to have received the information booklet within
24 hours of admission.

The research questions were to what extent family needs were
met during a restricted visiting policy (Group 1), to what extent

after implementation of an open visiting policy (Group 2) and to what extent after implementation of an open visiting policy and family information booklet together (Group 3). The instrument used in this study was developed by the principal investigator. It had three sections: a satisfaction scale, a knowledge evaluation, and demographic data. The first section was developed by an adaptation of Molter's needs inventory, identifying the needs of the family members, which in this case was used to show how satisfied were the members with the degree to which each of these needs was met.

The second section of the tool evaluated the members' ability to recall certain information such as physicians' and social workers' names, visiting hours and the ICU phone number. The last section for the demographic data included relationships, length of stay of the patient and any previous ICU admissions.

A panel of clinical experts established the content validity. Internal consistency using Cronbach's alpha was 0.97. Questionnaires were distributed between 24–48 hours after admission over a 6-month period with restricted visiting policy. 4 months after the open-visiting policy was implemented, data were collected from Group 2. The information booklet was given 6 months after the new policy began and, 2 months after that, data were collected from Group 3.

Over a total of 16 months, 180 questionnaires were distributed and 147 were returned (return rate 82%). There were 48 participants in Group 1, 50 in Group 2 and 49 in Group 3. In 86% of the cases this was the first admission to the ICU. No significant difference was found between the respondents' relationship to the patient, ICU experience or length of time in ICU.

Group 2 (open visiting) had statistically significant higher satisfaction for 9 of the 15 needs areas than Group 1 (restricted visiting policy) – $p < 0.05$ (average significance level $p = 0.0075$). Group 2 also showed a higher knowledge of details of the ICU, including visiting hours and unit phone number, but not the names of the personnel (average significance level $p = 0.003$). Group 2 and Group 3 did not have statistically significant differences in their satisfaction of the needs but they had significant (average $p = 0.03$) increases in their knowledge of specific details of the ICU, including the names of physicians and social workers. Group 3, finally, had significant increases in family satisfaction for 7 of the 15 need areas compared to Group 1 (average $p = 0.01$)

and also significant increases in knowledge about the ICU and the personnel (average p = 0.001).

Koller (1991) in a slightly different descriptive study tried to identify what family members use as coping behaviours to meet their needs, which of them are more effective, what the nurses can do to help them and the nature of the relationship between coping behaviour and need categories. In a 32-bed medical–surgical ICU in a 567-bed private tertiary hospital a convenience sample of 30 family members of 22 patients participated in the study. Criteria for relevance were: patient to be admitted for a minimum of 24 hours and maximum of 6 days; family members should visit the patient in the ICU, be older than 18 years, and be able to speak and write English.

80% of the sample were female; their mean age was 51.1 years and the mean age of the patients was 66.6 years. 63.5% of the patients were surgical patients and 36.5% were medical patients. Instruments used were the Jalowiec coping scale (Jalowiec 1989, cited in Koller 1991) to identify the coping strategies of the family members. This is a 60-item self-rating questionnaire divided into eight subscales of coping styles as follows: confronting, evasive, optimistic, fatalistic, emotive, palliative, supportive, and self-reliant'. Part A of the instrument asks the subjects to rate on a four-point Lifetree scale how often each strategy is used and part B asks the subjects to rate similarly how effective each strategy is. The instrument had previously obtained Cronbach's internal consistency alpha coefficient of 0.88–0.94 for the coping scale and 0.81–0.96 for total effectivenéss with cardiac transplant patients, and 0.64–0.85 with the elderly widows/widowers respectively (Jalowiec 1989, cited in Koller 1991). A seven open-ended questions structured interview – Family Member Structured Interview Guide (FMSIG) – was also used to obtain qualitative information about coping with critical illness.

The 10 coping behaviours with the 10 highest scores were: 'Hoping, talking problems over with the family, thinking positively, praying, worrying about the problem, think about the good things in life, look at problem objectively, keep situation under control, handle things one step at a time, think out different ways to handle the situation, keep a sense of humour'. The 10 most effective coping behaviours were identified as follows: 'talk the problem over with family or friends, think positively, pray/put trust in God, think about the good things in life, hope that things will get better, look at problem objectively, handle things one step at a time, keep the situation under control, think out different ways to handle the situation, worry about the problem'.

From the qualitative analysis of the interviews using the open-ended questions about coping in the ICU, responses were that the uncertainty of prognosis and the waiting were most stressful. Participants reported that social support (n = 16) and prayer (n = 11) helped them to overcome this situation. Suggestions for nursing interventions included provision of information, emotional support, frequent visitation, and competence and manners from the nurses.

Discussion

Information given through ICU booklets on domestic and patients' problems (Cray 1989, Henneman et al 1992) and educational classes (Cray 1989) has been beneficial and liked by family members (Table 6.1). Similarly, an education orientation programme (Chavez & Faber 1987) even though it did not produce a significant decrease in families' anxiety caused higher awareness of the patient's diagnoses.

Family support group sessions (Sabo et al 1989) decreased the factors that cause stress on the families. Open-visiting policies (Freismuth 1986, Henneman et al 1992) produced statistically significant improvement in the degree to which the needs of families are met. Koller (1991) found that the most effective coping behaviour of the family in the ICU is to 'talk the problem over with the family or friends' and this has implications for counselling the family, while the families themselves suggested that appropriate nursing interventions should be information, emotional support, frequent visitation, and competence and manners from the nurses.

Opening the visiting in ICUs allows the families to have a closer contact with the ICU staff and therefore receive appropriate and frequent information. Watching the procedures and the care that is provided to the patient, reassures them and their stress is decreased.

Information booklets are a way to provide information for the family and are a source for frequent reference on ICU issues as well as on the philosophy of the unit.

Table 6.1 Interventions to meet family needs in ICUs

Intervention	Evaluation method	Results
Cray (1989) Visitor teaching booklet Telephone call at home twice a week Visiting three times a week in waiting room Educational classes of 15 minutes on ICU procedures, equipment, respiratory failure, kidney failure and stages of awareness	Statements about the value of the programme Likert scale from 1 (disagree) to 5 (strongly agree) $n = 76$	Vast majority strongly agreed that the programme was helpful to them to cope better in the ICU
Chavez & Faber (1987) Education orientation programme and visitation Hand-out of unit policy	Experimental design Variables: heart rate, blood pressure, stress Instrument: Subjective Stress Scale by Kerle & Bialek $n = 20$ (control) $n = 20$ (experimental)	Statistically significant difference only in heart rate of experimental group $p = 0.016$ 85% of experimental group aware of diagnosis, 55% of control group
Sabo et al (1989) Family support group sessions (information, fostering hope, share and ventilate common concerns)	Experimental deisgn Variables: stress, social support, hope Instrument with 27 statements and five-point Likert scale Open ended questions $n = 36$ (control) $n = 31$ (experimental)	No statistically significant differences on stress, social support and hope 23% no change of stress 52% somewhat decreased 9% strongly decreased stress 71% increased support 45% increased hope

Table 6.1 (*Contd.*)   Interventions to meet family needs in ICUs

Intervention	Evaluation method	Results
Freismuth (1986) Open visiting	Quasi-experimental 30-item needs questionnaire to assess if needs were met $n = 24$ (control) $n = 20$ (experimental)	Statistically significant difference in favour of experimental group
Henneman et al (1992) Open visiting Family information booklet	Comparative design one way between subjects 15-item needs questionnaire to assess satisfaction of informational needs $n = 147$	Statistically significant higher satisfaction for 9 of 15 needs

Support groups bring people together and provide the opportunity for them to share their feelings, concerns and coping behaviours, and the giving and receiving of support among members. The feeling that they are not the only ones who have the same problem helps them to feel better.

In a literature review, Henneman & Cardin (1992) also found that education-oriented programmes, open visiting policy, orientation and follow-up programmes improve communication, understanding of the patients' diagnosis, and help to meet the families' needs more frequently.

It is necessary now to establish a wide strategy in meeting the needs of the relatives in the ICU and these strategies must be evaluated with more accurate research methods. The American Association of Critical Care Nurses (1987, cited in Henneman & Cardin 1992) have issued a booklet for the families in the ICU with the title 'It's Critical that You Know: A Resource for Families of Critically Ill Patients'. This and possibly other interventions must be evaluated to discover how effective they are in meeting the family's needs. Molter, in her interview with Leske (1991b), states that needs may evolve over time and researchers must investigate this issue so that we can have a variety of effective strategies to meet the needs of the families in different timeframes, as needs will differ from the immediate post-admission period to the long-term hospitalisation in the ICU.

With the patient's admission to the ICU an assessment of the family will be valuable for the preparation of the nursing care plan. Patterns of communications within the family will provide an understanding of the roles and relationships in the family, how decisions are made and how conflicts are resolved. Family's values, goals and aspirations during critical illness need to be assessed too. Family functioning during this time is another important thing for the nurse to assess. By observing the family and the interaction among its members, a nurse can understand whether the family's atmosphere is supportive or competitive in order to work with them during the crisis. Finally, an external factor that is important when supporting families is the availability of some other help, as with child care or some daily life help from friends or neighbours. All these are influential in assisting a family to cope during the crisis of a critical illness (Hartshorn et al 1993) .

Leske (1991a) states that helping family members deal with the stress of sudden critical illness has been recognised as an integral part of professional critical care nursing practice. Moreover, with earlier discharges, long-term critical illness and care the family may have to assume a greater burden for care. Critical care units continue to be the focus of critical care nursing but progressive areas of nursing practice or step-down units and home health care are becoming more common.

EVIDENCE OF RECOVERY OF PATIENT IF FAMILY IS SUPPORTED

Hartshorn et al (1993) highlight the need for the critical care nurse to recognise the influence of the family on the overall recovery of the patient. Serious illness brings a crisis within the family that can put a well-organised family into disequilibrium. The AACN (1989) standards emphasise the importance of assessment of the family and the continual involvement of the family in the care of the patient. The nursing role towards the family is to be sympathetic, to show understanding and to provide guidance throughout the experience (Hartshorn et al 1993).

Bouley et al (1994) have stated that if the needs of the family are not met the patient may not receive optimum support from the family. Nurses need to establish relationships with the families of patients in order to meet the needs of both patients and their families. The ability of nurses to convey warm, honest, caring and empathetic feelings toward both the patient and the family facilitates the development of this relationship. Because patients are usually too ill to be aware of the quality of care they receive, it is the family who realise that the care that the patient is receiving is of high quality and this leads to mutual trust between the nurse, the family and the patient.

Hartshorn et al (1993) state that patients admitted to the ICU are faced with several stressors. These include loss of privacy, artificial lighting 24 hours a day, lack of windows, noise from the various machines in the unit, and lack of meaningful stimuli to the patient. Ballard (1981, cited in Hartshorn et al 1993) stated that the top three stressors in the ICU were the feeling of being tied down by tubes, being in pain and being thirsty. The various life-support equipment attached to patients restricts their movements. Pain and being thirsty are a result of the treatment they receive in the ICU. 30–70% of the patients experience severe psychological stress, which results in developing powerlessness, anger and the ICU syndrome (Hartshorn et al 1993). The powerless patient has no control over events and situations, can not make decisions and control the environment. Physical care of the patient relies on the nurse; the patient has no knowledge of what is going on and what will happen and fears for the worst. A powerless patient is often frightened, anxious and frustrated. The frustration can lead to anger, hostility, withdrawal, or depression. These can prolong the recovery period (Hartshorn et al 1993). A derivative of powerlessness and anxiety is anger. Also a feeling of loss, such as of a bodily function or a limb, or the loss of one's former life due to illness, disability or disfigurement, leads to anxiety and frustration, which in turn cause anger (Hartshorn et al 1993). All these negative psychological responses contribute to the development of the ICU syndrome. It occurs on the third to the seventh day in the ICU. Common features are clouding of the consciousness, decreased attention span, disorientation, memory loss, and labile emotions. It affects 14–72% of patients admitted in the ICU and disappears 48 hours after transfer from the unit (Hartshorn et al 1993). Environmental factors that cause the problem are sleep deprivation, sensory deprivation and sensory overload. The lack of familiar faces such as the family constitutes sensory deprivation. It is therefore suggested that family should be encouraged to visit and bring personal items to place at the bedside (Hartshorn et al 1993).

The main contribution of families to the well-being of patients is visiting them. There has not been much research on this issue and more importantly no recent research. This kind of research commenced in the 1970s and was focused on patients' heart rate and blood pressure. Titler & Walsh (1992) reviewed the literature and stated that frequent visits caused more severe and frequent dysrhythmias in the patients than short visiting. However, in the ICU environment it is very difficult to control the many external factors that may have affected these results. In another study it was suggested that family members may transmit their anxiety to the patient. Allowing more time and having supported family members may decrease their anxiety levels and in turn this may decrease patients' anxiety. 5 minutes of visiting may not be long enough to allow complete processing of non-verbal cues (Titler & Walsh 1992). Zetterlund (1971, cited in Titler & Walsh 1992) found that heart rates of ICU patients increased 10% after visiting but returned to normal when nurses did not force the family members to leave when the 5 minutes of visiting allowance was over. In contrast, when the visiting allowance was strictly 5 minutes, patients' heart rates increased by 7% and did not return to baseline at the end of the visit. In another study, Mitchell (1977, cited in Titler & Walsh 1992) found that the number of premature ventricular contractions increased during the first 10 minutes of visiting but returned to below the baseline 20 minutes after visiting. Hansen (1982, cited by Titler & Walsh 1992) also found significant decrease in heart rate during 1 hour of visiting when compared with pre-visitation heart rates. Fuller & Foster (1982) measured the blood pressure and heart rate of patients and microtremor suppression (vocal stress) to assess the effects of visits of family and friends versus staff interaction on stress/arousal of ICU patients. Family visits studied over 15 minutes were no more or less stress/arousal-provoking than nurse–patient interaction as indicated by these parameters. The vocal microtremor suppression results suggested that lower patient stress arousal levels may accompany visits which include physical contact, ventilation of concern by patients and no ventilation of concern by visitors.

Bruya (1981, cited by Titler & Walsh 1992) found that intracranial pressures of patients with head injuries decreased when family members approached the bed. Restricting visits to short times and terminating visits prematurely contribute to adverse responses of the critically ill patients (Titler & Walsh 1992).

Titler & Walsh (1992) have also reviewed the literature on visiting preferences of patients and results show that they prefer flexible visiting hours guided by nurses in order to enhance the outcome of the care they provide. 50% of patients wanted more frequent family visits. They reported that the majority of visits were helpful. Visitors are seen by them as patient advocates, providers of a link with home and helpful by 'just being there'. Patients stated that they wanted from two to ten visits a day, preferably every 1–2 hours. Halm & Titler (1990, cited by Titler & Walsh 1992) found that 65% of patients surveyed preferred visits of 15–30 minutes. Simpson (1991) found that CCU patients preferred visits lasting 40 minutes, whereas SICU patients preferred 25-minute visits; the older the patient was the longer he or she wanted the visit to be. Patients preferred two or three visitors at a time and the more severe the condition the more visitors were required. Less than one-third of the patients stated that visiting was tiring. Generally, patients prefer individualised visiting policies.

Moseley & Jones (1991) described the use of a visitation contract in order to optimise the support patients receive from visiting. Visits are predetermined with the nurse in order to plan the care that the patient will receive during visits. After admission, the patient's and family's visiting needs are addressed and their preferences are discussed. Increasing the family's involvement in the care of the patient will decrease the feelings of powerlessness. Not only does the patient's health affect the integrity of the family, but the family's health can profoundly influence the recovery of the patient.

An open visiting policy would have some positive effects on patients' well-being. Patients are at risk of alterations in sensory perception. The several unfamiliar sounds interrupt the patient's sleep cycle and cause sensory overload. This can deplete the restorative energy available for adaptation to the disease. In addition, because of the lack of familiar sensory input and social isolation, sensory deprivation can occur. These factors may cause increased confusion, restlessness and other psychological problems. The presence of the family in the environment may decrease sensory disturbances, thus enhancing normalcy. Also, with open visiting hours, interruptions of patients' sleep may be reduced as they will feel more relaxed after having been with their loved ones for as long as they wish and whenever it suits them. Controlling their own visiting schedules is a step for patients towards minimising their dependency and improving their sense of well-being (Kirchhoff et al 1985).

Caine (1989) states that a person rarely experiences a crisis in isolation; rather what influences one person influences others with whom there is a close connection. Usually this is in the family context. Among the many needs of families, are relief from anxiety, information, being useful, getting help with family problems and acquiring support. Family members need to discover and recognise the significant role they play in the eventual recovery of the patient. It has also been shown that relatives with low anxiety levels may provide valuable psychological support as well as assist in the physical care of the patient (Caine 1989).

Curley & Wallace (1992) performed a quasi-experimental study to investigate the effects of a Nursing Mutual Participation Model of care on stress in the parents of paediatric ICU patients. It was found that when the Nursing Mutual Participation Model of care was implemented by staff nurses, parental stress was reduced in the area of parental role in the paediatric ICU setting. As parental stress is reduced, more energy will be available for the parents to support their child during this frightening time.

PREPARING THE FAMILY AND THE PATIENT TO GO HOME

Roe Prior et al (1994) state that after the introduction of diagnostic related groups and prospective payment systems in the 1980s, patients leave hospital quicker and sicker. Malloy (1989) named some other forces which contributed to the increased demand for home care. These are: (1) cost-containment pressures; (2) an increasing elderly population; (3) reduction in the number of caregivers (primarily women); (4) consumer health awareness; (5) advances in medical technology. With the increase of acutely ill patients and the shorter stay in hospital, some patients may require special equipment to support them in the home. Such equipment includes pumps for tube feeding and intravenous therapy, specialised catheters for total parenteral nutrition, ventilators, suctioning machines, cardiac and respiratory monitors, automated peritoneal dialysis systems and oxygen regulators (Noble 1988, Roe Prior et al 1994). Therefore advanced critical care expertise is becoming of ever greater importance to both hospitals and home health agencies (Noble 1988). If patients who are dependent on this equipment cannot be discharged home, they remain in hospital with great financial cost both to the patient and the institution. There is a great need for home health care agencies to be able to provide staff with knowledge and clinical skills relevant to acute-care nursing in order that patients who are dependent on high technology and have complex health care needs can be given the option of home health care (Malloy 1989, Roe Prior et al 1994). However, caring for patients at home is different from caring for them in hospital. In hospital the caregivers have total control of the situation, whereas at home nurses need greater expertise in decision-making, are more autonomous, have not only to access the patient but the whole environment, do not have the security of the institution and have to facilitate their clients and families to assume responsibility for the care of the patient (Malloy 1989).

Patients who are discharged earlier and require high-technology equipment at home can be medically safe. Two of the most important factors that will affect their care are an adequate number of follow-up visits and access to clinically expert health professionals (Roe Prior et al 1994).

Long-term home care patients, to be able to function, require critical care expertise and skill. Both patients and families need individualised teaching, emotional support, and guidance in the hospital and the community (Noble 1988). Ill patients often find it difficult to learn about their illnesses and their families may also be unable to learn how to care for them. The clinical nurse specialist can meet this important need by consulting with health and social agencies before discharge to arrange that both patients and their families will be informed. Sometimes, though, patients with cardiac problems or after cardiac surgery may not have had adequate time to adapt to the fact and its consequences. The role of the clinical nurse specialist in the discharge planning team is to alert the team to the fact that additional support or outside arrangements must be made before discharge, such as arrangements for family education, consultation, continuity of care with a home health agency and teaching programmes on diet, exercise, drugs and daily routine (Noble 1988).

Families in the community may often be in crisis and their physical and psychological strength as well as their financial resources can be limited. Sometimes having to care for a member of their family in the house does not permit them to work as much as they ought to. Other members of the family can also be affected by the situation at home, for example the children may have problems at school and the relationship between the couple may start to falter. The specialist nurse can intervene and guide and assist the nurses who regularly visit the home to offer emotional support and to refer to social agencies who can help to preserve the family integrity (Noble 1988).

Roe Prior et al (1994) conducted two surveys to explore whether there was a need for a critical care clinical nurse specialist (CCCNS) in high-tech, complex home care and to determine the characteristics of that role. Furthermore, the surveys sought to identify the necessary curriculum content a CCCNS graduate programme should include to prepare individuals for practice in home care. From 36 home care agencies in the Philadelphia metropolitan and New Jersey areas that responded to the first survey, 34 (94%) reported that they cared for patients requiring high-tech, complex home care. 81% of them had a diagnoses of heart failure, 78% respiratory failure and 72% neuromuscular disease. It was the family, with the assistance of the home health care nurse, that had the primary responsibility for the technological aspects of care. For 93% of the respondents the primary responsibility was patient–family teaching. Also, 78% of home care agencies reported caring for patients discharged home directly from a step-down unit, while 56% cared for patients discharged home directly from an intensive care unit. 83% of the respondents perceived a need for a CCCNS in the high-tech, complex home care field. There was little perceived need for a CCCNS in direct patient care. The areas where CCCNSs were needed were patient–family education, home care agency staff education, home care agency consultation, and hospital-to-home coordination. Also, some recommendations for the content of the course for CCCNSs included courses on technology, discharge planning, physical assessment, health policy and case management.

To the second survey that was sent to discharge planners, CCCNSs and social workers who were responsible for patient discharge, all of them (14) reported that they discharge patients with high-tech, complex home care needs. 43% of them reported discharging patients with ventilators and 64% reported patients with intravenous drug infusions. Answers to the question of who was responsible for educating the patient and the family on the technology of high-tech home care needs included: the primary registered nurse, the clinical nurse specialist and the respiratory therapist. A variety of individuals were responsible for coordinating the patient's discharge. These included the primary nurse, the discharge planning nurse, the social worker and the clinical nurse specialist. 12 of the 14 respondents reported having a patient's discharge home delayed because of the need for high-tech home care. 12 of the 14 respondents considered a critical care clinical nurse specialist (CCCNS) to be necessary for the high-tech, complex home care fields.

The role that was finally identified for the CCCNS was very interesting. It included consultant to the home care agency, patient–family education, hospital staff education, and hospital-to-home coordinator.

For complex home health care to be successful, access to clinically expert health professionals is of the utmost importance. Other things are appropriate patient selection, a psychologically stable family, a thorough education of the patient and family, a suitable home environment, adequate financial resources, the availability of equipment and supplies, and adequate patient follow-up visits (Roe Prior et al 1994).

ORGAN DONATION

With the improvement of surgical methods and more effective immunosuppressive drug therapy, the number and the type of successfully transplanted organs and tissues have increased (Martin & Crigger 1997). Critical care nurses can play an important role and maximise the availability of donor organs and tissues, as 95% of all donor situations occur in critical care units (Gill 1993). Special skills in identifying potential donors, mechanisms and methodologies for obtaining consent for donation, the referral process to organ procurement organisations and the clinical care of the donor are nursing's contribution to organ procurement (Gill 1993). Potential donors may at any time agree to donate organs by signing a donor card, but the family must give the final consent before the donor is declared brain dead (Martin & Crigger 1997).

Thus, the nurses in the critical care setting are often the first persons to have contact with family members of the patient who is declared brain dead. The ethical and legal responsibilities of the nurses have increased as they have developed more autonomy and their role has expanded. Nurses keep a high standard of care and are directly accountable for their nursing actions. Similarly, in the process of organ transplantation, nurses consider the rights and privileges of the donor, the recipient, and the family. Some of the most important ethical principles in ethical decision-making regarding transplantation are respect for persons and their autonomous choices, beneficence and non-maleficence, utility, justice and fidelity (Martin & Crigger 1997).

Organ donation has been perceived as the only positive event for the family after the loss of their loved one. It can help them during the process of grieving and provides altruistic feelings giving the opportunity to help another human being. Some families themselves start the discussion about the possibility for organ donation, but it is the critical care nurses who are expected to initiate the idea during this stressful time for the family (Gill 1993).

The participation of the critical care nurse in organ donation is by:

- providing supportive and factual information to the family of the brain dead patient
- participating in the request process
- providing clinical maintenance of the donor in order to ensure the viability of the donated organs (Gill 1993).

Critical care nursing is not only carried out within the traditional critical care units. Sole & Hartshorn (1997) state that acutely ill patients such as the ventilatory dependent are cared for in step-down units, in medical–surgical units, in long-term acute care hospitals and at home, while critical care nurses coordinate the care of these patients regardless of the setting.

McCoy & Bell (1994) state that less than 20% of individuals who meet the criteria to be donors actually donate organs. Therefore, more than 100 000 potential organs are not collected each year. The problem is extremely important, as in the USA for all types of transplantation the waiting lists are increasing by 200 monthly. Reasons for this lack of identification of potential donors are: knowledge deficits, poor documentation of patient condition, failure to notify procurement agencies and especially the high discomfort level of health care professionals when dealing with grieving families. Identification of potential donors and successful procurement are a solution to the problem and the role of critical care nurses is very important (McCoy & Bell 1994). McCoy & Bell (1994) conducted a study to examine the knowledge and attitudes of rural critical care nurses regarding organ donation. They found that most critical care nurses have positive attitudes toward organ procurement. Having positive attitudes, nurses can be very effective in providing support when approaching families regarding organ donation (McCoy & Bell 1994).

7

Dermatology nursing

Lynette Stone

INTRODUCTION

The skin is the largest organ in the body and forms the boundary between the person and the outside world. It has a variety of functions including protection against infections, infestations, trauma, irritants and ultraviolet radiation as well as controlling heat and water loss. The skin provides our sensory contact with the world, enabling us to feel touch, pain, itching, heat and cold and it is an important organ of social and sexual contact. Self-image can be altered by skin disease. Society today tends to categorise people according to their physical attributes and social credibility. Others' perception of an individual's appearance, rather than the appearance itself creates the problem which Goffman (1963) called stigma. The importance of having confidence in our appearance has become one of the requirements of daily life in the media and self-image conscious world of today. Helping people to cope with these pressures is one of the major challenges for nurses working in all areas of health care.

Although there are over 1000 skin diseases (Champion et al 1992), about 70% of the dermatological workload in primary and secondary care in the UK is taken up by only nine categories of skin diseases – skin cancer, acne, atopic eczema, psoriasis, viral warts, other infective skin disorders, benign tumours and vascular lesions, leg ulcers, contact dermatitis and other eczemas (Williams 1997). A study published by the Royal College of General Practitioners found that skin conditions were the fourth most common reason for people in England and Wales to consult their GP in 1991/92 (RCGP 1995).

Most people experience no, or few, problems with their skin. However, for some people with acute, widespread generalised conditions or skin diseases the situation can be extremely serious and even life-threatening. Damage to the skin may be as simple as a small cut that just needs to be healed or something such as generalised pustular psoriasis where problems with loss of protein and fluid can very quickly lead to serious illness. The challenge of caring for such patients can be considered similar to caring for someone with full body burns. Whatever the cause, people with skin failure are as entitled to care as are those with cardiac or renal failure.

PREVALENCE

The prevalence of skin disease is vastly underestimated. For example with common skin conditions such as eczema and psoriasis it is estimated that 5–10% of the population is affected by eczema (Williams 1997) and 1–3% by psoriasis (Nall & Farber 1977). It is accepted that skin disease affects 20–33% of the population at any one time (Rea et al 1976), seriously interfering with the activities of people in 10% of cases.

Market research and epidemiological evidence suggests that many people with skin disease do not even consult their GP or the local pharmacist (British Market Research Bureau 1987, Dunnell & Cartwright 1972, Wadsworth et al 1968). However, about 15% of the population do consult their family doctor about skin disease each year; 8% of these would then be referred on for specialist advice (Carmichael 1995).

For most people with skin disease it is a chronic disorder with acute exacerbations. After being diagnosed most people can cope well but often they require help and advice when their skin does flare up. It also should be borne in mind that minor skin complaints can frequently cause greater upset than most serious conditions, for example persistent itching of the skin in all age groups can be much more distressing than a major flare up of eczema or psoriasis. Mortality in skin disease accounts for 0.46% of all death (OPCS 1994). These are mostly from skin cancer, the most common form of cancer, but also from herpes and eczema in a few cases. It is estimated that 40 000 people in the UK contract skin cancer annually. Although melanoma, the most serious form of skin cancer, is curable if detected early enough it is now the second most common cause of death among people aged 34–35. Morbidity related to skin disease is high and can have major impact on the quality of life of both the sufferers and their families and carers. The impact on school and work should not be underestimated. It is one of the commonest reasons for certified sickness from work in the UK (DSS 1994).

THE CHANGING NHS AND ITS EFFECTS ON DERMATOLOGY NURSING

Dermatology care in the UK has been affected by the health care reforms, starting with those which were introduced with the government White Paper 'Working for Patients' (DoH 1989b) and followed by the introduction of the internal market, with its purchaser–provider split, the establishment of commissioning authorities with responsibility to purchase health care for their local area (NHSME 1990) and the development of hospital and community health services into self-governing trusts to become providers of health care. Additionally, with the higher-profile role of general practitioners as providers of primary medical care and purchasers of secondary care and the advent of fundholding GPs, dermatology services have been under review. The contribution of nursing to the shaping of health care services has continued to increase. In the government White Paper 'The New NHS: Modern, Dependable' (1997) it is proposed that in the primary care groups, which will replace GP fundholding, community nurses will take responsibility with GPs in commissioning services for the local community. Community nurses will therefore need to prepare themselves for dealing with the dermatology issues that affect up to 30% of their population at any one time. Inevitably, all these developments have had major implications for the role of the dermatology nurse. They have raised issues about who provides the patient care: should it be a nurse or a doctor; should its focus be in the primary or secondary care sector; and where should it be provided – in the hospital, GP surgery or in the home, or a mixture of all these options depending on the patient's condition and needs. The need for the patient's voice to be heard in discussions on these issues has led to the formation of the umbrella organisation, The Skin Care Campaign, which is a broad-based alliance including bodies representing patient support groups, health professionals and organisations such as the Health Education Authority.

WHY SPECIALIST DERMATOLOGY NURSES?

Patients with chronic skin disease value the role of the specialist trained dermatology nurses in providing their care, and the benefits of individualised nursing care taking into consideration all their needs have long been recognised (Jobling 1978).

Many people with skin diseases can be treated effectively in the community, and nurses in the primary care setting have a major role to play in improving the quality of life of people with skin disorders. The need for health care for people with skin disease is frequently unmet and when one considers that some 15% of consultations with the GP already are related to a skin disorder, it gives some measure of the size of the problem. The main reason for the demand for health care in skin disease is its high prevalence. There is an increasing incidence of some skin diseases such as skin cancer, which can be related to more frequent sunny holidays, atopic eczema, especially in children, and venous leg ulcers due to the ageing population. In addition, publicity and development of better treatments for conditions such as acne and psoriasis and publicity about moles and other skin growths have led to the general public becoming more aware and having increased expectations.

Most patients presenting with a skin problem do so for several reasons. They may feel that they have something contagious and perhaps very serious. They may be worried about the way they look and this can create tremendous psychological stress on the individual as well as affecting family life. It may be that they feel because it shows that they are socially unacceptable and are being treated as social outcasts. People with vitiligo, particularly among Afro-Caribbean and Asian groups, and psoriasis have been heard to say that they are made to 'feel like a leper'. Often patients or their carers are at the end of their tether as a result of just having to cope with the condition. The mother of a family having sleepless nights with a child with eczema, for example, needs support. Much help and support therefore is needed and the nurse is ideally placed to provide counselling, advice and education about treatments and to identify additional help that may be needed.

Dermatology nursing until fairly recently tended to be confined to the secondary care sector in the few large units within the UK and to the district general hospital dermatology department. There has been a gradual expansion of dermatological care in the community, particularly in the area of treatment of atopic eczema in children. Leg ulcers are regularly cited as a dermatological condition that is mainly managed now by the community nursing team. However, as the majority of leg ulcers are related to vascular disease rather than skin disease, this is not so much a dermatological condition as a basically vascular condition. Where an element of contact dermatitis is involved in ulceration, then it becomes a dermatologically related problem, often requiring referral to a specialist.

With the emphasis on care in the community and a primary-care-led health service, more is being done to raise awareness of the needs of patients with skin conditions. Specialist hospital-based dermatology nurses have been developing community liaison roles (Perkins 1994, Ruane Morris et al 1995b, Venables et al, unpublished work, 1995) and some practice and district nurses have taken a special interest in patients with skin problems, for example particularly families where children have eczema (Edwards 1997).

If people with skin diseases are to have access to dermatological nursing care, nurses must know how to examine and assess the patients' skin, be aware of common skin problems, how to prevent them or limit the likelihood of a 'flare up', the treatments that are commonly prescribed and how to apply them. Working with patients and their families or carers to teach them about these issues will help them develop greater understanding of their disease and independence. Nurses in the community may facilitate such activities by establishing nurse-led clinics which offer such services as skin assessment/screening, patient teaching and advice about therapy, application of topical treatments, promotion of healthy skin care and prevention of disease, and development of local support/self-help groups (Burr & Gradwell 1996).

If nurses are to expand their role into these areas for the benefit of patient care, as recognised in 'The Scope of Professional Practice' (UKCC 1992b) they need to equip themselves with the relevant knowledge and skills in dermatology.

EDUCATION AND TRAINING

In spite of the importance of maintaining a healthy skin and the common occurrence of skin disorders, little time is given in the undergraduate nursing curriculum to the theory and practice of nursing care and management in dermatology.

Practical experience is not always readily available and is dependent upon the opportunities that arise in clinical placements. Students attending colleges where there is no access to dermatology departments or wards will probably not gain any practical 'hands-on' experience in dermatology. For those who do have access to specialist dermatology services, experience is dependent upon allocation to a dermatology outpatient clinic as part of their community/hospital interface experience or to a dermatology ward as part of their medical nursing experience. Otherwise it is quite by chance if they have the opportunity to be involved in the care of patients with recognised dermatological problems.

The first recognised courses for dermatology nursing were the English National Board (ENB) Course 393 in Dermatology Nursing that was first run in 1985. Following the introduction of Project 2000 a subsequent academic dermatology nursing course at level 2 'Developments in Dermatology Nursing', ENB N25 was validated. Apart from these courses, dermatology nurse education has been limited to 'on-the-job' experience in clinical areas specialising in dermatology, attendance at ad hoc study days or planned 'in-house' courses at specialist dermatology units.

In 1989 the need for specialist dermatology nursing was recognised with the establishment of the British Dermatological Nursing Group (BDNG) which is affiliated to the British Association of Dermatologists and the Royal College of Nursing Dermatology Special Interest Group (SIG) and the publication of

'Standards of Care for Dermatology Nursing' (RCN 1995). The aim of both of these groups is to promote the specialist area of dermatology nursing, and membership is open to nurses working with patients with skin problems in both primary and secondary care areas. These groups provide an opportunity for education and training with national annual study days and, in the case of the British Dermatological Nursing Group, a programme of annual core educational modules has been developed. A recent initiative to support these developments further has been the publication of an annotated bibliography of dermatology nursing literature in conjunction with the Department of Health (Ersser 1997, 1998).

Further educational initiatives should include modules on dermatological pharmacology to equip specialist trained dermatology nurses for their role in prescribing the common dermatology treatments and Cox et al (1995) have demonstrated the benefits this can have for patient care.

DERMATOLOGY CARE SERVICES

The All Party Parliamentary Group on Skin in its report published in March 1997 recommended that more use should be made of nurse specialists in the provision of skin services, that specialist nurses should liaise between hospital dermatology departments and the community and recognised the need for more nursing support to be available in the primary care setting for patients. The All Party Group also recognised that nurses are an essential resource in providing dermatology care, whether it is in a specialist unit or the community. Nurses are able to educate and inform patients, not least about support groups, and they can be the key to patients continuing with their prescribed treatment. Community nurses who spend time in the homes of newly diagnosed patients can show them how to manage their disease and can help reduce the number of inpatient stays needed; they can be especially supportive where children are affected. Nurses have a vital role in the use of dressings and application of emollients and, with appropriate training, can help in the treatment and management of common skin diseases like eczema and psoriasis. They are also in an ideal position to do more to help patients plan a routine for maintaining skin health. The All Party Group also recommended that patients could make effective use of primary care if nurses and health visitors could prescribe or advise on the same terms as GPs in some circumstances. This obviously would also have benefits for the patients in having more ready access to their care. For day-to-day dermatological care most patients can be supported by the primary care team with advice, help with treatment, discussion of lifestyles and how to plan treatment or a skin care regime to prevent flare-ups. It is only when a condition flares up sufficiently severely to warrant referral to the hospital that patients will need to be seen there or if they are on a treatment regime which is only provided in a centralised service, for example with phototherapy equipment. Many patients, particularly those with eczema and psoriasis, will have variations in their condition and these patients may need sometimes to have hospital-based care, the rest of the time being maintained within the primary care setting.

For these patients there is a need for shared care, with continuity and seamlessness in their care programmes and liaison between the specialist nurses in the hospital and the nurses in the primary care setting.

MODELS OF NURSING CARE

The aim for most patients is to be independent and self-caring, and from this perspective Orem's model of care could be adapted for them (Hunter 1992). Other dermatology nurses have focused on the whole person and his or her reaction to stressors as well as nurse–patient interaction and developed their own model based on Neuman's and Peplau's (Ruane Morris et al 1995a). However, for patients who are seriously ill and requiring hospital care, initially, in their acute phase, their necessary nursing care would need to follow a model which supports all the daily activities of living until the patients' condition improves sufficiently for them to become independent and self-caring in preparation for their discharge home.

SPECIALIST DERMATOLOGY NURSES

The specialist dermatology nurse has a vital role to play in the future provision of dermatology care and within the domain of advanced practice which has recently been a major topic of discussion (Castledine 1996a). A possible way forward would be to develop the role of a dermatology nurse practitioner who is a registered nurse with specialist knowledge in general dermatology, who works in the hospital and/or the community and could be considered similar to a general medical practitioner with a specialist interest in dermatology. The nurse with additional expertise would be a dermatology clinical nurse specialist who is a registered nurse and who has specialised both in dermatology and a particular area of dermatology practice, for example phototherapy or the management of childhood eczema which could be in both the hospital and community. These specialists would be supported by a dermatology nurse who practises at an advanced level and who could be considered comparable with the consultant dermatologist. The nurse in this role should have a highly developed knowledge of complex nursing care, dermatology and dermatology nursing practice, and therefore be able to act as a consultant and a specialist dermatology nursing resource person for all the members of the multidisciplinary team both in the primary and secondary care sectors. Nurses fulfilling such a role would be expected to be educated to master's or doctorate level. For this to be achieved there must be more of a focus on nurse education and training in dermatology.

IMPACT OF SKIN DISEASE

Skin diseases affect all age groups, for example the baby and the school child with atopic eczema, the middle-aged sufferer with intractable psoriasis, and the elderly person with skin cancer all will have the problems of dealing with their skin condition and coping on a day-to-day basis. Cultural and social beliefs of different ethnic groups may introduce further issues for consideration when planning a programme of skin care for a patient, for example in bathing or showering (Fincham Gee 1992). So whether one is a health visitor, or a school, practice, district, occupational health or hospital-based nurse, the dermatology patients needing one's care will come from all age ranges and groups in the community.

The psychological and social impact of having a skin disorder can have a significant effect on the quality of life of an individual and should not be underestimated. Ramsey & O'Reagan (1988) reported their survey of a group of people with psoriasis and found that large numbers avoided sports, swimming and sunbathing, two-thirds felt limited in their choice of clothing, over half felt people stared at them and half of the group felt that the condition had inhibited their sexual relationships. Embarrassment and distress about a skin condition has been found to be significantly associated with younger age (Morgan et al 1997).

Among those in the adolescent group who are affected by skin disease there may be problems associated with emotional upset, effects of peer group pressures, feelings of altered body image and imperfect appearance. Acne can be a major problem for this age group and some people find it extremely distressing. The severity of the psychological effects of this condition on sufferers has been highlighted by Cotterill & Cunliffe (1997) in their report of suicide in 16 dermatology patients, of whom seven were acne sufferers between the ages of 16 and 24.

Nurses and health visitors are ideally placed to provide the reassurance and psychological support which is a fundamental element of the role of the nurse in dermatology and to liaise with colleagues to help any of these patients cope with this skin problem as well as help them in managing their treatment.

COMMON SKIN CONDITIONS IN PRIMARY CARE

Common conditions seen in primary care include skin cancer, eczema, psoriasis, infestations, infections and acne. Nurses in the primary care sector or even minor injuries units are well placed to advise patients about prevention, treatment and management of these conditions.

Skin cancer

Halting the year-on-year increase in the incidence of skin cancer by 2005 is a 'Health of the Nation' target (DoH 1993). The three most common skin cancers, basal and squamous cell carcinomas and malignant melanoma, appear most often in those people who have had too much sun exposure. Basal cell carcinoma (BCC) – also known as a rodent ulcer – is the most common form of skin cancer and occurs usually on the faces of the middle-aged or elderly. Early treatment when the lesions are small enables total removal without ugly scarring (Hunter et al 1989). Squamous cell carcinoma (SCC) is more aggressive and should be treated without delay. The increased incidence of skin cancer in organ transplant recipients is a cause for concern (Glover 1998) and a regular skin examination of these patients should be carried out as part of their routine health checks. Treatments for these non-melanoma skin cancers include surgical excision, cryosurgery, curettage and cautery and MOHs micrographic surgery (Vargo 1991).

Although malignant melanoma is less common it has attracted more publicity because it is a potentially fatal lesion with a 70% rise in the number of recorded deaths between 1972 and 1992 (Cancer Research Campaign 1994). Fair-skinned people with red or blond hair, those with a tendency to freckle and with a family history are more at risk of developing melanoma. As episodes of severe sunburn may also increase the risk, patients going out into the sun, even on a hot sunny day in Britain, should be reminded of the need to take precautions and protect their skin. As Perkins (1995) also says, there is a need for practice nurses to educate patients about prevention as well as supporting them following diagnosis.

The fashion for having a tanned 'healthy' look has contributed to the increase of skin cancers in recent years and the need for public attitudes to be changed underpins success of the 'Health of the Nation' strategy in reducing the incidence of skin cancer. Nurses need to be aware of how patients form their attitudes (Van der Weyden 1994) and of the importance of educating children and their families as soon as possible about preventive measures (Clore 1995, Kenning & Blackmore 1996, Pion 1996).

Prevention of sun damage has become a key component in the fight against cancer, and nurses have a huge role to play in public awareness and prevention of skin cancer by discouraging excessive sun exposure and promoting the use of sunscreens regularly and correctly (Butler 1997, Lamanna 1996, Morrison 1996, Rumsfield 1990) as well as the wearing of protective clothing. The role of the primary care team is an essential component of the health promotion strategy in reducing the incidence of skin cancer (Taylor & Roberts 1997).

Infective disorders

There are a range of common bacterial, viral and fungal infections which are seen in primary care. At least 4% of the population consult their GP about a skin infection other than viral warts each year (Royal College of General Practitioners 1995). Bacterial infections include boils, impetigo and folliculitis; other viral infections include molluscum contagiosum, herpes simplex and herpes zoster; common fungal infections include tinea corporis, tinea capitis and onychomycosis (fungal infections of the nails). Skin infections are also especially common in immunocompromised people such as those with AIDS (Stern 1994) or transplant patients on immunosuppressive drugs.

Bacterial infections

Impetigo. The most common organism responsible is *Staphylococcus aureus*. Although impetigo occurs mostly in children it is occasionally seen in adults. Skin care involves gentle removal of crusts and use of a simple bactericidal soap to help prevent recurrent infections. Patients must be encouraged to complete the course of prescribed antibiotics. Where scalp lesions are present it is worth inspecting for head lice as the skin broken from scratching may have provided the entry site for the infection. It is advisable to keep children at home from school until the infection has cleared.

Boils tend to affect the 18- to 34-year age group and are caused by a deep staphylococcal infection. Nurses need to remember that patients suffering with recurrent boils should have a urine test for the presence of glucose as the skin in diabetics is more prone to sepsis.

Consideration must also be given to the susceptibility of people with previous skin damage such as eczema, and ensuring that patients and parents are aware of the role that staphylococcal infection can play in atopic eczema (Atherton 1994) and the problems associated with antibiotic resistance.

Viral infections

Viral warts affect between 4 and 5% of children aged 11–16 in the UK (Williams et al 1993). Although 60–90% clear spontaneously within 2 years, many patients will seek advice from the local pharmacist, practice or school nurse about using one of the many over-the-counter (OTC) preparations to speed their clearance. In more persistent cases, liquid nitrogen therapy may be used to treat warts on the hand and this is an area where outpatient and practice nurses have gained the skills and competence necessary to expand their role (UKCC 1992b) and have developed nurse-led clinics to provide this service.

Herpes simplex ('cold sores') can be activated by stimuli such as heat, cold and sunlight. Those who suffer with recurrent outbreaks should be advised to keep a ready supply of an antiviral agent such as acyclovir so that it can be applied at the first signs of tingling, itching or burning. They should also be encouraged to apply a sunscreen during outdoor activities such as on the beach or the ski slopes.

Herpes simplex is contagious and those infected should always take care to follow 'safe sex' practices. Patients with genital herpes should be referred for specialist genitourinary medicine advice and treatment. The herpes virus can also be a serious complication in atopic eczema, known as Kaposi's varicelliform eruption, which can be potentially fatal if untreated. These patients are extremely ill and need urgent treatment with antiviral drugs in addition to their eczema care.

Herpes zoster ('shingles') tends to affect the older age group and can be quite debilitating. As well as treating the skin eruption it is important to try to prevent the extremely painful postherpetic neuralgia developing.

Fungal infections

The dermatophyte infections, normally called tinea, which are characterised by a round scaly lesion known as ringworm, and yeasts of the genus *Candida* cause the most common fungal infections of the skin.

Tinea pedis ('athletes' foot') is the commonest dermatophyte infection (Hay 1993) and may affect 3.9% of the population at any one time (Williams 1997). Most patients will try OTC preparations before going to see their GP. In addition to any prescribed treatment, patients should be advised to keep the feet clean and dry, and wear cotton socks and sandals or open-toed shoes where possible. Some people who work in wet conditions are more prone to fungal infections of the feet and will need to take extra preventive measures to protect their feet. Primary care and occupational health teams should help these people to adapt their foot care regimes appropriately.

Tinea capitis (scalp ringworm) usually affects children. These infections were uncommon until recently and, in Europe, were mainly due to the zoophilic fungus *Microsporon canis*, derived from cats or dogs. However, in the last 4–5 years there has been a reported dramatic increase in the incidence of tinea capitis in London, Birmingham, Bristol and South Wales and the emergence of the anthropophilic fungus *Trichophyton tonsurans* which was the predominant cause of tinea capitis in the USA (Leeming & Elliott 1995). Winsor et al (1997) reported on a study in South London where of 243 children screened 119 were mycologically proven cases of scalp ringworm due to *T. tonsurans*. Although the reasons for the current epidemic are not clear, it has been attributed to the use of tight braiding exposing the scalp to infection and the hair oils which may act as adherents for the spores long enough for them to germinate. Topical therapies are ineffective and griseofulvin, the only drug licensed specifically for tinea capitis, should be given in the recommended dose for at least 8 weeks. Health visitors, school and practice nurses can be instrumental in raising clinical awareness of the problem, encouraging compliance with treatment and by screening children at school and nursery help contain such epidemics.

***Candida* species** are normal commensals in the mouth, gastrointestinal tract and vaginal mucosa, and sometimes affect the skin or nails. Oral candidosis, or thrush, is a common infection in the elderly, denture wearers, infants and immunocompromised patients, being the most common infectious complication of AIDS (Hay 1993). Skin infections generally occur in the body folds. Groin candidosis is more common in diabetics, while patients with eczema or psoriasis in the skin flexures may develop a secondary candidosis. Most superficial candida infections respond to a topical treatment; however, in immunocompromised patients the infection will need an orally absorbed drug. Recurrent episodes of candida infection cause considerable distress and discomfort and nurses are well placed to assist patients in planning appropriate prevention regimes, to recognise the presence of infection, to ensure that patients seek medical help when necessary and to help them carry out the prescribed treatment correctly.

Infestations

Scabies is a common, extremely itchy and contagious disorder. Outbreaks of scabies have been increasing in the past 10 years (Price 1993) and the Royal College of General Practitioners which has been tracking the condition has seen a rise in cases since 1991. Severe itching at night is a classic sign of scabies; however, patients with compromised immune systems – cancer patients, the debilitated and AIDS sufferers – may not itch (Elgart 1993). Nurses need to be aware of the special care these patients require and the potential for the condition to develop into Norwegian scabies with the production of so many mites that health care staff – and other patients in institutions such as nursing homes – can be infected. Atypical distribution of lesions is common in the elderly and the diagnosis may be confused with senile pruritus, a drug eruption or eczema (Hicks & Lewis 1995). The psychological distress of people diagnosed with scabies should not be underestimated and nurses can make a major contribution in supporting their patients during the course of treatment. In cases where the condition seems to be resistant to treatment it is worth checking if the patient has a pet dog and ensuring that it is checked by a vet for scabies. The patient should be reminded that the pet's bedding should also be washed regularly.

Head lice continue to be a chronic problem in the community and the increasing incidence of the infestation has gained recent newspaper headlines (Boseley 1997). Traditionally it was the school nurse's role to inspect children's heads for head lice infestation. However, parents may now seek the advice of practice nurses and health visitors in checking children's scalps and the use of appropriate treatments. Nurses working with the elderly and adults may need to check scalps and suggest treatment if infestation is a possibility due to close contact with children or other infested people (Cook 1998). In some areas with an education programme and their cooperation, the role of monitoring has been passed to parents (Black 1991). Concerns about the emergence of resistance to prescribed medications and the toxic effects of organophosphates have led to a review of recommended treatments. An alternative way of treating head lice infestation has been encouraged using the natural method of wet combing. This method is used in 'bug busting' campaigns that involve parents, teachers and health professionals and can form part of an effective community health education programme (Duncan 1997). The 'bug buster' technique has been developed by the charity Community Hygiene Concern. Wet combing used on a weekly basis can also be used as a preventive measure against lice (Cook 1998).

Eczema

Atopic eczema is a common childhood inflammatory skin disease characterised by dry, itching, fragile skin, which consistently has some of the highest scores on the Dermatology Quality of Life Index (Finlay & Khan 1994). It currently affects between 5 and 20% of UK children by the age of 11 (Kay et al 1994) with differences between social classes (Williams et al 1994) and ethnic groups (Neame et al 1995, Williams et al 1995). The intractable itching associated with the disease can cause loss of sleep and such distress to children and their families that the physical and psychological stress becomes overwhelming. The need for liaison, communication and support for the home carers should not be underestimated (Spowart 1993) and recent research has demonstrated that nurses are an important source of advice to mothers and can help alleviate the burdens they experience by providing families with more support (Elliot & Luker 1997). Nurses in primary care are well placed to provide advice about treatments and educate their patients about how to apply the topical medications correctly (Stone et al 1989, Stone 1997). The topical management of eczema is centred on the regular use of emollients (moisturisers) to rehydrate the skin; they can be used in the form of creams, ointments and oils in bath preparations (Bullus 1997). When advising about or prescribing emollients, care must be taken to avoid preparations containing substances to which the patient is known to have a sensitivity (e.g. perfumes). It is also good practice initially to provide some samples of suitable emollients for patients to try, as they are more likely to use a preparation regularly if they like it. Topical steroids are the mainstay of treatment of eczema and should always be used in conjunction with a good emollient regime. The basic principle is to use the weakest steroid to control the eczema (Forsdyke & Watts 1994). The use of the 'wet wraps' technique (Turnbull 1994) to treat acute inflamed eczema can help reduce the degree of disturbed sleep at night, and nurses in the primary, secondary and community liaison areas continue to provide opportunities for parents and carers to learn to do these treatments. The social and psychological impact of skin disease must not be forgotten. Children with eczema may be teased or bullied, siblings may feel that they receive less parental attention, parents may be subjected to unhelpful comments about their child and there is a financial burden created by the need for extra non-prescription items, cotton clothing, special mattress covers, extra washing and ironing and frequent visits to the doctor (Herd et al 1994). The National Eczema Society, the patient support group, provides up-to-date information on benefits and respite opportunities available for those suffering with eczema (Jeyasingham 1997).

Reactions to food or additives are often suspected by patients as causing their atopic eczema; however, while the protein in cow's milk and eggs may cause an intolerance in young children this tends to be transient with only a few children retaining the allergy into adult life (Young et al 1994, Young 1998).

Complementary therapies have grown in popularity. Herbalism, Chinese herbs and aromatherapy are more frequently being used; however, it is important to ensure that patients understand that they complement the routine therapy and are not an alternative. Nurses are in an ideal position to discuss the use of complementary treatments with their patients (Frost 1994) and to advise them on seeing appropriately qualified practitioners in complementary therapies. Patients taking Chinese herbs should be monitored carefully as cases of hepatotoxicity have been reported (Sadler 1996).

Paediatric, school, practice, dermatology liaison nurses and health visitors can all offer practical help, support and education to parents and children in the community setting.

Dry skin and eczema is a common cause of intractable itching (pruritus) in the elderly. The three key principles of care are to treat the dry skin, the eczema and the complications (Perkins 1996) within an holistic approach to care. Patients should be encouraged to use emollients regularly and be reminded about using non-slip mats in the bath, especially baths containing emollients (Stone 1995). They may need encouragement and assistance with topical medications such as steroids, antiseptics and prescribed occlusive dressings. Patients whose pruritus remains severe in spite of regular use of emollients should be assessed to exclude scabies and then referred to the dermatologist for investigation of the underlying cause.

Contact dermatitis

Contact dermatitis refers to irritant contact dermatitis (e.g. frequent exposure to soaps as seen in hairdressers or nurses) or to allergic contact dermatitis where a delayed type of allergic response is developed to such potentially sensitising substances as perfumes, preservatives and rubber compounds.

Contact dermatitis is common in certain occupational groups (e.g. car, leather, metal, food, chemical and rubber industries). It has been estimated that eczema and contact dermatitis account for 84–90% of occupational skin disease (Emmet 1984, Mathias 1985) with skin diseases being among the top three reasons for occupational diseases in Northern Europe. Hand dermatitis is the form of eczema most frequently associated with work disability and practice nurses can play a vital role in helping this group of patients (Clare 1997) by taking the opportunities offered in the 1997 government White Paper to expand their practice to complement the role of the occupational health nurse.

Acne

Acne is a very common skin condition caused by abnormalities of the sebaceous glands and can range in severity from non-inflammatory open and closed comedones, known as 'blackheads' and 'whiteheads' to inflammatory papules, pustules and nodules, or 'cysts' (Gibson 1997). Patients should be assured that failure to cleanse the skin or diet are not responsible for causing acne (Leyden 1997). Although mainly seen as a teenage problem, around 3.5% of those aged 25–34 are also affected (Williams 1997). The physical and psychological effects of acne should not be underestimated. However mild or severe the condition, acne sufferers frequently experience shame or embarrassment and society today judges so much by appearance that the psychological impact of the disease can be so socially disabling as to affect their quality of life. Permanent scarring on the face, back or chest can contribute to poor self-image, social inhibition and depression and in some cases those affected can become suicidal (Cotterill & Cunliffe 1997). Nursing support and advice on management of treatment can be invaluable in helping patients not only to improve their skin but also their self-esteem, thus reducing the potential long-term physical and emotional damage.

Many people with acne use OTC preparations and do not seek medical advice. School and practice nurses can capitalise on opportunities to help those with acne by advising them on routine skin care, appropriate topical medications and the correct way to use them and the support available from The Acne Support Group. When seeing someone with acne it is an important element of the patient assessment to do a complete skin examination, as severe acne of the chest and back may be kept hidden by those who are extremely distressed by their condition. The nurse will need to be empathetic to the individual in discussing the condition, the range of available treatments and their side-effects (Black 1995). Topical treatments used in acne include antibiotics, azelaic acid and isotretinoin, and systemic preparations include antibiotics, isotretinoin, oestrogens and antiandrogens. Those who are more severely affected should be referred for specialist treatment. The development of the drug isotretinoin has revolutionised the treatment of severe acne but it needs to be carefully monitored because of its side-effects including xeroderma, eczema, dry eyes, arthralgia and raised serum lipids (Leyden 1997, Thiboutot 1997). Most importantly, as isotretinoin is teratogenic, any woman who is commencing treatment must not be pregnant and use effective contraception during the course of treatment and for at least 1 month after it has been stopped. Nurses should ensure that the patients understand the importance of these precautions and provide any necessary help and advice. Topical tazarotene and adapalene are new drugs that have been shown to be effective in the treatment of acne when applied daily. The development of effective new drugs to treat acne means that medical help can be sought early, and without waiting for the acne to clear spontaneously, so there is no reason for patients to endure physical and emotional scarring. Nurses in the primary care sector can be instrumental in helping their patients to achieve a better long-term outcome from treatment and an associated improved quality of life.

Psoriasis

Psoriasis is a common skin disease affecting around 1–3% of the population (Williams 1997). The exact cause of the condition is not known although there is a genetic predisposition. Currently several centres are involved in doing research into psoriasis and genetics and although studies agree that no single gene is responsible, a gene predisposing to psoriasis has been mapped to the distal end of the long arm of chromosome 17 (Guzzo 1997). A chronic inflammatory disease, it can be unsightly, itchy and painful. It is never infectious. When the hands and feet are affected or associated arthritis is present, it can be extremely disabling. Although it is rarely life-threatening, it can have a significant psychosocial impact on sufferers and their quality of life. Application of medications can be a time-consuming part of daily life, while choice of types of clothing, sporting, social and leisure activities can be affected by the sufferers feeling the need to keep themselves 'covered up'. At present there is no cure for psoriasis but there are many treatments which can help keep the condition controlled. All patients with psoriasis should be encouraged to use emollients regularly to moisturise their skin. Nurses can advise patients of the different types of emollients so that they can choose the most effective one for them. Other topical treatments include coal tar preparations, dithranol, vitamin D analogues, retinoids and in certain instances steroids (McClelland 1997, Watts 1997). Specialist dermatology trained practice nurses have an ideal opportunity to develop nurse-led services and clinics to provide support for psoriasis patients through education about the condition and the treatments available, explanations about how to apply their prescribed medication and advice about the patient support groups, The Psoriasis Association and the Psoriatic Arthropathy Alliance.

Scalp psoriasis is a particularly distressing form of the disease which patients find difficult to treat effectively themselves. Such patients could benefit greatly from expert help with their scalp treatment (Dawkes 1997) in the primary care setting enabling them to avoid hospital treatment, time off work or school and worrying about their appearance or visiting the hairdresser. Each person with psoriasis is affected in a different way and treatment needs to be tailored to suit the individual's own circumstances. The aim of the health care programme should be to assist the patient to be independent and self-caring. Participation of the patient and carers in developing the treatment plan is more likely to lead to success (Moore 1995) when the individual knows what type of treatment is to be carried out.

The availability of and easy access to a knowledgeable and understanding practitioner can be of enormous psychological benefit to the psoriasis sufferer in reducing feelings of isolation and helplessness.

Phototherapy and photochemotherapy which involve the use of specifically calculated doses of ultraviolet light are used to treat patients who do not respond to topical medications alone. These treatments are provided in specialist dermatology units as they need to be administered and monitored by specialist trained staff to ensure that correct doses are given and to reduce the side-effects of skin cancer and photodamage. Patients with more severe disease may need systemic therapy such as methotrexate, cyclosporin or an oral retinoid and must be closely monitored for side-effects of the relevant drug. This is also an area in which a practice nurse with specialist dermatology training could provide the regular patient care in the community in collaboration with the specialist secondary care dermatology medical and nursing team.

CONCLUSION

People with skin disease are as entitled to expert health care as any other group of sufferers. Nurses must take advantage of the opportunities to develop nurse-led clinics and services, particularly for those suffering with chronic or relapsing skin diseases. In a chronic disease such as psoriasis most individuals know what treatment works for them and early access to care with specialist trained dermatology nurses, who would be able to prescribe the appropriate medications and commence treatment in the primary care setting, would be a major improvement in quality of life. As the All Party Parliamentary Group on Skin stated in their report, nurses are an essential resource for dermatology at every level from specialist units to the community and nurses have a vital role to play in dermatology. Nurses must prepare themselves for their role in providing health care in the future for patients with skin disease.

USEFUL ADDRESSES

Acne Support Group
PO Box 230
Hayes
Middlesex UB4 0UT

Advice on the Prevention and Treatment of Head Lice
Department of Health
PO Box 410
Wetherby LS23 7LN

British Dermatological Nursing Group
19 Fitzroy Square
London W1P 5HQ

Community Hygiene Concern
32 Crane Avenue
Isleworth
Middlesex TW7 7JL

Dystrophic Epidermolysis Bullosa Research Association
DEBRA House
13 Wellington Business Park
Dukes Ride
Crowthorne
Berkshire RG11 6LS

National Eczema Society
163 Eversholt Street
London NW1 1BU

Psoriatic Arthropathy Alliance
PO Box 111
St Albans
Hertfordshire AL2 3JQ

The Psoriasis Association
7 Milton Street
Northampton NN2 7JG

Skin Care Campaign
163 Eversholt Street
London NW1 1BU

The Vitiligo Society
125 Kennington Road
London SE11 6SF

8

Community children's nursing

Mark Whiting

INTRODUCTION

In this chapter, I intend to explore the proposition that the nature of community nursing care needs for children within the UK at the end of the 20th century is such that those needs can best be met by the provision of a universal and comprehensive community children's nursing service. I hope to demonstrate that such a service is an essential component of the child health services whose continuing non-availability to the majority of the child population cannot be justified.

WHAT IS COMMUNITY CHILDREN'S NURSING?

The term 'community children's nursing' and the abbreviation CCN have recently been adopted to encompass a variety of alternative terms which have previously been used – and a number of which are still in use (paediatric community nurse (PCN), paediatric home care nurse, paediatric hospital-at-home nurse, children's home care nurse, community paediatric nurse). All of these titles relate fundamentally to the same area of nursing practice. In 1994, the UKCC formally adopted the term community children's nurse. For the purposes of the discussion which follows, a community children's nurse can be defined as: a registered children's nurse who has completed a programme of education in community nursing leading to registration with the United Kingdom Central Council for Nursing, Midwifery and Health Visiting and whose main focus of work is 'predominantly those children requiring treatment and care for acute and chronic ill health in a home setting.' (UKCC 1994a, p. 17).

The community children's nurse is one of many nurses who might be involved in the provision of care to children (Fig. 8.1).

Historical considerations

Much of the early work of the predecessors of contemporary district nurses (DNs) and health visitors (HVs) was concerned with the provision of nursing care to children and of health visiting advice/support to their parents. At around the time that community nursing services were first established in Liverpool (Rathbone 1890) and sanitary visitors first walked the streets of Manchester and Salford (Owen 1983), Charles West and Dame Catherine Wood, respectively the Medical Director and Nursing Superintendent of the Hospital for Sick Children, Great Ormond Street, London, were beginning to recognise the potential value of providing a community nursing resource for children who had already received care and treatment at the hospital:

Some consideration took place on the reference in Doctor West's paper to the training of nurses proposed by the Lady Superintendent and their employment in visiting out-patients at their own homes and supported by Doctor West and coincided in by the Lady Superintendent. The majority of the medical officers were in favour of the plan being made trial of for six months, but the lay members of the committee were unanimously opposed to the extension of the work of the hospital beyond the walls. (Minutes of a special meeting of the Joint Committee of The Hospital for Sick Children, 18 March, 1874).

Despite this initial lack of agreement between the joint committee members, archive material from the hospital confirms that children with a range of medical conditions were provided with continuing care in the community by nurses who were employed by the hospital, but whose salary costs were met

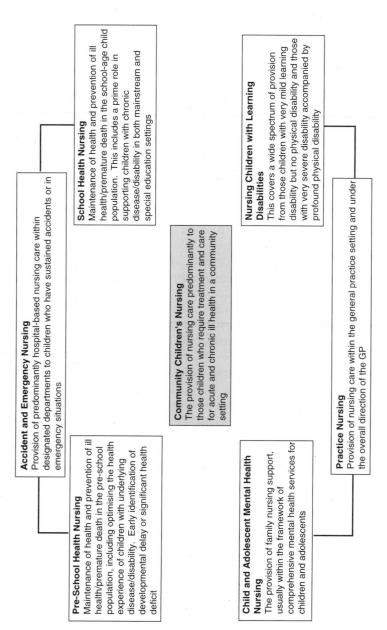

Figure 8.1   Community child health nursing.

predominantly by the parents of the children concerned. In some instances, and where parents were unable to pay, the services of the nurse were provided without charge to the family.

The period from 1870 to the inception of the National Health Service in 1948, saw very significant expansion and development of both district nursing and health visiting services. The requirements of the National Health Service Act 1946 for the newly created health authorities to 'secure the attendance of nurses on persons who require nursing in their own homes' (para. III, Section 25) and to 'make provision in their area for the visiting of persons in their homes by visitors to be called health visitors' (Part III, Section 24[1]) represented, in large areas of the UK, little more than the formal realignment of pre-existing services into the new structures of the National Health Service. However, at the time of the Act, it was not considered necessary to make separate arrangements specifically for meeting the nursing needs of sick children in the community. District nurses and health visitors continued to provide a valuable resource to children and families in the community but the numbers of children who required care were small.

From 1852, when the first children's hospital was established at Great Ormond Street, until the National Health Service Act of 1946, a considerable number of children's hospitals had been built, predominantly in the large metropolitan areas of the UK, and including 36 children's hospitals built between 1852 and 1899 of which 11 were in London alone (Kosky 1992). In addition, by the time of the NHS Act the majority of general hospitals contained one or more children's wards. During the first half of the 20th century, the admission of a sick child to hospital was considered as therapy in itself, and for many children discharge home was only permitted once the child was deemed to be fully recovered (Opeé 1971). Invariably, however, sick hospitalised children were separated from their families, hospital visiting was often restricted to a few hours each day (or sometimes only once per week) and parents were actively discouraged from 'rooming-in' with their sick child (MoH 1959).

The pioneering research of John Bowlby (1951) and James Robertson (1958), however, alerted both health care professionals and government departments to the potential damaging psychological impact of hospitalisation upon the young child in particular and prompted a fundamental re-think in attitudes.

This work informed the Ministry of Health's seminal review in the late 1950s of the welfare of children in hospital leading to the recommendation 'children should not be admitted to hospital if it can possibly be avoided' ('The Platt Report', para. 17, MoH 1959). Within the Platt Report, brief consideration was given to the small number of 'specialised nursing services for home care of children' (MoH 1959, para. 18), which had been established during the early years of the National Health Service. The NHS Act had required hospital and community sectors to work together in developing more integrated approaches to care provision and the schemes identified by the Platt Committee (in Birmingham, Rotherham and Paddington, North West London) represented clear examples of such 'working together'.

Despite this, from the time of the Platt Report until the mid-1980s, only a handful of new community children's nursing services were established (see Whiting (1988) for a detailed review of service development up to this time). During this period, the hospital experience of sick children improved dramatically, the average length of stay reduced from over 2 weeks to around 3 days (Audit Commission 1993) – though the numbers of children actually admitted to hospital has shown a steady and sustained increase every year since the 1950s – many surgical procedures which had previously required several nights in hospital were being undertaken in many centres within 'day-surgery' programmes (Thornes 1991), parental visiting and 'rooming-in' was actively encouraged by the hospital care team (Thornes 1988), the environment of care itself was becoming progressively more child (and family) friendly (Audit Commission 1993, DoH 1991b) and a new philosophy of partnership and family involvement in care began to emerge (Casey 1995, Cleary 1992, Darbyshire 1994, Smith 1995).

Community children's nursing in the 1990s

Each of these trends in hospital care of children continued throughout the 1990s. In addition, during the period from 1985–1996, the number of community children's nursing services expanded dramatically (Whiting 1996) (Fig. 8.2). However, services are far from universally available within the UK. The House of Commons Health Select Committee reported in 1997 that:

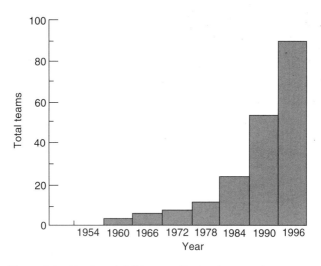

Figure 8.2 Number of CCN teams (England): generalist teams.

It is a cause for serious concern that only 50% of health authorities purchase CCN services and only 10% of the country's children have access to a 24-hour CCN service. We regard it as highly undesirable that there should be such local disparities in the provision of CCN services and are not convinced that there is any logical explanation for this. (House of Commons Health Select Committee 1997, para. 48).

The Health Select Committee further observed (para. 49): 'For many years there has been a community nursing service available to all adults in their own homes. We consider that, as a matter of principle, sick children need and deserve no less.'

The analogy with district nursing services will be considered a little further presently.

For the approximately 50% of the country within which CCN services are available, a wide range of models of CCN provision exist (House of Commons Health Select Committee 1997, Tatman 1994). Some are based in hospital wards, others in special care baby units, others in outpatient departments. A number of teams are based in office premises away from the main hospital site. Many schemes are based in community health centres or in child development centres. Many of the services make arrangements to see children on hospital wards, in accident and emergency departments, in outpatient departments, in schools or nurseries, in health centres, in GP premises.

In order to ensure that a comprehensive service is provided to the local child population, it is vital that CCNs work effectively at the interfaces between the primary and secondary care sectors (BPA 1993, Cash et al 1994, House of Commons Health Select Committee 1997, NHSE 1996a, Thornes 1993).

Figure 8.3A provides a much simplified diagrammatic representation of the main interfaces between the CCN team and hospital/community-based staff. Figure 8.3B provides a comparative diagram relating to interfaces between a typical district nurse team and the hospital/community-based staff. A number of factors account for these quite dramatic differences in the relationships which CCN teams have established, including:

- The small number of children within a typical GP practice population who might require input from the CCN team at any

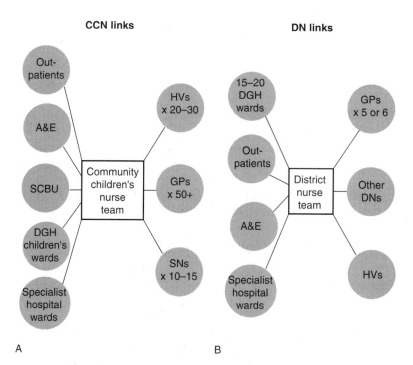

CCN links   **DN links**

A   B

Figure 8.3   Typical links between CCNs/DNs and hospital/community-based staff: A&E = accident and emergency; CCN = community children's nurse; DGH = district general hospital; GP = general practitioner; HV = health visitor; DN = district nurse; SCBU = special-care baby unit; SN = school nurse.

one time – this would probably amount to no more than 10–15 children, even within a multi-handed GP practice. At any one time, a CCN team caseload of 200 patients might be drawn from 60 or 70 different GPs. A DN team could reasonably expect that most or all of its patients would arise from a very small number of practices.

• Major referral sources to CCN teams are hospital-based wards and departments, whereas for DNs the main source of referral is likely to be the GP.

• A typical CCN team will regularly link with no more than two to four hospital wards/departments, and team members will often visit those wards on a daily/weekly basis. A DN team might reasonably expect that its patient base could be drawn from a multitude of different wards and departments. Arrangements for linking with such an array of departments on a regular basis are less common than for CCNs, and where regular contact is maintained, this will often relate to specific patients.

• Most CCN teams provide a service to a population based upon a total health authority commissioning locality or the population served by a community trust, whereas a DN team would usually cover a much smaller locality or neighbourhood.

Many of these differences arise because of the nature of the practice of the CCN team and it would now be useful to consider that practice in a little more detail.

COMMUNITY CHILDREN'S NURSING PRACTICE

The practice of community children's nursing (CCN) is concerned with the provision of care to children from birth, throughout childhood and adolescence and sometimes into young adulthood. The provision of a CCN services has a number of potential advantages and also a number of potential disadvantages (see Box 8.1).

On balance, there is general support for the view that the potential advantages of care in the child's home outweigh the potential disadvantages. It would perhaps be useful to now consider in detail the range of nursing need to which that practice relates.

Box 8.1   Potential advantages and disadvantages of providing nursing care in the child's home rather than in hospital

Potential advantages
- A reduction in the potential negative psychological impact of hospitalisation upon a young child by avoidance of hospitalisation or by facilitation of early discharge.
- Reducing the frequency of readmission to hospital for children with chronic health problems.
- Reducing the demand for hospital inpatient beds by:
  - prevention of admission
  - facilitation of early discharge
  - support of day-care/day-surgery programmes.
- Potential reduction in hospital-acquired infection and other iatrogenic problems.
- Reduced disruption to family life arising from the demands placed upon the family by the unscheduled admission of a child to hospital.
- Reduced expense to the family (as a result of travel to the hospital, parking charges, loss of earned income, etc.).
- Improved communication between primary and secondary health services.

Potential disadvantages
- Parental concerns/anxieties/fears when caring for a sick child at home and when medical/nursing help and advice is not immediately available as would have been the case if the child were in hospital.
- The child's own fears/anxieties at the loss of 'security' which hospital might represent.
- Potential morbidity (or even potential mortality) as a result of inadequacies in care, inappropriate care or arising as a result of delay in gaining timely access to medical or nursing care.
- Disruption to/restrictions on family life as a consequence of the child's care needs at home.
- 'Medicalisation' of the home environment.

Neonatal and post-neonatal care

In the mid 1940s, a community special care baby service, staffed by community midwives, was established in Manchester, specifically because of concerns regarding the high infant mortality rate in that part of the country. At that time, most babies were born at home and many of the infants cared for by the service were either premature or of low birth weight (Couriel & Davies 1988). By the provision of support services to such babies and their families in the community and by closely monitoring their progress, it was possible to avoid admission of such babies into hospital, as was the norm in other parts of the UK at this time. In the more recent past, advances in neonatal care have resulted in a growing population of young babies with long-term complications of extreme prematurity. These babies have often spent several months in hospital, have attained a position of relative medical stability but are expected to require respiratory and/or nutritional support for several more months. Close collaborative working between hospital neonatal units, health visitors, general practitioners and CCN teams can facilitate and support discharge of many of these babies into the care of their parents in the community. A number of CCN teams have taken on these specialised roles, supporting, for instance, small babies who are oxygen dependent, who require enteral or parenteral nutritional support or who require phototherapy at home.

Infancy and childhood

The work of Bowlby (1951) and Robertson (1958), to which reference was made earlier, and subsequent research by Douglas (1975) and others, identified young children as being particularly susceptible to the potential psychological ill-effects of hospitalisation. Children under 5 years of age, however, are very significant users of the health services and in particular of hospital-based services (see Box 8.2).

Young children present with a range of problems, many of which are potentially amenable to intervention and support

---

Box 8.2 Morbidity experience in childhood

- Over 1 million children per year are admitted to hospital for a stay of at least one night (House of Commons Health Committee 1997) of which over 80% are emergency admissions (Audit Commission 1993).
- Over 3 million children attend accident and emergency departments each year (House of Commons Health Committee 1997).
- Around 5 million children are seen each year as outpatients (Thornes 1987).
- General practitioner consultation rates (per 10 000 person years at risk) are higher among under-5-year-olds than for any age group other than the 85-and-overs (OPCS 1994).
- An estimated 360 000 children in Great Britain – just under 3% of all children under the age of 16 are considered to have a disability (Bone & Meltzer 1989).

from community children's nursing services. These may be conveniently considered as either short-term or long-term needs.

Short-term nursing needs

Children may present within the general practice or accident and emergency setting with problems such as gastroenteritis, acute infections of the urinary tract and respiratory tract (including pneumonia), otitis media, febrile convulsions and meningitis. The availability of skilled nursing resources in the community has much to offer in support of family general practitioners. Furthermore, from the hospital perspective, access to such resources can both facilitate early discharge and potentially prevent hospital admission, as well as reducing 'ward-attenders' and the need for outpatient follow-up (BPA 1993). As the number of paediatric hospital beds continues to reduce and the emerging speciality of ambulatory paediatric medicine develops (Heller 1994, Meates 1997), the potential implications for expanding CCN practice are very considerable indeed.

Follow-up and support of children requiring emergency treatment of surgical, trauma and orthopaedic problems is another area where CCN involvement has tremendous potential (Dryden 1989, Whiting 1995). In addition, for children undergoing planned surgery, involvement of the CCN in the child's care can help to streamline the hospital episode, ensuring that the period in hospital is kept to an absolute minimum and, by maintaining good liaison with both the hospital and primary health care teams, maximising opportunities for effective preoperative preparation, making maximum use of day surgery facilities, and ensuring continuity of care between hospital and home (Atwell & Gow 1985, Gow & Ridgway 1993, Thornes 1991).

Long-term nursing needs

Under this heading can be considered three particular groups: children with chronic physical illness; children with disabilities and children who require palliative care.

The first group will include children with a range of problems such as asthma, diabetes mellitus, tracheostomies, cancers and leukaemias, cystic fibrosis, chronic nutritional failure, endocrine disorders, cardiac and renal disease, constipation and enuresis. The range of nursing intervention required by children in this group is very broad, and the role of the CCN team is wide ranging. It often involves practical caregiving, drawing upon a range of clinical skills, and these are often skills which will be taught to one or more family members in order to facilitate independence. The nursing role will invariably include the provision of psychological and emotional support to families, offering positive reinforcement and reassurance that practical skills, which are often quite complicated, are being executed well by the family. This might also involve supporting families through periodic exacerbations of chronic illness, when visiting might be very intensive, for instance in supporting the family of a child with cystic fibrosis who is receiving a course of intravenous antibiotics for a chest infection at home. A further dimension of the nursing role is in acting as an advocate, a resource, a facilitator on behalf of the family, linking between various agencies involved in the child's care, coordinating care management meetings, organising urgent outpatient appointments, arranging for a domiciliary visit by a hospital-based registrar or consultant (and transporting them to and from the child's home!) (Cash et al 1994, Smith et al 1996, Thornes 1993, Whyte et al 1995).

This group of children with long-term physical ill health form the mainstay of CCN practice; the elements of these multifaceted roles pertain to all aspects of the work of the CCN.

There are approximately 360 000 children with disability in the UK (Bone & Meltzer 1989), although CCNs are likely to be involved in the provision of services only to those children whose disabilities are the most complex and where discrete, ongoing nursing needs can be identified. This is an area of expanding work, particularly as many children with complex problems which have historically lead to death in infancy are now surviving. This group of children present many potential challenges to CCN teams, particularly because their nursing needs are often very extensive and very long term (Beresford 1995).

Around 10 000 children die each year in the UK (Royal College of Paediatrics and Child Health et al 1997), including approximately 400 with cancers and around 200 with heart disease. There is a growing body of evidence that for many of these children and families, if the choice were available, they would prefer the child to die at home rather than in hospital (RCN 1996, While et al 1996). However, there are also significant concerns that without adequate support, and that is primarily nursing support, this can not be achieved (Thomas 1994, While et al 1996). CCNs are developing a range of strategies in caring for this population of children, including collaborative working between paediatric departments, hospice and respite care facilities and the provision of home-based respite care.

Adolescence and early adulthood

Many of the problems of chronic ill health in children outlined above will continue as the child approaches adolescence and becomes an adult, though it is worth noting at this point that for some children, the impact of chronic ill health can significantly impede physical, emotional, social and cognitive development. Clearly many of the children with long-term nursing need will become adults and for many their medical conditions are life-long. For some medical conditions, such as diabetes mellitus, cerebral palsy or muscular dystrophy, survival into adulthood represents a well-established pattern of disease; however, for other medical conditions such as cystic fibrosis, or congenital cardiac problems increased life-expectancy presents a new range of challenges in terms of the transition from children's health services into adult-based services. Community children's nurses need to play a central role in ensuring that this transition is smooth for all children with whom they have been involved and in making the necessary arrangements for the continuing provision of adult-based nursing services.

KEY ISSUES

I would now like to briefly turn attention to a number of key issues facing the future development of community children's nursing. These issues are:

- Education for the practice of community children's nursing
- Generalism and specialism in practice
- Working 'in partnership' with parents and children
- A generic community child health nurse?

Education for the practice of community children's nursing

There is widespread acceptance of the view that the nursing of sick children should be undertaken by nurses who possess a registered children's nurse qualification (Audit Commission 1993, DoH 1991b, MoH 1959). These 'official' endorsements have equal validity in both hospital and community settings. A survey undertaken by the author in 1995 sought details of the professional and academic qualifications of CCNs working within the North and South Thames Regions (Whiting 1997). Of the 139 staff identified within the survey, all were qualified as registered children's nurses – at the time of the study, all staff were registered on Part 8 of the UKCC Register (RSCN). A number of staff registered on Part 15 of the Register (Project 2000 Child Branch) have since been appointed to posts in CCN teams. Many of the nurses have undertaken additional studies, often related to areas of more specialised practice such as diabetes nursing (ENB course 928), cancer nursing (ENB course 240), asthma (the Asthma Training Diploma), HIV disease (ENB course 934). 71 staff (51%) had completed the ENB course 998, ('teaching and assessing in clinical practice').

In an earlier study by the author (Whiting 1988) – in effect at the time of the study, a national census of CCNs – concern was raised because almost 50% of the nurses did not possess a community nursing qualification. In the second study within the Thames Region (Whiting 1997), the percentage of staff who had completed a community nursing qualification was barely 30% (25 staff (18%) were DN qualified, 15 staff (12%) were HV qualified and 1 nurse possessed both HV and DN certificates). Until recently, community education programmes which were available to prospective CCNs fell a long way short of recognising and meeting their specific learning needs. At best, and in a very small number of institutions, they were based upon partly modified DN programmes (ENB 1990) which allowed for students to both gain practical experience in and submit theoretical work based upon the practice of community children's nursing. At worst, programmes failed completely to recognise the particular educational needs of RSCNs who wished to gain a community qualification of relevance to their future practice in the care of children in the community (Whiting et al 1994). The introduction of 'specialist practitioner' education programmes (UKCC 1994a), is likely to result in a significant increase in the numbers of CCN staff who possess a community nursing qualification. Considerable interest has been generated in these exciting new programmes, though the House of Commons Health Select Committee (1997) has identified a number of concerns in relation to the low numbers of students entering the courses, primarily as a result of uncertainty about the funding and sponsorship of places on the courses.

The Department of Health has advised (NHSE 1996a) that CCN services should be: 'led and predominantly staffed by nurses who possess both registration as a children's nurse and experience of community nursing' (para. 11.7) and have 'sufficient children's nurses with post-registration community training to provide leadership, advice and training to nurses who have not yet proceeded beyond children's branch registration' (para. 11.8).

Earlier in the chapter, some comparisons were made with district nursing services. The current ratio of qualified 'district nurses' to 'other qualified nurses within district nursing' is approximately 1.5 : 1 (NHSE 1986b). In the absence of any clear guidelines on the ratio of CCNs, who should possess the specialist practitioner qualification, to other nurses working in CCN teams, a similar ratio might be considered appropriate. However, as the size of CCN teams is generally much smaller than that of DN teams (Tatman 1994), a slightly higher ratio (of 2 qualified CCNs to 1 other qualified children's nurse) might be required. The Royal College of Nursing Paediatric Community Nurses Forum (1996) has argued that an approximate ratio of 1 nurse per 10 000 child population is required in order to provide a comprehensive service. The potential breadth of nursing need identified earlier in this chapter is such that CCN teams ought to include staff who possess a wide range of practice skills (and appropriate educational preparation). Children who are increasingly technology dependent are requiring care in the community (see below). In addition, the scope of professional nursing practice (UKCC 1992b) is expanding rapidly, incorporating new technical and other skills, such as the prescribing of medicines. CCN teams must be configured in a way that maximises the opportunity for ensuring that the range of practice skills and professional knowledge available within the team can meet the challenges of developing nursing practice.

In considering the subject of education in CCN practice it is important to draw attention to a number of additional challenges.

In respect of pre-registration education, there is a clear expectation that CCN teams will provide educational placements for student nurses undertaking Child Branch programmes (Cash et al 1994, UKCC 1986). Evidence would suggest, however, that potential demand for placement experience is far greater than CCN teams can currently provide. Cash et al (1994), in a study undertaken on behalf of the English National Board, expressed concern that 'Community paediatric nurses are thin on the ground and the demand for places is high' (p. 164). Whiting (1997) reported an average of 8.7 days' placement experience with CCN teams for 475 students placed within the Thames Region during 1995. This situation is unlikely to improve without considerable expansion in CCN provision and, whilst it is important to acknowledge the value of the broad range of community placements provided within Child Branch programmes (for instance within health visiting or school nursing), the shortage of specific CCN placements remains a major concern (ENB 1997).

For students undertaking post-registration specialist practitioner CCN programmes, placements are at a premium. These programmes require a 50% practice element and logic would suggest that much of this practice experience ought to be gained within CCN teams. The situation is further compounded by the small number of suitably qualified practice teachers in CCN teams (Whiting 1997). Recent proposals from the UKCC (1997b) are unlikely to provide an early resolution to this problem and the use of flexible and imaginative practice teaching/supervision arrangements such as those examined by Neill & Muir (1997) offer a range of solutions.

With less than 300 generalist CCNs in post by mid-1996 (Whiting 1996), and over 4200 students enrolled on programmes leading to registration on either part 8 (RSCN) or part 15 (Project 2000 Child Branch) of the UKCC Register (ENB 1996b), and increasing numbers of students entering specialist practitioner CCN programmes, the pressures on this particular part of the education system are potentially overwhelming.

Generalism and specialism in practice

Some might consider that the nursing of children in the community is an area of specialist nursing practice (Brocklehurst 1995); however, from the earlier discussion, it is evident that community children's nursing is largely concerned with the provision of a range of 'generalist' nursing care services to children in the community. Whilst many CCNs do develop areas of particular practice expertise, for instance in the management of children with tracheostomies or in the care of children with cystic fibrosis, usually these nurses retain a practice role which involves the provision of care to children with a wide range of nursing need in addition to their particular focus area (Hughes 1997). Such practice is most appropriately described as 'generalist'.

Some CCNs develop their practice in such a way that they no longer retain a 'generalist' caseload and for many of these nurses, the title 'specialist' is entirely appropriate. Many of these nurses are based in hospitals and are managed as part of a hospital service (Hunt 1995). In some CCN teams, one or more members of the team have developed exclusive specialist roles, whilst other team members retain responsibility for the generalist workload. In the main, the work of CCNs who have a generalist role and those who are specialists are complementary to each other. Beardsmore & Alder (1994), for instance, examined the work of the nurses in the symptom care team based at the Hospital for Sick Children, Great Ormond Street, supporting children with cancer who require palliative care in the community, who have established close working relationships with many of the generalist CCN teams within the Thames Regions. Joint visiting of children at home by members of the symptom care team and the local CCNs occurs on a regular basis. In addition, where no local CCN service is available, the symptom care team will often work with district nurses, health visitors and school nurses. In general, the problems of hospital-based specialists working in the community which were identified as a major cause for concern in the Cumberlege Report (DHSS 1986a), have not materialised in community children's nursing practice though some concerns still remain (Perkins & Billingham 1997).

Before closing this discussion on generalist and specialist practice, it is important to return briefly to consider the particular needs of medically fragile and technology dependent children in the community. In the USA, there is a large and growing population of such children to the extent that the Surgeon General has overseen the workings of a 'medical task force' on the subject and entire text books have been written concerning the 'home care' needs of technology dependent children (Wagner et al 1988). In the UK, the numbers of medically fragile/technology dependent children seem to be increasing, including small babies who require long-term oxygen therapy or parenteral nutrition, children who require gastrostomy feeding, peritoneal dialysis or management of central venous lines, children with tracheostomies and a small but increasing number of children who require long-term home ventilation. In order to provide for the nursing care needs of such children, it is important to recognise the value of clinical nursing knowledge and skills developed within hospital settings. This expertise must be harnessed if opportunities for application and transfer into the community setting are to be optimised. Hospital-based clinical nurse specialists and generalist CCNs have much to learn from each other.

Working 'in partnership' with parents and children

The term 'partnership' was introduced to children's nursing in the UK by Anne Casey (1988) following its development and implementation at the Hospital for Sick Children, Great Ormond Street. It has been widely adopted within children's nursing in the UK both in hospitals and in the community – see Casey 1995 for a more detailed discussion. Philip Darbyshire (1995) has analysed many of the problems associated with establishing the partnership philosophy within the hospital environment and suggests that 'parenting in public' places significant pressures upon the parents to deliver care to their children in the full view of the nursing team whom many parents perceive as 'experts'. As a consequence, parents often feel under intense scrutiny not only in relation to the nursing care responsibilities which they have taken on following negotiation with the nursing team but even of 'basic mothering: doing "the natural mother thing"'(Darbyshire 1995, p. 93). The extent to which parents can escape from this 'goldfish bowl' by virtue of their child's care being undertaken in the community is unknown; however, once in the community, partnership presents a whole series of challenges, requiring the building of trusting relationships between the nursing team, the child and family. In many instances, the CCN sees the child and family for only 1 or 2 hours per week; at all other times, the nursing care plans negotiated between the nurse and family are largely followed out by the family, predominantly the child's parents. Successful implementation of the plan of care requires the careful compliance of the family with the plan of care which has been negotiated and agreed with them. The burden of responsibility taken on by parents, who are often very keen to extricate their child from the hospital, can be enormous and, without adequate support, the notion of partnership can become meaningless.

A generic community child health nurse?

The provision of a fully integrated nursing service to children in the community is an essential element of a comprehensive child health service (BPA 1991). The principles which ought to underpin such a service were outlined over 20 years ago in the Court Report (DHSS 1976). Whilst much has been achieved in the intervening years, the House of Commons Health Select Committee (1997) found much cause for concern, perhaps best summed up in the following quotation: 'A recurrent theme in the evidence we have taken in community child health services is the problem caused by fragmentation of responsibility for such services between differing groups of health care professionals: in particular community children's nurses, specialist "outreach" nurses, practice nurses, health visitors and school nurses.' (p. vii, para. 9).

In response to the problems identified, the Health Select Committee has argued that: 'The creation of an integrated children's community nursing service with responsibility of the whole range of children's nursing including health promotion, health assessment and "hands-on" care would provide a simpler and more cost-effective service and would end the present confusion of categories.' (p. liii, para. 30).

There is, however, nothing new in this suggestion, the Court Committee (DHSS 1976) had argued for the development of health visitors with a specialist interest in children (child health visitors, CHVs); the Cumberlege Committee (DHSS 1986a) had criticised professional tribalism, arguing for the disentangling of 'professional demarcation lines' in order that 'staff would exploit more flexibly and fully those skills they have which at present go unused' (p. 20). The arguments for combining the roles of child health visitor, school nurse and community children's nurse would appear to have considerable merit. Perhaps, the aspirations of Project 2000 have much to offer the community child health services of the future. Such initial preparation would appear to be highly relevant for a children's nurse who, with further appropriate professional development and education, could take on any one or perhaps several of the nursing roles identified earlier in Figure 8.1.

If what is really required is the combining of several of these roles within one post it is important to consider elements of the current configuration of community child health nursing services and how they might fit such a model.

Health visiting services to children are provided within the context of a 'cradle to grave' approach and although much health visiting practice is focused upon young children, a significant element of the health visitor's work is targeted specifically at the adult and/or elderly population. All health visitors are registered general nurses, and only a small minority are also registered as children's nurses. Recruitment into health visiting courses is predominantly from the registered general nurse base, with small but increasing numbers of Project 2000 diplomates (from both Adult and Child branches). The extent to which health visitors might be able to assimilate the care of children with complex health needs into their roles has been the subject of considerable debate in recent years, and for many health visitors this would be impractical.

School nursing is also predominantly staffed by registered general nurses. The number of school nurses who are also registered as children's nurses is unknown. Although some school nurses do undertake home visits, in the main, they provide for 'the health needs of school age children' (BPA 1995) during school hours and within school premises. Their work is predominantly focused within health surveillance, health education and health promotion, but also includes significant involvement with children who have health problems. When such problems are complex, school nurses will often work closely with both CCNs and hospital-based clinical nurse specialists.

Such arrangements apply both within the context of mainstream and special school education.

The work of the CCN is generally restricted to involvement with children who have pre-evident health problems. Their role as health educators is very much an opportunistic one, for instance providing general guidance on home safety to the family of a child who is being visited at home because of a specific nursing need. However, CCNs are also involved in health-promotion activity on a more structured basis. As an example, a CCN may coordinate and lead a session on healthy eating for a group of teenagers with diabetes mellitus. As has been discussed earlier, large numbers of CCNs do not possess a community qualification. It has been argued (Perkins & Billingham 1997, p. 47) that in striving to 'promote the need for RSCNs in the community there is a risk of neglecting the specialist skills and knowledge required to work in community/primary care setting.' Whilst this is a legitimate concern, the recently introduced 'specialist practitioner' programmes discussed earlier ought to ensure that the future preparation for practice of CCNs is fundamentally based upon a primary care philosophy.

From this short discussion, two key questions seem to be emerging:

1. Is it possible (or even desirable) to combine the various elements of health visiting, school nursing and community children's nursing practice within a single post – a comprehensive community child health nurse?

2. Is it realistic to talk about comprehensive child health services when, at the present time, responsibility for the provision of primary care and secondary care often falls to separate provider entities? (House of Commons Health Select Committee 1997). The notion of a primary care-led (NHSE 1996a) child health service will surely stand or fall on the answer to this second question.

The future of community children's nursing also lies in the answer to these questions.

9

Community nursing services for people with a learning disability

Owen Barr

INTRODUCTION

The development of services for people with learning disabilities in the local community, as distinct from hospital provision, is now a key component of the 'care in the community' policies (DHSS 1991, DHSS NI 1990). A major focus of change in the last 15 years has been the closure of many hospitals for people with learning disabilities and the development of community-based services.

Such facilities include residential and nursing homes, respite care services, and group homes for people with learning disabilities. During the day people with learning disabilities may work within full- or part-time jobs, attend open social education centres, outreach and supported employment schemes, attend further education courses or a combination of the above. Not all people have full-time day services and therefore may spend a considerable amount of time at home.

Interdisciplinary community learning disability teams have now replaced the majority of single discipline teams which used to exist (e.g. specialist nursing or social work teams for people with learning disabilities). Team membership varies depending on the needs of the locality it serves. A considerable variation between the membership of teams and the structures around which they are organised has been noted within the UK (Ovretveit 1993). The membership of the community learning disabilities team usually includes the community nurses for people with learning disabilities, social workers, psychologists and psychiatrists as core members. In addition to this, extended team members may include occupational therapists, physiotherapists, speech and language therapists, and representatives from voluntary organisations.

The rationale for the development of community learning disability teams was the provision of a more coordinated and comprehensive service to people with learning disabilities and their families. This anticipated outcome has been realised in relation to some aspects of services but is by no means a resounding success (Brown 1992, Hadley & Clough 1996, McGrath 1991).

In 1992, approximately 25 000 adults with severe or profound learning disabilities continued to live in hospitals or National Health Service community residential facilities. A further 35 000 lived in local authority community-based residential facilities, and 65 000 at home. These figures represent a considerable shift in services from 1969 when 60 000 people with learning disabilities lived in hospitals or National Health Service community residential facilities and only 6000 lived in local authority community-based residential facilities (DHSS 1992, cited in Williams 1995). (See Wright & Digby (1996) and Mansell & Ericsson (1996) for a detailed historical review of service development.)

Following a brief consideration of the concept of learning disabilities, this chapter will consider the growth of, and some major challenges that now face community nursing services for people with learning disabilities.

A BRIEF REFLECTION ON TERMINOLOGY

The changing terminology used to refer to people now described as having learning disabilities is noticeable when reviewing the literature from health, social care and education, and within social policy and legislation. It clearly illustrates the recurring but elusive desire to identify a term which is considered acceptable by all to describe a specific group of people.

'People with learning disabilities' is the most recent of a long list of terms used in Britain and internationally (Gates 1997). The term is relatively new within Britain, it was introduced to replace the term 'people with mental handicap' in England, Scotland and Wales policy documents in 1990, and subsequently in Northern Ireland in 1995 (DHSS NI 1995). The rationale for its current use, in preference to previous terms, is that it is considered to most accurately identify the nature of the concept being described, namely a disability associated with learning.

Some degree of confusion has been generated by the growing use of the term 'learning difficulties'; this is, in the main, used to refer to people who have difficulties with learning but do not have an impairment of intelligence. However, it is increasingly being used within social services and education services, and is the term of choice of self-advocacy groups (although it is disputed if a term is required at all). This is a vague and more imprecise term than 'people with learning disabilities'; indeed, this is its attraction to many people who see it as less stigmatising. People with learning difficulties could include people with sensory impairments, physical disabilities, or conditions such as dyslexia. In the absence of significant impairment of intelligence and social functioning, such people do not have learning disabilities as recognised within the current mental health legalisation.

Terminology and labels do have important positive implications such as gaining access to specialist services. The risk of an overemphasis on terminology and the need to be politically correct can detract from the most important task of increasing the social value and role of people with learning disabilities (Shanley & Starrs 1993).

In conclusion, although frequent attempts have been made to quantify the nature of learning disabilities, it is apparent that the diagnosis of learning disabilities is not an exact science. It has historically been, and continues to be influenced by medical, legal, psychological and social considerations. However, the term 'people with learning disabilities' is at present the term most frequently used.

NORMALISATION – A MODEL FOR CURRENT SERVICES?

The first issue is again one of terminology. In 1983 Wolfensberger proposed the term 'normalisation' be replaced with the term 'social role valorisation'. This new term was proposed to highlight that normalisation was not about making people normal as it had been misinterpreted by many, but was about 'the creation and defence of socially valued roles' (Wolfensberger 1983). The term 'social role valorisation' was not widely taken up across the UK, but is used by some services (Emerson 1992). As normalisation is the most recognised term used to describe the philosophy of services, it will be used in this chapter. A more recent development is the philosophy of 'inclusion', this will be discussed at the end of this section.

Normalisation has its origins in the late 1950s and early 1960s in Scandinavia. This approach has had major impact on services in the USA since the early 1970s and became an emerging force in the UK in the late 1970s and early 1980s (Brown & Smith 1992).

Definitions of normalisation have evolved over this time from process-focused definitions such as 'letting the mentally retarded obtain an existence as close as possible to normal' (Bank-Mikkelson 1969) to more outcome-based definitions such as 'the use of means which are valued in our society, in order to develop and support personal characteristics, behaviours, and experiences which are likewise valued' or put into four words 'to revalue devalued people' (Tyne & O'Brien 1981). The application of normalisation to services for people with learning disabilities highlighted the need for people to have the opportunity to live independently, use local community services, and become more involved in decisions which affected their daily activities and their life overall.

Five services accomplishments for people with learning disabilities that should be visible in services incorporating normalisation have been identified (O'Brien 1992). These are:

- having a *presence* in the local community and using the local facilities
- *making choices* about their lives which are informed by the provision of appropriate and accessible information
- *developing competence* and socially valued skills
- receiving *respect* in the services provided

- being enabled to *participate* in the activities and in developing a range of relationships inside and outside of services.

The work of O'Brien has been developed by the addition of three further accomplishments to produce eight 'user-led' accomplishments which reflect 'positive life experiences that we all seek to increase' (Wright et al 1994, p. 15). The three additional accomplishments are:

- awareness of opportunities and constraints
- self-determination
- personal continuity (in relationships with people, places and possessions).

Despite being a central concept in services for people with learning disabilities, many staff and informal carers are not familiar with the practical applications of normalisation (Box 9.1). It involves a wide range of aspects of day-to-day living and to be successfully applied must be evident in the actions of staff as well as in policy statements and decisions.

The greatest current challenge is to guard against the risk of 'window dressing'. This occurs when people and policies have the right words, photographs and images, but these are not

---

Box 9.1 The main practical components of normalisation (adapted from Barr 1995)

N normal = typical, conventional, valued
O ordinary living principles
R rhythm of life – daily, weekly, seasonal, yearly, life cycle: responsibility and risk taking
M mainstream society
A age appropriateness
L learning is possible, learning occurs through involvement in daily activities of life
I integration – physical, functional, and social
S specialist help if/when needed, socially valued provision
A attitudes in staff, people with learning disabilities, and the general public
T tradition/culture specific
I independence–dependence continuum
O opportunities – planned, presented, developed, valued, increased, individualised
N not an all-or-nothing concept, not making people normal

matched by action. This is particularly evident in services, in which the language is one of normalisation but the decisions about interventions are primarily financially driven.

Challenges to normalisation

The concept of normalisation has not been without its challengers. Two categories of challenge exist: firstly, challenges to the concept of normalisation; and secondly, challenges to the application of normalisation in services. The concept of normalisation has been increasingly criticised over the past few years on several fronts. Dalley (1992) claimed that it contains conflicting social welfare ideologies, in so far as it argues that people should be viewed as valued and seen as an equal part of society, but yet at the same time argues for extra assistance and exemptions due to the presence of learning disability. The lack of a sociological basis has been highlighted by Chappell (1992), and a failure to acknowledge materialism was presented by Gilbert (1993). This is particularly relevant when one considers the impact of poverty on the life of people with learning disabilities and the emphasis on financial decisions and cash-releasing measures (often cutbacks in reality) in the current health and social services structures. A lack of a scientific basis has been highlighted. Although the appropriate application of normalisation may support the hypothesis that normalisation will improve the quality of life of people with learning disabilities, there is an absence of any testable theory of normalisation to explain this effect (Rapley & Baldwin 1995).

On the second count, the application of the concept has been criticised by several authors. Jackson (1988) highlighted what he referred to as 'pseudo-normalisation'. This occurred when the components of normalisation are interpreted literally and, for example, almost any expression of choice is accepted as an informed choice and therefore acceptable within normalisation, even when it leads to reduced social value and reduced social roles for people with learning disabilities.

Gilbert (1993) argues that normalisation is essentially a professional philosophy which treats people with learning disabilities as a homogeneous group of people and fails to recognise their uniqueness, leading to the overall consequence of interventions being 'philosophy driven', not client centred.

Wolfensberger & Thomas (1994) have levelled much of the responsibility for the failure of normalisation in practice at the influence of professional culture. They identified several key obstacles to the successful implementation of normalisation within professional culture. These were as follows: professionals are deeply distrustful, pessimistic and sceptical of ordinary citizens; professionals are unrealistically prideful of their supposedly specialised knowledge, education, training and expertise; they are less likely to seek integrative experiences for people with learning disabilities; 'a social worker in every pot' mentality; professionals are poorly integrated into ordinary society; lack of theory, presence of notional consensus and no clear agreement as to what constitutes normalisation; and finally a lack of common sense often leading to meddling in people's lives.

Some policy documents are now highlighting the need for 'inclusion'. This is noted within the recent 'Review of Policy for People With a Learning Disability' (DHSS NI 1995) which stated:

'*Normalisation* is today regarded by many clients and carers alike as patronising and not appropriate for the 21st century. Their aspirations now extend beyond the normalisation of integration and focus on **inclusion** which stresses citizenship ... The Review Team accepts that now is the time to set aside normalisation as a policy aim and recommends that hitherto **the aim of government policy for people with a learning disability should be inclusion**. It is for the Government and society to include people with a learning disability as they would any other member of society and to accept them for who they are and the way they are.' (DHSS NI 1995, p. 44, original emphasis).

Although many would argue that there is little if any difference between well-implemented normalisation and inclusion, it is important to consider one key distinction. Within normalisation-based services people with learning disabilities often have to argue (with some professionals and legal institutions) for their rights and the freedom to express these rights. However, within inclusion, people with learning disabilities have rights and freedom to exercise these because they are citizens. The focus is now more than ever on the professionals (as individuals and collectively as organisations) to justify the overt and covert obstruction and removal of the rights of people with learning disabilities.

The consistent challenge across normalisation/social role valorisation and inclusion is to make them a reality for people with learning disabilities and their families. They must become more than the rhetoric of service mission statements and posters of services objectives on office walls. These principles must be evident in all our interactions with people with learning disabilities and their families.

COMMUNITY NURSING SERVICES FOR PEOPLE WITH LEARNING DISABILITIES: AN OVERVIEW

Origins

In the early 1970s there was an increasing recognition of the need to provide nursing support to people with learning disabilities and their families in their own homes. In addition to visiting people with learning disabilities and their families at home, community nurses also visit people in settings such as a variety of day-care facilities, schools, residential and nursing homes and maintain a close liaison between hospital- and community-based services.

Community nursing services were developed to support people with learning disabilities who had always lived at home, as opposed to people who had been discharged from hospital. The majority of people with learning disabilities visited by community nurses continues to be those without a history of admission to hospital. Therefore the rate of discharge of people from hospital should not be considered to be a key indicator of the need to increase the number of community nurses. The need to develop services has more to do with the number and the abilities and needs of people who remain at home.

Community nursing services have developed from an uncertain beginning in the 1970s into services which are now integral to the work of community teams for people with learning disabilities. Their numbers have grown from a few in the early 1970s (Hall & Russell 1985) to 1396 by 1988 (RCN 1988). It is not known exactly how many community nurses for people with learning disabilities are in post at present, owing to the lack of centrally collected data on services. However, the rate of growth in Northern Ireland between 1988 and 1996 has been approximately 200%, with nurses increasing from 18 in 1988 to approximately 60 in 1996. An estimate of 2500–3000 community nurses for people with learning disabilities in the UK is not unrealistic.

The organisation of community nursing services has evolved from nurses working in specific teams of community nurses for people with learning disabilities, which were often located in hospital-based offices. At present the majority of community nurses for people with learning disabilities work within multi-disciplinary community learning disability teams with office accommodation within locally based community services (Jenkins & Johnson 1991).

The evolving role

Initially the role of the community nurses for people with learning disabilities was ill-defined and a lack of consensus existed on how services should evolve. The early expectations of the community nurses for people with learning disabilities was that they would provide similar care for people with learning disabilities at home as was provided in hospital. A recorded qualification recognised by the UKCC for community nurses for people with learning disabilities was introduced in 1985 to meet the growing need to prepare nurses who had originally trained to work in a hospital setting. Since October 1995, this course has been taught at degree level, similar to other recorded and registered qualifications in community nursing.

Although the recorded qualification for community nurses for people with learning disabilities is not a mandatory requirement at present, the majority of nurses working as domiciliary community nurses have undertaken additional education to prepare them for working in the community.

Since 1985, several studies, at both local and national level, have identified a number of reasons for community nurses to visit people with learning disabilities (Table 9.1). These studies provide clear evidence that community nurses for people with learning disabilities are an important resource for people with learning disabilities and their families. However, it was also noted that considerable regional variation exists in caseload size and the use of waiting lists for services. The average caseload size for the UK was reported as 24.3, but regional averages ranged from 17.4 (North Western) to 34.3 (Northern Ireland). Higher caseload numbers have been consistently noted in Northern Ireland-based studies with figures of 40 and 42.7 reported by Carson (Mackay 1989) and Parahoo & Barr (1996) respectively.

The early 1990s witnessed major changes in the funding and philosophy of health care provision. The focus on financial

Table 9.1   Reported reasons for community nurse involvement

Authors/year	Reported areas of involvement (in hierarchical order from each study)
Mackay (Carson) 1989	Behavioural problems Epilepsy Physical handicap Psychiatric illness Problems of Adolescence
Jenkins & Johnson 1989	Challenging behaviour Mental health needs Physical disability Sensory disability Ageing-related problems Forensic issues
Parahoo & Barr 1996	Physical care Epilepsy Aggression Mental health Other Withdrawn Sexuality Ageing

accountability appeared paramount (Hadley & Clough 1996), and all professionals had to re-examine their role. Two documents published in 1992 helped clarify the role and function of the community nurses for people with learning disabilities and the overall standards for the nursing care of people with learning disabilities (RCN 1992a,b). Within the framework of individualised services the following areas were identified as central to the role of the community nurse: individual collaborative life planning and care management; meeting health-related needs; functional skills assessment; interpersonal skills development; family support and support services; supporting people with physical and sensory handicaps; promoting socially appropriate (valued) behaviours; promoting independent lifestyles; developing and exercising political and professional awareness; education (nurses and other team members, general public) (RCN 1992a). In addition, standards which specified structure, process and desired outcomes of nursing care were published pertaining to the role of all nurses for people with learning disabilities in relation to: philosophy of care; professional development; research and evaluation; management of care; multidisciplinary teamwork; health promotion; personal relationships; advocacy and influencing social policy (RCN 1992b). Together these documents provide a clear framework for community nurses to remain responsive to the abilities and needs of people with learning disabilities and their families in the current climate within health and social services.

CHALLENGES FACING COMMUNITY NURSING SERVICES FOR PEOPLE WITH LEARNING DISABILITIES

Community nurses have become a major component of community services for people with learning disabilities and their families. Despite several challenges to the need for nurses for people with learning disabilities, they have clearly demonstrated their ability to deliver high quality individualised services, which are valued by people with learning disabilities, their families and other team members (Brown 1990, 1994, Cullen 1991, Clifton et al 1993, Kay et al 1995).

A separate identity distinct from hospital-based nurses for people with learning disabilities and other community nurses has emerged for this group of staff. Their work is an illustration of how the skills of nurses for people with learning disabilities are adaptable to new situations and the changing climate within health and social care. This characteristic was recognised by Cullen (1991) when he described the skills of nurses for people with learning disabilities as 'facility independent'.

Despite the progress made in the past 20 years community nursing services for people with learning disabilities still have major challenges to further enhance the contribution they make to services for people with learning disabilities and their families. Challenges arise in five key areas, namely:

- becoming more visible and recognised
- responding to market-led services
- collaboration with people with learning disabilities and their families
- interdisciplinary teamwork in services
- facilitating service development.

The challenges highlighted for discussion do not form an exhaustive list and overlap to varying degrees with each other. They have been selected because they should now be priorities for action, and practical responses are possible.

Becoming more visible and recognised

The increased numbers of community nurses for people with learning disabilities now in post compared with the early 1980s is often not apparent in recent important service documents and reports (Brown 1994, Cullen 1991, DHSS NI 1995). It appears at times that they are grouped together with other nurses for people with learning disabilities, other community nurses, or collectively included in references to the interdisciplinary team.

Unfortunately, community nurses for people with learning disabilities are relatively unknown outside of specialist learning disabilities services. In particular, members of the primary health care team (PHCT) may not be aware of who the local community nurses for people with learning disabilities are. This is particularly important in relation to developing health promotion opportunities and the inclusive use of mainstream health and social services for people with learning disabilities. The additional challenges faced by people with learning disabilities in maintaining an acceptable level of health have been outlined in 'The Health of the Nation. A Strategy for People with Learning Disabilities' (DoH 1995c). Considering the key role general practitioners and other team members are now undertaking in respect of purchasing and coordinating services, their lack of knowledge on the role of community nurses for people with learning disabilities has major implications. On other occasions community nurses for people with learning disabilities are confused with community psychiatric nurses, an occurrence that most community nurses for people with learning disabilities have probably experienced.

Lack of visibility and reduced recognition of the role of community nurses increases the risk that they will not be included in packages of care designed within the PHCT, or individual client-centred care-managed packages. Opportunities for shared learning and referrals for intervention may also be reduced, particularly in relation to infants and young children. When community nurses have a limited profile in a locality the effectiveness of any open referral systems will be greatly reduced if they are less accessible to family members and people with learning disabilities.

Several reasons contribute to the reduced visibility of community nurses. Organisational factors include: a limited number of community nurses for people with learning disabilities compared to other staff groups; a tendency of these nurses to be based in specialist facilities such as resource centres as opposed to local health centres and therefore having less social contact with other professionals; a philosophy of care more aligned to social models of intervention than medical interventions; a closer relationship with hospital-based services than PHCT services; and large caseloads making visits to people the priority with less time for networking.

Personal factors also have an influence and include aspects such as: a belief that other staff do know who the community nurses for people with learning disabilities are; lack of confidence in asserting the role of the community nurse, or indeed a lack of clarity about one's own role; a belief that visibility is not important in services, or a desire to keep out of the spotlight and avoid increased pressures on resources.

Community nurses for people with learning disabilities must take action now to enhance their visibility and recognition. This could involve the provision of leaflets within local services for people with learning disabilities, in public places such as health centres, post offices, and local shops. Information about community nurses should be included in local information leaflets about health care, and not be restricted to leaflets about services for people with learning disabilities. Liaison with national and local voluntary groups, schools and self-help support groups provides valuable opportunities for the exchange of information. Involvement of the people at whom the information is targeted in the preparation of the leaflets can be an effective means of increasing the relevance of the information included. Unfortunately, many current leaflets contain information that professionals alone think people need. The usefulness of producing different information leaflets which target specific groups of people should be weighed against the practice of producing broad-ranging and often superficial leaflets which are intended to cover all people. Recent research reporting feedback from people with learning disabilities highlighted the lack of available information in relation to health care decisions (Greenhalgh 1994, Mental Health Foundation 1996). The leaflets produced should contain real and significant information which assists people to make informed decisions – jargon and buzz words should be avoided. A leaflet full of terms such as 'individualised client-centred packages of care', 'targeting those in greatest need', 'holistic services', 'facilitating client empowerment', or their equivalents, does little to provide clear and significant detail to assist people make decisions. Such terms are often used to reduce the amount of words, but their limitations must be recognised. It would be more productive to clearly state in day-to-day language exactly what people can expect. Information should be made available in a variety of forms (written, audio, video, Braille, several languages, photographs, symbols) to make it accessible to people with learning disabilities, their families, and people with sensory impairment. A further complication is that, owing to the speed of changes in services, leaflets can quickly become inaccurate. The use of loose-leaf formats, allowing single pages to be replaced, and stickers with up-dated information to be added, assists in maintaining the currency of the leaflets.

There is a need to increase the visibility of community nurses for people with learning disabilities on the conference and publication level. Although there has been an increase in the number of publications in relation to work of community nurses for people with learning disabilities, they continue to have a limited profile in both conferences and publications. Practical steps towards achieving higher visibility include obtaining guidelines for contributors from journals, the setting up of a local learning disability nursing or multidisciplinary journal club, and sending outlines of articles to, or discussing them on the telephone with, journal editors. It may be reassuring to know that the people who review your submitted article do so anonymously and are required to be constructive in their feedback. Conferences and publications should not be the domain of educationalists or a selected few presenters. They need to have input from many community nurses who can illustrate through their work that they have major contributions to make.

Therefore, it is important that people are given the opportunity to prepare for public presentations and eased into it if possible. An onus also rests on experienced authors and presenters to assist people develop these skills and demystify the publication and conference process (remembering how traumatic their first conference presentation or submission for publication was). To be successful, the importance in promoting increased visibility must become part of the 'culture' of community nurses and be valued, rather than viewed as a luxury or something to be undertaken by someone else.

Responding to market-led services

The move towards a more market-led service in community nursing has been clear over the past few years. This is noted in the emphasis on the cost of services, accountability for budgets, cost-effectiveness, and the language of consumerism. Community nurses are now contracted to make a certain number of visits on a monthly basis and have to log in to a computer system the nature and outcome of these visits.

Purchasers of service are primarily health and social services agencies at board level, and increasingly general practitioners, either single practices or multi-fundholding arrangements (Norman 1996). Most contracts at present operate on a quantitative basis with a focus on the number of contacts between nurses and clients, and give consideration to the purpose and duration of these contacts. In such a contract, unfortunately, less attention appears to be given to the qualitative aspects of the intervention. As increased pressures are placed on nurses to meet numbers of contracted visits, what are considered less important aspects of the job may receive inadequate attention. In particular, the delayed recording of nursing notes following contact with people with learning disabilities or their families needs to be addressed. Nursing notes are not an optional extra and their legal and professional importance must not be underestimated. Concern over the quality of recording by nurses led to the production of clear guidelines for nurses on reporting and recording of information (UKCC 1998a).

Nurses must remain vigilant to the quality of the service they provide as professional practitioners and refer regularly to the guidance from the UKCC (1992a,b, 1996a). The need to meet contract requirements is no justification for poor practice. If standards of care, safety or professional conduct are jeopardised, nurses have an obligation to inform the responsible managers. These managers must then respond appropriately and acknowledge their responsibility and accountability (UKCC 1996b).

Nurses who take on extra work and jeopardise the health of their clients and their own health will find little support from managers if a complaint about the service arises. Community nurses must also be very specific about their objectives of intervention with clear competencies to be achieved, and conditions and criteria for success identified for each client. The key focus with client-centred and needs-led services is not how many times the person was visited and what services were provided, but the success attained in achieving client-based outcomes (Braye & Preston-Shoot 1995).

Although services may be purchased in consultation with people with learning disabilities and their families, they do not have full consumer status as they are often lacking in accurate information, accessibility, choice, representation, and redress (Braye & Preston-Shoot 1995). However, the development of direct care payments and service brokerage models of care provision will enhance their role. Consumers buy products, and will seek out what they perceive to be the best value for money. In this case the product is the interventions of the community nurses for people with learning disabilities. It may not be a pleasant thought when described in that way but it is necessary to recognise the principle involved. Therefore the key questions to be addressed are what is the 'product' offered by the community nurses, at what cost and why should people buy it as opposed to another service?

A considerable amount of time and energy has been expended by community nurses over the past decade but to little avail, in debating what it was that made the role of the community nurses for people with learning disabilities so important. Each time a specific skill was identified as unique, another professional group would argue that they also practised these skills. Despite being referred to as specialist within the new post-registration education and practice framework (UKCC 1994a) the majority of community nursing services do not possess a single elusive skill that makes them totally unique. The strength of the community nurses is the combination of skills that they possess. The package of skills present in nurses for people with learning disabilities is recognised as integral to their provision of holistic care (Brown 1990) and is reflected in the varied nature of their role as discussed earlier in the chapter. These skills are not fragmented but are integrated into their practice, providing a sound basis for high quality interventions (Clifton et al 1993). In the current climate of cost-effectiveness and the desire for continuity in interventions the package of skills held by community nurses for people with learning disabilities is a very significant 'product'. Community nurses need to recognise the importance and practical significance of their skills and build on this foundation.

A valuable package of skills alone is not enough in the market-led climate; their importance needs to be made known to purchasers of services. A key strategy in this process is the production of accurate and accessible information as discussed previously. However, the information provided to purchasers needs to be further developed to incorporate details about the practical benefits of nurses for people with learning disabilities as team members. A recent example of this was produced as a result of the Learning Disability Nursing Project (Kay et al 1995). This document is concise in its use of models of good practice to illustrate the practical contributions nurses can make across a variety of settings; it is colourful and uses photographs to assist in its impact. It has been produced free of charge and would be a very useful document to give to prospective purchasers, and also to design a local information document around. Unfortunately, this document is not familiar to a large number of community nurses and consequently is not being utilised (see Bibliography for further details).

The provision of value for money is a central principle in the NHS and Community Care Act (1990) and the Personal Health and Social Services (NI) Order (1991). Therefore community nurses must become aware of the costs associated with their service and the other community nursing services that are more visible and therefore may be utilised. New services are emerging, such as community children's nurse, specialist health visitors, practice nurses, voluntary and private providers of services, all of which are expected to undertake some of the work undertaken by community nurses for people with learning disabilities. Nurses must also have an up-to-date knowledge of the services provided by colleagues such as social workers, physiotherapists, and occupational therapists.

For many community nurses the thought of their work as a marketable product is inconsistent with how they view their role. However, the climate of current services needs to be reflected upon, and provision can not be left to chance or the belief that, because community nurses for people with learning disabilities have always undertaken certain aspects of care, they will continue always to do so. The notion of clearly defined boundaries and agreed demarcation of roles and 'territories' is no longer strictly possible.

For some time now the blurring of roles within multidisciplinary teams has been recognised. It has been viewed at times as a challenge to be overcome. It has also generated concerns about the future of some professional roles and the frameworks of professional and managerial accountability (Cullen 1991, McGrath 1991, Ovretveit 1993). In particular, the need to reformulate the interface between nurses, doctors, and social workers has received attention. Community nurses for people with learning disabilities are becoming increasingly recognised as valuable team members in their own right. The idea that they only follow the instructions of the doctor is no longer consistent with the view of the nurse as an autonomous practitioner.

Considerable overlap has been identified between the role of nurses for people with learning disabilities and social workers in community learning disability teams (McGrath 1991). This has also been noted in the development of joint educational programmes for professional qualification as nurses for people with learning disabilities and social workers. In addition some attempts have been made (largely for financial reasons) to identify separate health and social components of care (Cullen 1991, Social Services Inspectorate 1991). However, this lacks any clear theoretical basis and may act against a holistic approach to services. The impact of these developments on the quality and individuality of services available to people with learning disabilities and their families remains to be evaluated over the next 5–10 years.

The costing of services provided by community nurses must include the actual time in contact with the people with learning disabilities and their families. It should reflect travelling expenses, preparation and recording time and any associated work in relation to the intervention, such as liaison with other professionals or the provision of equipment. It will also include a proportion of the costs of the administrative and managerial support involved in providing the service. It is not desirable to sacrifice quality to save money (a lesson still to be learnt in some aspects of community care), instead it is necessary to clarify why a service which costs more is worth the extra expenditure.

It has been suggested that community nurses for people with learning disabilities developed in response to gaps in community support for people with learning disabilities and their families in the 1970s (Hall & Russell 1985). The ability to continue to identify gaps and provide an effective response is a necessary part of remaining an integral part of current services. Community nurses have already demonstrated their ability to respond to gaps such as the need for health screening and the provision of personal development education for people with learning disabilities (Meehan et al 1995). The development of specialist roles for community nurses is also evidence of the ability to identify and respond to gaps in services. A number of community nurses have developed specialist roles based on additional recordable nursing courses, for example in relation to behavioural approaches to working with people with learning disabilities. Other community nurses have developed further skills by completing additional courses (not recorded by the UKCC) in a variety of areas such as in work with people with epilepsy, counselling, family therapy, people who are elderly, people who have been abused, aromatherapy, and reflexology. In addition to this, yet more community nurses have developed enhanced skills on the basis of their experience and special interest in working with people with particular abilities and needs; such areas include, personal development, working with children, people with additional physical and sensory disabilities. Finally, the reorganisation of services into teams which are specific to age groups has resulted in some nurses working with a specific client group.

The variety of different routes in developing roles can be confusing for people who use services and people who will purchase services. Therefore the information published about services must clarify if people have additional areas of skill and what this is based on. The attainment of additional recognised qualifications can be an advantage when marketing services.

Three further issues need to be considered. Firstly, if the service wishes nurses to undertake additional training which will increase the marketability of the service, then nurses should be supported in undertaking such courses. This support should be financial and in respect of the time needed to complete the training involved, including study outside of lectures. The recognition of additional practice skills should also be acknowledged in the nurse's caseload and clinical grading, particularly if an increased level of autonomous practice is required. Nurses who undertake additional roles normally hold a smaller caseload to facilitate additional time with clients.

The second issue is the need to prevent fragmentation of services. A clear vision of the developing service is required so that nurses undertake courses which assist in achieving the planned service. Community nurses undertaking additional courses based purely on personal interest reduce the likelihood of being given the opportunity to integrate their skills into the community nursing service provided. This can lead to resentment, frustration and disillusionment among nurses and is wasteful of potential resources.

Finally, a careful balance must be maintained between the needs of a service in a given locality and the skills of the nurses and other team members. It is also important that an attitude of elitism does not creep in with additional courses; all nurses within the service are valuable to its success. People could not work effectively in specialist areas of practice without the cooperation of their colleagues; this should always be remembered. Successful community nursing is a team effort.

Working in partnership with people with learning disabilities and their families

A stated priority in many community nursing services is the need to make decisions about interventions in partnership with people with learning disabilities and their families. Relationships between community nurses and people with learning disabilities and their families should be based on as equal a partnership as possible. Nurses are obliged to work in partnership with people with learning disabilities and their families (UKCC 1992); this is also consistent with the concepts of inclusion and citizenship (DHSS NI 1995). It is impossible for much to be achieved without partnership; a lack of consistency and the refusal of cooperation from people with learning disabilities or their family will often scupper even the best formulated care plans.

It is recognised that, at times, tensions may exist between the desires of people with learning disabilities and those of other family members. This is often not a straightforward matter to resolve, but the greatest promise for an acceptable solution lies in partnership and negotiation with all involved, as opposed to making unilateral decisions. The issues raised below in relation to partnership have relevance when interacting with people with learning disabilities, and their families or colleagues.

Partnership is a much-used word 'but simply paying lip service to the notion of working in partnership is not enough to make it a reality and to bring new practices into play' (Wide 1996, p. 14). All involved need to reflect on the definitions of partnership available and identify the components involved (Dale 1996). Despite the amount of talk there is about partnership it is an aspect of services which continues to be widely identified as in need of further development (Dale 1996, Dyer 1996, Hornby 1994, Mental Health Foundation 1996, Wide 1996).

The potential benefits of partnership with people with learning disabilities and their family members include increased knowledge and skills for all involved, feedback to evaluate current services and assist in future services planning, fresh ideas, and greater satisfaction in the interpersonal interaction. The benefits need to be considered in relation to the costs associated with partnership, the greater time needed for negotiation, increased resource implications, the challenge of working in partnership and the tensions, and managing the shift in responsibilities between professional, parents, and other family members (Wide 1996). Families and people with learning disabilities form an elaborate interactional system, which must be acknowledged when working in partnership (Barr 1997).

Empowerment and collaboration are terms regularly used in services. At times they are used interchangeably with each other and used to imply partnership. This can be misleading; although overlap exists, subtle distinctions are also present. Collaboration does not always mean partnership. Family members and professionals may interact within an expert model in which the professional always knows best. Or in a transplant model where, although professionals may assist family members to develop new skills, the professionals decide which skills and control the pace. Although these models could be described as collaboration, they are not partnership. This is a key feature in distinguishing expert and transplant models from the consumer, empowerment and negotiation models of collaboration (Dale 1996). Partnership requires a shared involvement in the decision-making process and a recognition of the strengths and limitations of all involved (Hornby 1993).

Empowerment has been defined in several ways, with each definition having a slightly different emphasis (Braye & Preston-Shoot 1995, Gibson 1991). The consistent themes across the definitions used are the sharing of power, and the need for mutual understanding and the respect of differences in people. The foundation to facilitating people to become empowered in services is a recognition of the importance of agreed values and clear models for understanding the experiences of people with learning disabilities and their families (Braye & Preston-Shoot 1995).

The process of becoming empowered has been described as being characterised by frustration, commitment to change, gradually gaining insights into oneself and one's situation, eventually taking charge of one's situation and then actively participating in decision-making (Gibson 1995). Feeling respected and trusted are important antecedents to becoming empowered and working in effective partnerships. Various avenues may be used to increase the degree of empowerment achieved by people with learning disabilities, their families and professionals. These include increased understanding of clients' experiences, changes in legislation, increased resources and financial support for clients, access to independent representation and advocacy and teaching assertiveness skills to people (Laxton et al 1997). The past 5 years have witnessed an increase in the number of people with learning disabilities who have opportunities to become involved in service evaluation, the education of professionals and make independent or assisted presentations at conferences (McNally 1997).

The previous simplistic conceptualisation of advocacy within nursing services as 'speaking up for someone' has been challenged by refinements and distinctions now made between differing levels of advocacy (Table 9.2). Advocacy can no longer be viewed as a single entity, but involves a number of levels that present different opportunities and challenges for people with learning disabilities, their families and professionals.

Obstacles that exist to successful partnership with families have been grouped into several main categories, namely, issues arising from the family, the health and social care system, and professionals (Bjorck-Akesson & Granlund 1995). Obstacles in families may include limited knowledge/skills, attitudes inconsistent with negotiation, limited resources or other family characteristics, such as increased family vulnerability due to additional stressors (Mathias 1992). At the level of the health and social care

Table 9.2   Variations in the types of advocacy (Conlan & Day 1994, McNally 1995)

Type	Characteristics
Self	Person speaks on own behalf. Confident in own ability, adequate knowledge and skills to make informed decisions
Citizen	Volunteer/friend (unpaid) develops a relationship with the person wishing to have an advocate. Volunteer speaks on behalf of the concerns of the other person. Defends these concerns as if they were their own. Does not have to agree with specific concerns/wishes but respects and defends the person's right to have his or her views heard and appropriate action taken
Legal	Demonstrated by lawyers, is concerned with the exercise and protection of legal rights/entitlements
Peer	Support from advocates who have had personal experiences of using similar services (e.g. mental health services)
Crisis	Also referred to as 'short-term' advocacy. Time limited with specific client-determined objectives to be achieved. Often urgent in nature and does not involve a long-term relationship
Collective	As for self-advocacy, only exercised by a group as opposed to individuals. Concerns expressed may relate to an individual or a group of people
Family	Provided by family members, based on knowledge of the individual. There is a risk of conflict between the wishes of the individual and those of the family
Formal	Emerging term in the UK, refers to schemes run by voluntary groups, often not user-led, but use the 'expert' model – giving advice, prioritising options, counselling and mediation
Professional	Provided by staff within services, based on knowledge of the person, professional education and skills, knowledge of the structure and function of the service system. Potential for conflict as 'advocate' is part of the system

system, obstacles may include restrictive routines and procedures which have the effect of limiting opportunities for joint decision-making and action. Limited resources can result in the language of partnership being used to create the illusion of progress and conceal a service-led decision-making process. This is becoming increasingly visible within care management as it moves away from the promise of a needs-led service based on individual need to a service in which decisions are made almost exclusively on the basis of financial considerations.

User-managed participation has been contrasted with managed user participation (Braye & Preston-Shoot 1995). At a glance both may appear the same thing, but considerable differences exist. In the 'user-managed participation' services people with learning disabilities have real opportunities to influence decisions, are provided with information and time and their contribution is recognised. Conversely in managed user services, users may be hand picked and not representative, provided with little information, time, or opportunities to develop the necessary skills. The priority is for the service to present the outward picture of working with user groups, while at the same time professionals maintain a 'we know best' approach to service planning, implementation and evaluation.

Among professionals there is a strong desire to maintain the status quo in relationships with people with learning disabilities and their families. This 'professional protectionism' (Sines 1995a) perpetuates the expert model of intervention and seriously restricts opportunities for developing partnership and achieving empowerment.

Limited knowledge of their subject area or more specifically of partnership and a corresponding gap in skills can impede the development of partnership. Fear of the unknown, lack of preparation, lack of confidence, aloofness and arrogance in staff, people with learning disabilities and their families are some of the factors which may contribute to a reluctance to move away from the status quo in relationships.

Attitudes of professionals which view family members as problems, adversaries, vulnerable, less able, needing treatment, causal of the problems or needing to be kept at a professional distance restrict the degree to which partnership can be developed (Hornby 1994). These attitudes may be reflected in the unnecessary use of jargon, poor listening, stereotyping people with learning disabilities and family members, and an unwillingness to accept the holistic nature of learning disabilities and their impact on the family.

Obstacles to partnership rarely arise from one side of the partnership; the old adage 'it takes two (or more) to fight' is particularly relevant when considering failures in partnership. More often than not partnerships fail to develop because people involved in the interaction are not prepared to seek a resolution to conflict.

There are no simple answers to overcoming the challenges associated with establishing and maintaining effective partnerships. However, a series of important characteristics of successful partnership have been identified primarily by parents and professionals working together in an attempt to clarify what they need from each other to establish, develop and maintain

> **Box 9.2** Recommendations for 'building bridges' in partnerships between parents, people with learning disabilities, other family members and professionals (Hornby 1994, Maxwell 1993, Wide 1996, p. 13)
>
> - Be clear about the principles and values that underpin the provision of services.
> - Be succinct, honest and to the point, and present complex information and difficult choices clearly and accurately.
> - Have good listening skills, and the ability to communicate sympathetically.
> - Be honest with family members about what individual practitioners and agencies can and cannot do.
> - Be conscientious, and have the determination to 'do what you say'.
> - Be aware of, and respect, racial and cultural differences and work with these issues openly.
> - Be able to cope in an ever changing environment.
> - Be open to complaints, comments and suggestions backed by effective and accessible procedures.
> - Ensure that making a complaint does not carry a threat (implicit or explicit) of victimisation or labelling and that comments and suggestions are taken on board.
> - Be able to cope with, and accept, strong emotions, and do not be overwhelmed by what parents, relatives and carers feel and express.
> - Have caring attitudes and values, and the ability to demonstrate them, acknowledging that good intentions are not enough.
> - Build on existing positive family coping strategies and support networks rather than dismantling them or reducing their effectiveness.
> - Be involved in the lives of parents, relatives and carers, as well as in the lives of individuals with learning disabilities.
> - Empower family members to act to enhance their own abilities and needs as well as those of the person with learning disabilities, and the family as a unit.
> - Be willing to keep learning and training. Never get to the point of 'knowing it all'.
> - Be realistic and have a sense of when it is right to push the limits. Anticipate problems and do not lurch from crisis to crisis.

partnerships (Box 9.2). These provide practical and realistic targets for all community nurses. Crucial to the achievement of real partnership with people with learning disabilities and their families is a commitment by all involved to engage in what will at times be a difficult process.

Developing interdisciplinary teamwork

Community learning disability teams, of which community nurses for people with learning disabilities are members, are focused 'locality based' multidisciplinary teams. It is clear that no single model of effective teamwork or team leadership exists; instead several models have been shown to be effective (Ovretveit 1993). Multidisciplinary teamwork holds many anticipated benefits including: increased coordination of services; more effective communication between professionals; greater speed and accuracy of response to client needs; increased appreciation of colleagues' roles and the breakdown of divisive professional barriers; increased learning opportunities for team members to enhance skills and knowledge; and reduced costs through the sharing of offices and other equipment (Pritchard 1995, Rawson 1994).

However, despite the almost universal need for multidisciplinary teams within the UK health and social services, their effectiveness has been questioned recently by several authors. Brown (1992) asserted that 'in some teams, members appear to be working alongside each other with only the most rudimentary cooperation' (p. 374). This is a phenomenon which he described as 'separate but parallel teams'. Brown went on to state that 'our studies of community learning disabilities teams point inexorably to one perplexing conclusion. It is that the work undertaken by staff in teams is not for the most part highly specialist' (p. 384).

A similar issue was identified by Carrier & Kendall (1995) when they stated that multiprofessional work 'is a co-operative enterprise in which traditional forms and division of professional knowledge are retained'. Braye & Preston-Shoot (1995) conclude on reviewing the evidence on multidisciplinary teamwork that 'the track record of multidisciplinary teamwork remains unimpressive' (p. 147). Hudson (1995) goes further and questions if a seamless service and effective teamwork is realistically attainable. The obstacles to effective teamwork may be viewed as arising from within organisational, professional and interpersonal levels (Box 9.3).

A wide variety of important areas have been highlighted as needing consideration if the effectiveness of teamwork in health and social care is to be increased (Brown 1992, Hattersly 1995, Hudson 1995, Ovretveit 1993, Sines 1995b). In particular five issues are consistently highlighted as requiring urgent attention, namely, clarifying team membership, agreement on the team values and priorities, a comprehensive operational policy, the

---

Box 9.3   Possible obstacles to effective teamwork (Sines & Barr 1998)

Organisational
- Differences in pay and conditions between team members
- Inadequate time made available for team members to get to know each other
- High staff turnover and long periods of reduced staff numbers
- Lack of autonomy (actual or perceived)
- Lack of support and commitment from team members and outside managers
- Lack of resources
- Lack of feedback/recognition for individual members and the team as a unit
- Competitive individual performance appraisals
- Peer pressure or management pressure to conform
- Having no choice about joining the team
- Over-control by managers/professional advisors outside the team

Professional
- Differences in values and philosophy
- Professional (and/or personal) defensiveness
- Development of professional cliques
- Unnecessarily complication and exclusive language or jargon
- Felt need to keep a professional distance
- Desire to retain exclusive control over professional knowledge and/or skills

Personal
- Varying expectations of one's own role in relation to the degree of acceptable client involvement
- Struggles to assert personal power within the team
- Sabotage of team effort due to perverse incentives (such as maintaining previous status, making others look ineffective)
- Previous limited or negative experiences of teamwork
- Lack of confidence in one's own ability to function as a team member
- Lack of interpersonal communication skills, in particular assertive skills
- Fear of reducing autonomy

---

recognition and management of conflict, and the evaluation of team effectiveness.

This may appear to some people such an obvious first step that they feel it does not need attention. However, that assumption is the very reason why issues around team membership needs to be addressed. Most professionals within health and social care belong to more than one team and often perform different roles in these teams depending on the nature of their involvement and the dynamics within the team (Ovretveit 1993). It may be that one person is a core member of one team and a member of an extended team in another part of the service. Even when individuals are clear about what teams they belong to, other team members may not be so sure. If this first step is not clarified the prospects of effective teamwork will be diminished. Team membership will vary depending on factors such as the locality, the purpose and priorities within the team, resources and the level of cooperation between agencies. Nevertheless one consistent aspect that should be clear to all team members is who belongs to the team. If team members also provided details of what other teams they belonged to this could assist networking across services, reduce overlap and enhance the understanding of individual contributions.

By definition, teams can be distinguished from groups by the fact that teams have shared values, aims and objectives and structures (Carrier & Kendall 1995, Pritchard 1995). Differences over priorities for action is one of the major factors that impedes effective teamwork. A main aim of interdisciplinary teamwork is to increase the available resources and to be able to respond flexibly. Therefore it is essential that no single member, nor one group of members (based on professional background, previous relationships, hierarchical position or the same major interests) makes all decisions. Teams take time to become effective and move through stages before becoming fully functional. Tuckman (1965, cited in Mullins 1996) proposed the four stages of forming, storming, norming, performing. This model has been commented on by many authors since, but has remained largely unchanged (Baron & Byrne 1991, Blair 1995, Mullins 1996, Robards 1994).

Team values should be agreed after a period of settling in, during which team members will have an opportunity to develop relationships with each other. It is necessary to recognise that reaching a consensus on values and priorities can often be a stormy process, during which debate should be encouraged. People with learning disabilities and their family members should also be provided with opportunities to influence team priorities. Team members should consider how they will integrate service philosophies such as normalisation and inclusion into team values and priorities.

Providing opportunities for shared learning among team members in relation to people with learning disabilities and their families often assists all concerned to develop a clearer understanding of each other's values (Wide 1996). This increases the prospect of reaching agreement on shared values and priorities in teams.

Team values and priorities must be evident in the individual practice of team members and the team as a unit, they must be more than a few words on paper. For effective teamwork there should be no inconsistency between the documented team values/priorities and the 'operational culture' of the team. Brown (1992) stressed the importance of acknowledging and responding to the pervasive influence of team operational culture, which he defined as 'the routine and often unspoken ways that team members define their roles and their professional relationships'. He concluded that even when strong operational procedures are present, teams can be severely restricted in their effectiveness and brought to the point of breakdown because of failure to recognise the importance of operational culture.

Operational policies are to some degree the rulebook for teamwork in that team. The operational policy should clarify among other things issues such as: aims, priorities of the team, team membership, team structure, the position and authority of the team leader, referral and caseload management issues, sharing and recording of information, and suggested strategies for the management of conflict within the team. Operational policies also require to be updated regularly to adapt to the changing nature of services.

Most teams have operational policies somewhere. However, the familiarity of team members with operational policies can vary greatly. Copies of these policies may be freely available to all members of the team, or available only to a few members on the basis of their role, status, or contacts. Alternatively, the operational policy may be available to only one team member who uses it as a strategy of control. Indeed, it may not have been influenced by any current team members because it was written by previous team members or service managers outside the team. A useful measure of team structure and coherence is to determine how many team members have access to the team operational policy. Policy documents which lie idle on shelves and with which staff are not up to date have no real positive impact on team functioning, and are of no real value.

One of the few certainties in teamwork is conflict. By its very nature interdisciplinary teamworking generates different perspectives on issues under discussion. This in turn leads to the exchange of points of view, which can be mannerly or on some occasions heated. Operational policies will provide information on the boundaries of acceptable degrees of conflict and the procedures for responding to conflict.

Critical factors to the effectiveness of teamwork are the beliefs about conflict and its contribution to team functioning. The most effective teams view conflict as a positive aspect of teamwork, recognising it as part of teamwork and developing procedures to assist in its constructive resolution. This in turn will, it is hoped, lead to more informed decisions and more innovative and holistic interventions. Assertiveness, confidence and a clear belief in one's own ability and role are necessary for open debates to take place.

Viewing conflict as a negative aspect of teamwork can result in it being suppressed, becoming covert, and ultimately destructive to team effectiveness and services provided. A team in which members never disagree openly or rarely discuss their differences gives the outward appearance of functioning effectively. On closer inspection it is likely that such a team lacks innovation, has limited cohesion and supports a culture in which obedience to authority is the rule.

Finally, in addition to the review of the work of individual team members, the effectiveness and achievements of teams needs to be evaluated. Even when teams consist of a collection of skilled individuals, there is no guarantee that they will gel together as a cohesive unit. Indeed the most effective teams are recognised as containing people with qualities that complement, as opposed to compete with, each other, whereas 'teams' of experts have been shown to be less effective (Belbin 1993). If only individual effectiveness is evaluated, then reduced opportunities will be available to highlight team successes as well as areas for development. Teams are major investments and like any other investment in services need to be monitored carefully.

Facilitating the development of community nursing services for people with learning disabilities and their families

The preceding sections have identified specific areas in which community nurses for people with learning disabilities could enhance the services available. Developing services will require community nurses to have a vision of how they wish services to evolve. This vision should take cognisance of the views of people with learning disabilities and their families, other members of the interdisciplinary team and the current economic and cultural influences within the health and social services. While acknowledging the views of these people, nurses must work hard to articulate the specialist nursing contribution to the vision of future services for people with learning disabilities. This was emphasised in the conclusions of the Learning Disability Nursing Project (Kay et al 1995) which emphasised the need 'to ensure that the health focus of the nurse's role is clearly articulated' (p. 36). There is a great danger that in an attempt to be seen to be willing team members, nurses will fit into other visions of services instead of articulating a nursing vision. Different ideas are the essence of teamwork, whereas conformity and 'sameness' will block innovation and promote inertia.

Nurses must become more aware of the politics involved in services and how these influence decisions that are made. Once such an understanding has been gained, nurses will be in a better position to influence the decision-making process. It is also necessary to be aware of wider social issues such as the impact of poverty, gender, discrimination and social structure (Philpot & Ward 1995). Responses to these issues need to be reflected in community nursing services. Influence will also be gained by having a sound research-based knowledge of our interventions. This means reading regularly from the key journals and books which exist, discussing and critiquing the information gained and taking steps to integrate this into daily practice. Nurses must read specialist as well as broader professional journals. All nurses should consider subscribing to a journal, and if this were coordinated within a team and members subscribed to separate journals, several important titles could be covered.

Research awareness also means involvement in research. This may be in the form of assisting in an on-going project, or undertaking a research project into community nursing services for people with learning disabilities. This information must then be disseminated if it is to be worthwhile on more than a local basis. An increased use of networking and the use of professional organisations can assist in learning new information and skills, disseminating information to others, understanding how services are developing elsewhere. These factors may help in reducing the isolation felt by many community nurses. Networks can be of several different types, they may include only nurses or may be interdisciplinary, involving people with learning disabilities and mixed economy of care. These must also include members of the primary health care team. They may be relatively local, national or indeed international. The ability to pass information and keep in touch nationally and internationally is becoming easier with increasing access to e-mail and Internet facilities.

CONCLUSION

The future development of community nursing services for people with learning disabilities and their families will be influenced as much by the practical actions of community nurses individually and collectively as members of interdisciplinary teams, as by any government policy. Key focus in the development of future services must be to establish the most effective means by which community nurses can facilitate people with learning disabilities to make use of mainstream inclusive services. This will involve an increased liaison by community nurses for people with learning disabilities with mainstream health and social care services and vice versa. It will also require action to increase awareness among mainstream services of the contribution community nurses and other members of the community learning disability team can make to the holistic health of people with learning disabilities.

The greatest challenge to be overcome is getting community nurses to realise that action is needed. This action is required at the level of individual practitioners, local, regional and national levels. The argument often put by community nurses that they are too busy to reflect and act on the major challenges is no longer adequate to explain the inaction of many nurses in response to the areas highlighted. The challenges facing community nurses for people with learning disabilities face all of them to varying degrees, and equally require a response from all of them.

10

Education for practice

Linda Burke   Debbie Harris

INTRODUCTION

The role of the nurse in the community is undergoing a period of rapid and intense change. The demand for more nurses working within primary care is increasing, yet the nature of the responsibilities and activities they will be expected to take on remains unclear and much debated. Discussions are ongoing within primary health care concerning the increasing importance of professional autonomy and accountability (Champion 1991), the definition of advanced practice (Jasper 1994), the utilisation of nurse practitioners and the introduction of nurse prescribing.

Additionally, the impact of external factors, notably the end of the internal market, the devolution of resources for non-medical education to education and training consortia (Jarrold 1995) and the introduction of the 'post-registration education and practice project' (PREPP) (UKCC 1997a) have yet to be fully appreciated.

In 1996, the White Paper 'Primary Care, Delivering the Future'

(DoH 1996b) emphasised the importance of developing continuing education programmes that meet the needs of community nursing.

'Nursing, Midwifery and Health Visiting Education: A Statement of Strategic Intent' (DoH 1994d) stressed the importance of continuing education that is relevant to practice, appropriate and of value to patient, employer and practitioner.

In the words of the Department of Health (1994d) 'education is the bedrock of professional practice', yet the educational needs and requirements of practising community nurses have not yet been looked at within a national coherent framework. Where continuing education courses or programmes of study exist they are usually localised, ad hoc or short term, and information about them is rarely disseminated beyond the immediate group of nurses who undertake them. This is true for both registered specialist community nurses and for the many non-specialist trained nurses practising in the community.

One of the fundamental questions that will be addressed in this chapter is what kind of education, training and learning experiences will be required by specialist and community nurses so that they are enabled to make the most of the opportunities that are presented as a result of this unprecedented period of change?

The chapter will focus mainly on three key areas:

- the structure of education and training consortia and the specific issues that have arisen from them for specialist and community nurse continuing education
- a needs assessment of the education which will assist nurses working within primary care to take on the challenges inherent within 'The New NHS: Modern, Dependable' (DoH 1997)
- professional learning requirements of community nurses – ways in which the community nurse can meet the five focus areas for study in relation to PREP.

ONGOING ISSUES FOR COMMUNITY NURSE CONTINUING EDUCATION

There are a number of key issues that have a particular impact on continuing education for community nurses.

Firstly, the range of knowledge and skills possessed by the nurses that work in the community is enormously varied. As a result of the skill-mix reviews that have occurred over the last 10 years, many of the nurses working in the community have not undertaken the specialist community nurse courses but are working at D and E grades (the two lowest staff nurse grades), with some supervision from specialist community nurses. They have usually been practising in acute clinical areas or have just graduated from Project 2000 diploma courses. The education needs of the nurses that have come straight out of either pre-registration diploma courses or from hospitals, who are working at D and E grades, are very different from those of experienced specialist nurses (Hennessy 1995).

In the same way that health care resources are directed disproportionately towards secondary care in preference to the primary care sector, so it is the case that most post-registration continuing education courses are also aimed at nurses working within acute clinical settings. As a result, many of the nurses working at D and E grades in the community have ENB qualifications that are of little relevance to the environment in which they are now working.

With the advent of Project 2000 diploma courses, which had greater emphasis on primary health within their content, it was claimed that newly qualified nurses would be able to work in the community immediately after qualifying, and a number of nurses do take on community nurse posts as their first jobs. However, there is still some controversy as to whether all, or even most, Project 2000 diploma courses contain enough primary care content and placement time to adequately prepare nurses to work in such an environment, where nurses are expected to work alone and make decisions independently, and where the amount of supervision they receive may, in reality, be minimal.

Equally, because of the changes that have taken place in the curriculum preparing specialist community practitioners, nurses who did their specialist training several years ago may have completed courses which did not include the level three research and critical thinking skills which are essential for today's practitioners (DoH 1994d).

There is also a particular problem in identifying educational needs for each of the eight areas of specialist community practice. It was only in 1993 that it was recommended that all the specialist pathways should be brought together in one curriculum. This has meant that core learning and practice outcomes have been identified which should, in the long term, enable both shared and specific continuing education units of learning to be built onto this framework. It will, it is hoped, also enhance understanding and sharing of skills and knowledge across specialities, enabling more patient-focused working. This is of particular value in the community where patients' problems are multifaceted and rarely relate to just one area of speciality. Unfortunately, as this is relatively new, although in most education institutions it is now up and running, there will be difficulties for some years to come in identifying common educational needs across areas of speciality.

Community nurses have different working practice from those in the acute sector. Although they work in teams, most of their day-to-day activities are carried out independently. It is, therefore, more difficult to arrange times and cover so that they can take up the education opportunities that are available to them. They also tend to stay in their area of practice for long periods of time and, whilst this has many benefits, one of the potential problems is that there may be fewer chances for them to update their knowledge and skills. Changes in the length of stay of patients in acute hospitals mean that patients are being discharged into the community much earlier with more acute conditions, and the skills needed to care for them have changed considerably (Littlewood 1995). Therefore, it is essential that community nurses are given the opportunity to update skills and knowledge.

EDUCATION AND TRAINING CONSORTIA
Structure and organisation of consortia

In April 1998, resources for the education and training of community nurses, along with all other non-medical health care professionals, were placed in the hands of education and training consortia (ETCs).

This was the culmination of a process of restructuring the resourcing of nurse education which began with the implementation of 'Education and Training: Working Paper 10' (WP10) (DoH 1989a) which was an integral part of 'Working For Patients' (DoH 1989b) and as such was alleged to embrace the same fundamental principles (Box 10.1). ETCs are also featured in 'The New NHS: Modern, Dependable' (DoH 1997).

WP10 was intended to remove training costs from service pricing decisions so that a level playing field exists as far as possible in the competition for health care services. Costs associated with non-medical training do not give one trust an unfair advantage over another and education and training are protected (Rogers 1990). NHS trusts are required to participate in the training of professional staff, and their staff continue to have access to nationally recognised training.

WP10 was also an attempt to rationalise what was believed by many to be a confused system of funding for nurse education. Historically, such money had been distributed from the DoH between the English National Board for Nursing and Midwifery Education (ENB) and the district health authorities (DHAs), from where it was distributed to colleges and students. There was little effort to relate cash flow to workforce planning and money designated for education could fall prey to district health authorities who found themselves short of resources. The system of financing in WP10 was intended to rationalise the system. Most importantly, the supply of nurses would now be closely linked to local demand.

The purchaser–provider split is clearly defined, with the responsibility for providing education in the hands of colleges or higher education (HE) institutions and the clinical units identified as purchasers. Purchasers of education can choose from a variety of providers and thereby achieve the presumed market advantages of increased efficiency and value for money. Employers are responsible for ensuring that their training arrangements are of the scale and quality needed to meet the needs set by the local labour market.

Box 10.1   Main proposals of WP10

- To introduce the market and competition to non-medical education
- To reduce central control and improve local responsiveness and flexibility
- To increase consumer choice
- To maintain quality by protecting education and training within the internal market
- To improve efficiency by linking education to workforce planning

Resources for nurse education were originally given to the regional offices (ROs) to act on behalf of clinical units to purchase education. However, it was made clear that they should be passed to education and training consortia (ETCs) (see Box 10.2), made up of education purchasers (NHS and non-NHS), GPs and health care purchasers by April 1998. They should take responsibility for holding the budgets for non-medical education and training (NMET), commissioning NMET and contracting with providers (Jarrold 1995). Regions must then establish regional education and development groups (REDGs) to advise on the acceptability of education commissioning plans. REDGs include representation from each ETC, the regional office, the Postgraduate Dean and an independent education expert.

ROs and ETCs decide the appropriate level of funding to be top-sliced and utilised for education. ROs and ETCs can also choose what to do with any potential surplus or extra money or decide to offer financial incentives to students to train in a particular area. Increasingly, the student is no longer seen as the purchaser within this equation, as the needs of students are believed to link into those of the clinical units for which they will provide the workforce. Student numbers should relate to service requirements for qualified staff to ensure regional self-sufficiency, thus preventing overtraining and reducing the possibility of wage inflation (Burke 1997).

Issues for community nursing

It is clear that ETCs are powerful bodies in that they have control of the resources that fund education and training, with considerable budgets. The most important issues for community nurses relate to three key areas: knowledge and information, representation and equitable distribution of the resources.

Box 10.2 Membership of education and training consortia (Jarrold 1995)

- A representative of each trust
- A representative of each NHS purchasing authority
- Representatives of GPs, including fundholders
- A representative of each social services authority
- Representatives of the non-NHS public sector and the independent and voluntary sector

---

Community nurses are not always represented on the consortia (see Box 10.2). In fact, the Department of Health does not insist that any nurses are members of consortia but does say that the consortia member should be from the executive board of the hospital (Jarrold 1995). In reality, many acute trusts do send a nurse, usually the Director of Nursing, as their representative to the consortia but this often is not the case with community nurses.

It can be argued that community nurse interests could be brought forward by the GP representatives. However, there are a number of problems with this. Consortia often find it difficult to find consistent GP representation, particularly as GPs may not see it as of immediate relevance to them. Because GPs work as independent practitioners, they may only represent the interests of one practice. Furthermore, many nurses may not feel that GPs are the best people to look after their professional education needs and may also not be clear about the requirements of the eight different community nurse specialists.

One positive development is that a number of community trust chief executives have taken on the role of chair of the consortia and, although they may not be there as nurses, some have backgrounds in nursing and, therefore, have a considerable understanding of the implications for them. Another potential solution to this problem is the development of primary care groups (DoH 1997). If, as expected, nurses take on leading roles within these organisations, they would be ideally placed to represent the nurses within their group on the education consortium. In addition, it is hoped that education strategies will link in with the new health improvement programmes (DoH 1997), which should emphasise the importance of primary care and of pathways of care, and which primary care nurses should be active partners in devising.

The way in which resources are distributed within consortia is based on a number of factors. For pre-registration training, resources usually follow the number of commissions. However, in post-registration the budgets are allocated to regions and then to consortia, often on historical patterns with some scope for flexibility depending on the nature of the contracts. Within consortia there is, therefore, the possibility of negotiating for resources not only from the existing budget but also from extra funds that are, on occasion, allocated centrally.

As yet there is no indication that purchasing patterns are changing from the traditional ENB courses and as there are so few ENB courses for community nurses, this means that they receive a small share of the consortia resources. Whilst there are local initiatives in education and training – for example, part-time courses preparing hospital nurses to transfer and adapt their skills, enabling them to work in the community – these tend to be funded by individual trusts rather than by the consortia.

In addition, individuals are often unaware that they can access finance from the consortia, which means that a number of community nurses who do undertake further education pro-grammes such as master's degrees, are usually self-funding. The reasons why this is the case are not altogether clear but there are a number of possibilities. Firstly, it may be that the consortia or higher education institutions are unwilling or unable to change historical purchasing patterns and divert monies into new courses which may not prove popular or financially viable; also short-term contracts are not conducive to investment in innova-tive courses (Booth 1992). As stated previously, there may not be a representative of primary care nurses on the consortium. It may also be the case that community nurses are unaware either of the potential of the consortia to purchase education on their behalf or of extra resource allocations. There are exceptions to this, for example some of the Action Agenda monies have been allocated to community nurses for training in dealing with clients with mental health problems (Miller 1998), but it is probable that community nurses are not receiving an equitable share of educa-tion and training resources.

It is, therefore, essential that community nurses ensure that their educational needs are represented to the consortia. Locally, individuals have a responsibility to be informed of policy devel-opments and initiatives and must be assertive. This may entail devising programmes of education that are tailored to their own needs, which is not easy for individuals who work indepen-dently, and it may be that professional organisations and educa-tion institutions can be of assistance in enabling community nurses to access a more equitable share of resources.

One positive feature is that all trusts should have equal power on the consortia, which gives community trusts the opportunity to put forward their interests. However, a number of the trusts have concerns that when consortia sign the collateral agreement with respect to legal and financial responsibility for the resources that are devolved to the consortia, the consortia budget may be as large as the trust budget. They may, therefore, feel that their risk is greater than that of the larger trusts.

Nationally, there is likely to be a review of the funding distribution, and primary care nurses' views must be part of this. A national database, providing information both about extra resource allocations and perhaps a step-by-step guide to accessing consortia funds or identifying community representatives on consortia elsewhere, could be of immense value.

From a wider perspective, it seems that there are a number of innovative and interesting local modules of education developing (South Bank University 1997b), but that there is not yet a national strategy or programme of continuing education for community nurses of varying levels of grade, experience and knowledge. Whilst there will always be a need for local flexibility, there are clearly a number of national educational needs that nurses share. Greater coordination and planning at a national level could be of value, perhaps developing learning outcomes or minimum standards for continuing education, and could help ensure that there is some national coherence, that good practice is shared and resources are not wasted.

'THE NEW NHS: MODERN, DEPENDABLE'

The long-awaited White Paper – 'The New NHS: Modern, Dependable'– outlining the Labour Government's plans for the health service appeared in November 1997. As predicted, primary care was identified as a key area for continued development. Perhaps a little less expected, however, was the emphasis within it on the role of community nurses as not only essential and equal members of primary care teams, but also as *leaders* of such teams. In the words of Health Minister, Baroness Jay, 'primary care groups will create a new leadership role for community nurses', and she went on further to say that, 'this government is guaranteeing nursing a seat at the decision-making table in every town and city across the NHS' (Jay 1997).

Thus, for community nurses it is very clear within the White Paper that they have an unprecedented opportunity to play an active and leading role in shaping the 'New NHS' from all levels of the organisation.

There are four areas in particular where they will be expected to take on new roles:

- as key members or even partners within primary care groups (PCGs)
- as part of teams looking at improved methods of quality monitoring
- in developing joint working arrangements with social services
- getting involved in NHS Direct, a nurse-led 24-hour advice and information helpline.

Primary care groups

The Government intends to establish primary care groups which will bring together GPs and community nurses in each geographical area to work together to improve the health of local people (DoH 1997). Their structural development should be evolutionary and they will gradually replace the variety of organisational arrangements under which GP practices currently function. Some PCGs may, in the short term, merely support health authorities in their role as commissioners of health care. However, it is intended that eventually many will become free-standing bodies which take over completely the commissioning function from the health authorities and may even merge with community trusts to become primary care trusts.

Community nurses of all specialities and levels are identified as essential members of PCGs (DoH 1997). However, one of the most important changes for community nurses will be the development of the new roles that some nurses will take on as leaders of the PCGs. The pilot schemes that have resulted from the 1997 NHS Primary Care Act may provide some models for practice from which lessons can be learned. Of the 95 successful schemes to run Primary Care Act pilots, 10 include nurses in the leadership teams and they are focusing particularly on providing services for vulnerable groups (Queen's Nursing Institute 1998). There are, however, a number of important issues to be clarified with regard to nurses' future roles as partners in PCG governing bodies:

- How will their employment and salary status be affected? If nurses are not employed by PCGs but by community trusts, how can they be part of the governing body? If nurses *are* employed by the PCG, what will be the implications for nursing autonomy and accountability?

- What will be the financial and legal responsibilities of nurses who are partners in PCGs?
- Will it be compulsory for all PCGs to have nurse representation and, if so, what percentage of them will there be in relation to doctors? What will the nurse's role be if GPs have problems working together or refuse to join a PCG?
- What effect will PCGs have on ongoing practice developments such as nurse prescribing and the introduction of nurse practitioners?
- How can the nursing profession ensure that community nurses have the knowledge and skills to enable them to grasp these opportunities and thereby influence the future development of primary care?

The education needs of nurses taking on these leading roles will be different from those required in the past. Financial management and budgetary proficiency have not traditionally been part of the curriculum in basic or post-basic training. Equally, whilst some 'people'-management competencies have been introduced to newer courses, these have been concerned mostly with leading teams of nurses. For nurses to manage teams which may include administrators, accountants, other health care professionals and doctors, additional input will be needed, not least assertiveness and decision-making, business planning and resource management skills. It will also be essential that such nurses learn more about the law and their legal and financial responsibilities. To do this they will need assistance, not only from educational institutions but also from the professional bodies and the Royal College of Nursing.

Quality assurance

The Government is committed to making quality assurance part of 'every aspect' of the NHS and, once again, states that nursing will play a major part in this process. Quality assurance or 'clinical governance' will involve the NHS executive, professionals, academics, health economists and patient representatives and will drive clinical and cost-effectiveness and disseminate best practice throughout the health service.

'The New NHS' has outlined a structure for quality which begins at the top with four national bodies:

- the National Performance Framework, which will develop indicators for health improvement, outcomes, efficiency, effective and appropriate care and fair access
- National Service Frameworks, to establish evidence-based pathways of care for major care or disease groups
- the National Institute for Clinical Excellence, which will draw up guidelines on best practice and on clinical audit;
- the Commission for Health Improvement, which will support and oversee the quality of clinical governance and clinical services. It will support local developments but also have the power to 'spot-check' to ensure that care is of good quality and to intervene to resolve serious or persistent problems.

All of these bodies will include nurses and community nurses, and their input is vital if a quality, seamless service from hospital to home is to be achieved.

The underlying principle of the quality framework is that national standards will be enforced and improved upon locally. In order to accomplish this, 3-year health improvement plans will be drawn up locally between health authorities, PCGs and trusts, which will give detailed plans of what the needs of the population are and how services will meet them.

In addition, 'clinical governance' in trusts will ensure that national and local standards are met. The White Paper (DoH 1997) actually suggests that nurses are the ideal professionals to lead clinical governance teams in trusts. If trusts are failing to meet required standards, the Commission for Health Improvement will have the job of stepping in to rectify the situation.

The details of how each of these organisations will operate have yet to be decided so it is vital that community nurses are involved at the early stages, to make sure that realistic and practicable systems and targets are devised that are as appropriate to primary care as to acute services.

These systems will only work if the professionals closest to the patients, the nurses, are able to understand and apply the standards. It will be a priority to ensure that community nurses at all levels have knowledge and understanding of auditing and of implementation of protocols of care. In addition, nurses are likely to be the most appropriate people to measure the effectiveness of care and feed in information about the quality of care that is delivered – why there might be problems or where there are examples of excellent practice. Therefore, they need evaluation skills and knowledge of research critiquing, application and basic methodologies, so that they are enabled to do this effectively and clinical governance does not just become a paper exercise but a real system that is owned by practitioners and permeates the whole organisation (Whitfield 1998).

Working together – health and social services

One of the key principles of 'The New NHS' is that of working in partnership by breaking down organisational barriers and forging links with local authorities (DoH 1997). In this way, patients are put at the centre of the care process and are no longer subject to the ongoing debates about which organisation – health or social services – is responsible for resourcing care.

Community nurses have been working with social workers since the implementation of the NHS and Community Care Act 1990 in assessing their clients' needs and devising care packages for them (Sloman 1995). They have also been involved in working out if the care clients need is 'nursing' or 'social', deciding whether patients fit the eligibility criteria for the appropriate service area and then evaluating the resulting budget implications. In all the specialist areas, community nurses have been active in dealing with the problems and pressures that arise from the division of resources between health authorities and local authorities, particularly in relation to continuing care and mental illness.

Community nurses are, therefore, ideally placed to take a lead in setting up partnerships and joint working arrangements with local authorities. They have a head start on doctors who have often left liaison with other agencies to the nurses. Initiatives, which already involve nurses in this way, are the health action zone pilots. Health action zones have been set up by the Government to bring together consortia of organisations both within and external to the NHS to develop and implement locally agreed strategies for improving the health of local people. The first 10 pilot schemes began in April 1998. Many of the bids involve community nurses in key roles.

One of the principal ways in which education institutions can assist community nurses to facilitate joint working arrangements is by developing more interprofessional education programmes between nursing and social work. In a number of institutions this is already happening. For example, in pre-registration training (South Bank University 1997a) and on master's degrees (South Bank University 1992). Such courses should be made more widely available and perhaps targeted specifically at community nurses. It may also be possible to set up local arrangements for units or modules of education that can be run in-house around issues which will be relevant for both groups of practitioners. Examples could include: writing contracts; resource management; clinical governance and standard setting; policy analysis and implementation; organisational psychology; team management; workforce planning and information technology.

Interprofessional education is one of the best ways to ensure that practitioners from different agencies gain mutual understanding, appreciate the difficulties that each of them faces and work together effectively.

POST-REGISTRATION EDUCATION AND PRACTICE

Professional issues in relation to the education of qualified practitioners have, since the early 1990s, taken a complete change in response to the instigation of the UKCC's mandatory updating of staff in the form of PREP. In 1991, Professor Margaret Green – who was the chair of the project – stated that it was trying to inculcate in the profession a truly professional approach to development. 'It is about individuals sitting down and thinking through what they want to do' (Green 1991, cited in Friend 1991, p. 24). The Project Group that was made up of representatives of the four national boards and the Educational Policy Advisory Committee of the UKCC, set out to produce a coherent and comprehensive framework for education and practice beyond registration. It was perceived that these requirements would help to address issues relating to the changing focus of health care.

The background

During the course of this century, and especially since the inception of the National Health Service in 1948, patterns of health and disease have changed significantly – the major influences being the 'germ theory' in the early part of the 1900s where advances in laboratory medicine meant that immunisation and vaccination became the most dominant form of health care provision. Consequently, this increased child care services and school health and vaccination programmes. In the 1930s, based on the continuing success and advances in research and technology, the 'therapeutic era' developed. This was gained by a marked shift towards more hospital-based care services. This resulted in the decline in the power and influence of public health departments, and health policy was now dominated by an orientation towards treatment and cure (Tinson, cited in Cain et al 1995). In the 1970s, another shift in perspective has resulted in the return to a community-based assessment of need. This was due to the rising cost of health care, the ever increasing demand for medical care, as well as the changing pattern of disease. 'Environmental lifestyle' is in relation to four major factors: heredity, the health service, individual lifestyle and the environment (Lalonde 1974). The NHS and Community Care Act of 1990 produced the required radical overhaul of the National Health Service in the social programmes for health, creating a new climate for practitioners functioning in a market economy for health care.

In the light of this, it was felt that the professions would be affected by the environment of rapid change and that practitioners needed a strategy to cope with this uncertainty (UKCC 1991). The two key issues that were seen as paramount in the framework for education and practice beyond registration were:

- meeting the needs of patients, clients and the health service
- maintaining and enhancing standards of education and practice.

Therefore, nurses, midwives and health visitors will become explicitly accountable for their practice and for their own development. Equally, the professional body will have the facility to monitor the activity of their members to ensure that standards in both education and practice are maintained.

The historical background to the context of professional practice

Several factors were seen to affect the future of the nursing, midwifery and health visiting workforce and the requirements of professionals within a health care setting. These were based on five major elements:

- *Demographic trends.* At the instigation of this project it was seen to have two central factors, the first that the elderly population was increasing in number and would continue to do so. As a result, the demands of caring for more very elderly people would require innovation in practice underpinned with research so that this growing section of the population could maintain their optimum health (UKCC 1991). Secondly, it was thought that the number of school leavers entering the labour market was set to decline (DoE 1990). This potentially meant that there were not enough 17- to 18-year-olds to provide recruits for pre-registration education. The implication of a declining workforce was seen as enormous and strategies would need to be set in place both to encourage mature entrants into nursing and midwifery, and also to maintain the existing workforce.
- *Lifestyles and health inequalities.* It was felt that despite major technological advances and increased clinical skills, there were still many people who had limited or virtually non-existent access to health care. Those at the bottom of the social scale have a higher death and morbidity rate and chronic sickness; disabilities have been linked to unemployment and poverty (Black 1980). Equally, the higher proportion of single parents in today's society has led to inequalities in employment opportunities.
- *The NHS and Community Care Act 1990.* This involved the change of emphasis from secondary to primary care. The throughput of patients from the acute centres was being increased in response to the instigation of new general managers who were concerned with efficiency of resources. Therefore, the community services were seen to be needing further developments to deal with the increased patients/clients who were being discharged sooner from hospitals and needing intensive care (Enthoven 1991). Alan Maynard further influenced the change in health care by arguing that the GPs would be in a much better position if they could purchase health care on their clients' behalf (Maynard 1991). This gave a high status role to the GP and guaranteed a prominent place on the Government's agenda for primary care.
- *Health promotion.* The implementation of the World Health Organization's 'Health for All' and the government's 'Health of

the Nation' strategy launched in 1992, set the nurse in the key role of health promotion. This is because, to be able to undertake the key targets such as coronary heart disease and stroke, a community assessment of the population's health status, using available data and current medical knowledge, would be required, which would then be able to influence health care provision and practice.

• *Changing nursing and midwifery education.* Owing to the ethos of the purchaser–provider split and the introduction of the self-governing trusts, contractual arrangements have been made in terms of the provision of education at pre- and post-registration levels with appropriate faculties or colleges of health care that are now integrated within universities. This has been looked at in light of the output of the workforce skill-mix and individual consortia projected business plans.

All of these factors reiterated the need for qualified practitioners who are informed, credible and accountable for their practice. The Project Group, therefore, developed a framework that would incorporate these elements whilst maintaining standards of education and practice which reflect in the outcome of patient/client care.

Maintaining registration

As such, qualified staff would need to continue to develop throughout their professional careers. Updating and maintaining registration would be vital to ensure that specific learning has taken place within the continuum of practice. The approach was seen to allow proposed standards for education and practice to be interwoven logically and progressively in a way that could be applied throughout the professional life of the practitioner (UKCC 1990a). The four key elements to maintaining registration are:

- completing a notification of practice form at the point of re-registration every 3 years and/or when the area of professional practice changes to one where it will be a different registerable qualification
- a minimum of 5 days or equivalent of study activity every 3 years
- maintaining a personal profile containing details of your professional development

- a return to practice programme for those who have not practised for a minimum of 750 hours or 100 working days in the 5-year period leading up to the renewal of the registration (from 1 April, 2000) (UKCC 1997a, p. 6).

The document 'Post-registration Education and Practice and You' (UKCC 1997a) also states that if the practitioner is working in a capacity where a registered nursing, midwifery or health visiting qualification is used in some way, then it will be necessary to maintain the registration with the UKCC – even if a nursing, midwifery or health visiting qualification is not a requirement for the post but the qualification is being used in the context of the description of the work. This is a matter of keeping options open and knowledge and skills up to date.

The PREP timetable

1 April, 1995. All practitioners were notified of the new requirements as they renewed their registration. All practitioners must complete a notification of practice form each time they renew their registration. After renewing registration for the first time, the requirements relating to study activity and completion of a personal professional profile must be met by the end of that 3-year period and every 3 years thereafter.

September 1995. New UKCC requirements for programmes of specialist education were introduced.

September 1998. All programmes of specialist education had to meet UKCC requirements.

1 April 2000. Statutory return to practice programmes for nurses and health visitors start.

1 April 2000. All practitioners have to meet all the PREPP requirements.

Support for practitioners

There is also one final recommendation that was put forward by the Project Group which was seen to be key and vital for qualified practitioners and that is support for the first 4 months following a professional registration to consolidate the competencies or learning outcomes achieved. This facility is extended to all practitioners entering a new field of practice, be that another professional registerable qualified role or a more senior appointment. This is to be offered regardless of previous experience. The rationale for this decision is that practitioners need support in a new role, and even though they may be experienced or even an expert in another area of nursing, midwifery or health visiting, initially they are beginners in the field they have chosen. Benner (1984) underlines this, stating that the practitioner will be operating at 'novice' level in the beginning of any new experience and additional support is required in what is likely to be a stressful period. It was also acknowledged that the care and protection of patients and clients will be strengthened by the development of more confident and supported practitioners.

The support is provided by an experienced nurse, midwife or health visitor who is known as a preceptor and will act as a role model for the new practitioner in the day-to-day practice of the job.

These recommendations were seen as statements of good practice by the UKCC and as such it was expected that employers would have implemented them by January 1993. At present the majority of employers within the NHS and private sector have instigated this support system. For self-employed practitioners this remains a problem and also for staff who work within agency settings. However, some far-sighted agencies are in the process of formalising a preceptorship model based on the preceptor being a member of the full-time agency staff.

Return to practice

From 1 April 2000, any practitioner who has a break in practice of more than 100 working days or 750 hours over the 3-year period will have to complete a return-to-practice programme and demonstrate that she or he is able to provide safe and competent care before the registration will be renewed. Generally, the returning practitioner will have to pay to undertake the course that will be at least 5 days long and will include relevant supervised practice. Some trusts who have a problem with recruitment may, however, in trying to employ staff, offer the return to practice programme free of charge and state that although they cannot guarantee a position on completion of the course, they would consider the applicant as a result of a successful outcome from the period of study.

Study activity

Looking at what constitutes study activity, the UKCC is asking its registered practitioners to develop the habit of lifelong learning. This is important in today's health care as increasing growth of knowledge, research and evidence-based practice, together with the development of new technology, means that knowledge and skills are not static and can, over time, be no longer appropriate. It is vital that practitioners keep up to date with the latest developments so that they can keep pace with the changing health care arena. Education that fits nurses, midwives and health visitors for practice now may not be relevant in 5, let alone 10, year's time. Practitioners need to be able to access knowledge and develop skills and attitudes to upgrade consciously, systematically and continuously, their existing repertoire. This in turn allows for practitioners to extend and expand their practice to the benefit of the patient/client, the profession and the practitioners themselves.

In the UKCC document, 'The Scope of Professional Practice', it states that 'Practice must remain dynamic, sensitive, relevant and responsive to the changing needs of patients and clients' (UKCC 1992b, p. 3).

The minimum of 5 days (or 35 hours) of study activity over a 3-year period is very little; not even constituting 1 day per year, this can be undertaken as a block of activity or undertaken in an individual timeframe. Flexibility of learning should be the key to this requirement as it is not going to be expected that every qualified practitioner will undertake a formal experience of learning such as another professional qualification, specialist course or 'in-house' course which is given a certificate. Learning, however, must be needs related, that is the needs of the individual, the patient/client group, the profession and finally the workplace. To help the practitioner focus on areas of activity, the UKCC has established five categories of study. They are designed to be broad and flexible to 'enable personal growth without being over-prescriptive' (UKCC 1994c, p. 4). They are as follows:

1. *Reducing risk.* This incorporates health problem identification, protection of individuals, risk reduction, health promotion, screening and heightening of awareness.

Examples of study in relation to these areas are practitioners who set up teaching schemes around differing aspects of health promotion with a variety of client groups, or nurses or health visitors who undertake health promotion exercises within such areas as shopping centres or comprehensive schools. These activities should be documented as part of their personal study. Developmental learning is where the practitioner has carried through an idea, either on an individual or a collaborative basis, that has been researched and planned for the benefit of other individuals to expand knowledge, skills or understanding.

2. *Care enhancement.* This incorporates developments in clinical practice and treatment, new techniques and approaches to care, standard setting and empowering consumers.

This is a very key role for specialist practitioners who are at the forefront of standard setting within their own field of expertise. The instigation of new methods of undertaking care and treatment for client groups is an area that can be documented as part of advanced learning and study activity. Within all of the eight specialist roles in community nursing, this category has relevance and is undertaken in the practitioner's everyday practice.

Many nurses, midwives and health visitors are initiating and leading practice developments to enhance and contribute to the quality of client care. They are innovators of care which is individual to the client and which also acknowledges the needs of the client and/or carer(s), as well as the resources available. All of these factors are considered as priorities by the practitioner to produce the optimum package of care. These types of developments are extending the role of the professional because of the complex nature of the required outcome and as such need to be researched and formulated, utilising a range of health and social agencies.

3. *Patient, client and colleague support.* This includes counselling techniques, leadership for professional practice and supervision of clinical practice.

Evidence of this would be provided by practitioners documenting how they clinically direct a professional team to ensure the implementation and monitoring of standards of care. They may also advise staff and develop support networks and systems in relation to clinical supervision and these strategies should be accounted for as part of study activities.

4. *Practice development.* This includes external visits, exchange arrangements, personal research/study, briefing on health policy change and service audit.

In today's health care arena, evidence-based practice is the 'buzz' phrase and practitioners are encouraged to undertake relevant research either at macro or more often at micro level to support practice initiatives. These projects are an indication of professional development. As nurses, midwives and health visitors visit other practitioners to learn about new developments, or to collaborate on designing or setting up new systems for client care, all are involved in their own personal growth and this is vital to study activities.

5. *Education development.* This includes external visits, exchange arrangements, personal research/study, educational and clinical audit and teaching and learning skills.

Practitioners are often involved in learning activities on an individual or group basis with colleagues, peers, clients and carers. This may be a one-off formalised teaching session or undertaken as a series of informal unstructured sessions in relation to an aspect of client assessment and need. Skills of teaching require a knowledge base both of the subject area and of appropriate teaching styles which require preparation and planning and, as such, constitute a learning activity.

As can be seen from the above descriptions, the UKCC have been very broad in their interpretation of the areas for evidence of study, and it is perceived that all practitioners will be able to acknowledge elements of activities which incorporate these categories. Equally, collaboration between peers and colleagues over developments and innovations should be used to support evidence of study activity.

If practitioners have dual or more professional qualifications, they will be required to show evidence of study activities in all areas to be retained on the professional register. This, however, will not require them to undertake more than the statutory 5 days if they can integrate the activities to reflect the differing professional roles.

An example of this would be for a practitioner who is working as a specialist nurse within the community as a community children's nurse and who has a dual professional qualification as an RGN, RSCN and has undertaken district nursing. The practitioner would have to demonstrate that within the study activity she or he worked as an adult practitioner and as a children's nurse – part of the role would be working in partnership with the family to provide optimum care of the child. Evidence of the practitioner setting up a support group for parents, giving counselling and guidance as well as providing an individualised package of care for the child in relation to possibly a new treatment for the condition, would be seen as integrating both professional roles.

All of the activities have to be evidenced and submitted within the personal professional profile when practitioners renew their registration.

Profiling

The UKCC states that 'a profile is a record of career progress and professional development. It is not a CV, a daily diary of events or your whole life history' (UKCC 1997a, p. 13). The profile has two main functions:

- to contribute to practitioners' professional development by allowing them to recognise their abilities, achievements and experience
- to provide an information source of material to evidence standards of education following registration.

The profile should contain evidence of what the practitioner has undertaken over the 3-year period and how this will lead into future developments following the renewal of the registration. Therefore, a clear career pathway should be recognised or a rationale for the practitioners' personal and professional development.

The second element in the profile is self-appraisal based upon the practitioner's performance and the standards used to support the educational development. This involves focusing on one event and critically analysing the issues raised from the experience, therefore expanding the practitioner's knowledge base and learning skills. There are several ways in which this can be undertaken and one of the most commonly used in the educational setting is Flannagan's (1954) critical incident technique. He starts by describing the incident and the persons involved, which leads into the nurse debating the successes or problems raised by the situation. These can be related to the practitioners themselves, the other individuals involved and/or the organisation. This technique will encompass an element of self-reflection and analysis which allows the community nurse to look into a situation from several differing perspectives. Finally, the technique identifies what has been learnt from the event and how this will impact on the practitioner in the future and as such outlines the learning experience.

The third part of the profile is to set goals and action plans; this requires practitioners to evaluate their learning and to identify what future learning needs it would be appropriate to develop over the next 3 years.

There are no set procedures for putting together a profile and the UKCC has not provided an official document. However, it states that the main factor to be considered is confidentiality in terms of identification of clients' and/or carers' names and addresses, surgeries and hospitals in relation to the use of critical incidents. The profile can be submitted in a paper presentation or on floppy disc.

From 1 April 1998, practitioners applying for renewal of their registration have had to make a formal declaration that they have met the statutory obligations, although they are not required to submit any documentation at this time.

Future developments

In the early part of 1998, the UKCC advertised for tenders from appropriate institutions to develop a pilot study of this scheme. A series of studies will be undertaken between now and the start of the formal audit system on 1 April 2000. At present, there is no definitive format for these studies and no clear-cut guidelines have been given for the audit system. Practitioners are waiting with bated breath to discover how their professional body is going to orchestrate this mammoth task.

This is due to the fact that it is acknowledged by the UKCC that they probably cannot look at all of the professional profiles of practitioners who wish to renew their registration. So what proportion will be seen and how these will be chosen remains debatable. It is possible that a selection from those submitted will be inspected but the decision of how these are picked will be made during the pilot studies. Also, the major question of who is going to assess the profile and declare its evidence as acceptable has not been answered. Many practitioners have fears that this will be undertaken by administrative staff who will be cheaper to employ for what will essentially be a paper-pushing job. However, the problem with this is surely that these administrators, unless they have prior or recent experience in nursing, have neither the expertise nor credibility to assess the value of the documentation. It has been suggested that if very strict criteria were produced then anybody could assess these profiles but this could penalise nurses who wish to produce innovative and unusual evidence of their personal development. A question raised at one of the UKCC's roadshows in relation to PREPP was: 'How would the professional body be aware of or respond to practitioners who have lied in the production of evidence?' The UKCC's reply was that it did not anticipate that a practitioner who is bound by a code of conduct and worked as a professional would choose to falsify evidence.

It has not been decided either what constitutes an unsuccessful profile. All the UKCC will state at present is that the practitioner will be informed of the requirement to submit the profile at least 3 months before the submission date and that if it is unsuccessful, the practitioner will be required to re-submit a reviewed profile within 6 months of the original submission date.

The maintenance of professional standards and competence, however, is firmly in place. Practitioners now and in the future will have to provide evidence of learning and study. No longer will qualified staff be allowed to think that at the point of registration they have undertaken enough education for lifelong professional practice. 'Everyone must expect constant change, and with it new goals to be achieved and new understanding and skill to be mastered' (Houle 1980, p. 128).

CONCLUSION

As a result of PREP and of the changes to the NHS initiated by the new Government, there are unprecedented professional and personal development opportunities available for community nurses. Community nurses should work with colleagues in the professional bodies and in higher education to ensure that their educational needs are considered so that they make the most of such opportunities.

As stated by the UKCC (1997a), learning is a continuous process which will be undertaken by practitioners throughout their professional life. It is, therefore, essential that community nurses begin to influence the type of educational experience that is available to them and appreciate how flexible education programmes can be. Higher education institutions are now much more responsive to the needs of different groups of practitioners. For example, there are departments within most universities which can assess students' learning needs and the level at which they will be able to study – from certificate through to diplomas and degrees and on to master's and doctoral programmes. Community nurses' prior learning and experience will be taken into consideration through 'Accreditation of Prior Learning' or 'Accreditation of Prior Experiential Learning' schemes. Such establishments are often willing to deliver courses at a variety of levels and in different modes: part-time, evening classes, short blocks of study, distance learning, through the Internet and as computer-assisted learning packages.

PREP has identified that learning takes place not only in formal settings but also within the clinical area and can be part of the practitioner's day-to-day activity. Community nurses will often be undertaking new dimensions to their practice which can be utilised as educational experiences and as part of their own professional development.

Lecturers from higher education institutions can be invaluable in facilitating learning within the practice area. Ways in which they might do this include:

• Enabling staff to have the confidence and skills to assess, become involved in, and implement practice-based research. The teacher, with access to higher education expertise and resources is ideally placed to initiate practice-based research and development projects.

• Assisting practitioners to make the best of the existing learning resources in the clinical area – not least by enabling nurses to share their own knowledge and expertise.

• Supporting community nurses in their roles as supervisors, so that they both feel supported and can benefit from the supervision process as a learning experience.

• Developing clinical supervision programmes. Such programmes can take place in the classroom or in the clinical area and can often lead to the formation of peer support and education circles which continue after the formal supervision by the teacher has ended.

- Validating, that is giving academic credit to in-house training courses or units of learning which can be specifically tailored to the particular needs of the primary care nurses in that locality.
- Helping staff to formulate practice frameworks and extend problem-solving skills, which can be then used to improve client care.
- Giving practical advice and assistance with such matters as implementing PREP and utilising information technology.
- Encouraging the development of the critical thinking, reflecting, evaluating and assertiveness skills of community nurses.
- Defining the educational needs of all levels of staff, or assisting them to identify their *own* learning needs in conjunction with the needs of the organisation. The teacher can often help to provide staff with a wider perspective on the definition of learning and on the context or environment in which it can occur (Burke 1995).

In order to take on this role, lecturers involved in teaching community nurses will also need to be fully aware of the changes that are happening in national policies and their potential impact on the practice area. Teacher preparation courses must, therefore, enable lecturers to work in all environments where learning takes place and give them the skills to offer educational programmes in a variety of modes of delivery. Furthermore, more emphasis should be placed on recruiting potential lecturers from primary care settings. Equally, a post-registration curriculum should be designed so that it is appropriate for nurses from all settings and no longer focuses mainly on acute health care.

There is clearly a need for a more structured approach to the continuing education of community nurses. Without this, there is a danger that their specific educational requirements could be ignored and that the only available programmes may be inappropriate in both focus and content. In addition, there is the possibility of fragmentation, duplication and wasting of resources. The way to prevent this could be the introduction of a national, coherent strategy or framework which addresses the needs of community nurses at all levels of the organisation, whilst allowing room for local flexibility.

One of the most important questions will, ultimately, be that of control. It is essential that education programmes are not imposed by external bodies or other professionals who believe that they have greater experience and ability in this area. Community nurses take charge of their own destiny by defining their own educational needs and then determining the type of learning experiences which they believe to be of most value and use to them.

References and further reading

Access to Personal Files Bill 1987 HMSO Bill 20 49/4. HMSO, London

Advisory Committee on Alcoholism 1978 The Kessell report. HMSO, London

Advisory Council for the Misuse of Drugs 1982 Treatment and rehabilitation. HMSO, London

Advisory Council for the Misuse of Drugs 1984 Prevention. HMSO, London

Advisory Council for the Misuse of Drugs 1988 Drugs and AIDS Part 1. HMSO, London

Advisory Council for the Misuse of Drugs 1989 Drugs and AIDS Part 2. HMSO, London

Advisory Council for the Misuse of Drugs 1990 Problem drug use: a review of training. HMSO, London

Advisory Council for the Misuse of Drugs 1994 AIDS and drug misuse: update. HMSO, London

Advocacy Alliance 1986 Annual report. Advocacy Alliance, London

Albarran J 1992 Advocacy in critical care – an evaluation of the implications for nurses and the future. Intensive and Critical Care Nursing 8(1): 47–53

Albarran J W, Fulbrook P 1998 Advanced nursing practice: a historical perspective. In: Fulbrook P, Rolfe G (eds) Perspectives on advanced nursing practice. Butterworth Heinemann, Oxford

Albarran J W, Whittle C 1997 An analysis of professional, specialist and advanced nursing practice in critical care. Nurse Education Today 17(1): 72–79

Alcohol Concern 1994 National alcohol training strategy. Alcohol Concern, London

Alcohol Concern 1995 What about alcohol? Alcohol Concern, London

Alcohol Concern 1996 Pop fiction? The truth about alcopops. Alcohol Concern, London

Alexander J S, Younger R E, Cohen R M, Crawford L V 1988 Effectiveness of a nurse managed programme for children with chronic asthma. Journal of Paediatric Nursing 3: 312–317

All Party Parliamentary Group on Skin 1997 An investigation into the adequacy of service provision and treatments for patients with skin diseases in the UK. HMSO, London

Alsop A 1997 Evidence-based practice and continuing professional development. British Journal of Occupational Therapy 60 (11): 503–508

American Association of Critical Care Nurses (AACN) 1989 Standards for nursing care of the critically ill, 2nd edn. Appleton & Lange, Norwalk, CT

American Nurses' Association, Drug and Alcohol Nursing Association & National Nurses' Society on Addictions 1987 The care of clients with addictions: dimension of nursing practice. American Nurses' Association, Kansas City, Missouri

American Nurses' Association & National Nurses' Society on Addictions 1988 Standards of addictions practice. American Nurses' Association, Kansas City, Missouri

Anderson J 1988 Coming to terms with mastectomy. Nursing Times 84(43): 41–44

Anderson M, Smereck G 1989 Personalized nursing light model. Nursing Science Quarterly 2(3): 120–130

Anderson P 1987 Early intervention in general practice. In: Stockwell T, Clement S (eds) Helping the problem drinker. Croom Helm, London, pp 61–62

Anderson P 1990 Management of drinking problems. WHO Regional Publications, European Series, 32, WHO, Geneva

Andrews I, McIntosh V 1992 Patients' charter, standards, respect for religions and cultural beliefs. AM Enterprises, London

Andrews S 1988 An expert in practice. Nursing Times 84(26): 31–32

ANSA 1997a Substance use – guidance on good clinical practice for nurses, midwives and health visitors. Working with alcohol and drug users. Association of Nurses in Substance Abuse, London

ANSA 1997b Substance use – guidance on good clinical practice for nurses, midwives and health visitors. Working within primary health care teams. Association of Nurses in Substance Abuse, London

ANSA 1997c Substance use – guidance on good clinical practice for nurses, midwives and health visitors. Working with children and young people. Association of Nurses in Substance Abuse, London

Arena D M, Page N 1992 The impostor phenomenon in the clinical nurse specialist. Image: the Journal of Nursing Scholarship 24(2): 121–125

Asen K E, Tomson P 1992 Family solutions in family practice. Quay Publishing, Lancaster

Ashworth P D, Longmaate M A, Morrison P 1992 Patient participation: its meaning and significance in the context of caring. Journal of Advanced Nursing 17: 1430–1439

Association of Cancer Physicians 1994 Review of the pattern of cancer services in England and Wales. Southampton General Hospital, Southampton

Atherton D 1994 Eczema in childhood: the facts. Oxford University Press, Oxford

Atwell J D, Gow M A 1985 Paediatric trained district nurse in the community: expensive luxury or economic necessity? British Medical Journal 291(6489): 227–229

Audit Commission 1993 Children first: a study of hospital services. HMSO, London

Austoker J 1994 Cancer prevention: setting the scene. BMJ 308: 1415–1420

Babor T F, Ritson E M, Hodgson R J 1986 Alcohol related problems in primary health care setting: a review of early intervention strategies. British Journal of Addiction 81: 23–46

Bailey J, MacCulloch M 1992 Characteristics of 112 cases discharged directly to the community from a new special hospital and some comparisons of performance. Journal of Forensic Psychiatry 3(1): 91–112

Bank-Mikkelson N E 1969 A metropolitan area in Denmark, Copenhagen. In: Kurgel R, Wolfensberger W (eds) Changing patterns in residential services for the mentally retarded. President's Committee on Mental Retardation, Washington

Baron R A, Byrne D 1991 Social psychology. Understanding human interaction, 6th edn. Allyn and Bacon, Boston

Barr O 1995 Normalisation. What it means in practice. British Journal of Nursing 2(2): 90–94

Barr O 1997 Interventions in a family context. In: Gates B (ed) Learning disabilities. A handbook of care, 3rd edn. Churchill Livingstone, Edinburgh

Bates B 1970 Doctor and nurse: changing roles and relations. New England Journal of Medicine 283: 129–134

Beardsmore S, Alder S 1994 Terminal care at home – the practical issues. In: Hill L (ed) Caring for dying children and their families. Chapman & Hall, London

Beattie A 1991 Knowledge and control in health promotion. In: Gale J, Calnan M, Bury M (eds) The sociology of health service. Routledge, London, pp 162–202

Beedham H, Wilson-Barnett J 1995 HIV and AIDS care: consumers view on needs and services. Journal of Advanced Nursing 22: 667–686

Belbin R M 1993 Team roles at work. Butterworth Heinemann, London

Bendall E, Raybould E 1969 A history of the GNC for England and Wales 1919–1969. Lewis, London

Benner P 1984 From novice to expert: excellence and power in clinical nursing practice. Addison-Wesley, Menlo Park

Beresford B 1995 Expert opinions: a national survey of parents caring for a severely disabled child (on behalf of the Joseph Rowntree Foundation). Policy Press, Bristol

Bien T H, Miller W R, Tonnigan J S 1993 Brief intervention for alcohol problems: a review. Addiction 88: 315–336

Billingham K, Boyd M 1996 Developing clinical expertise in community nursing. In: Gastrell P, Edwards J (eds) Community health care nursing, Baillière Tindall, ch 4.1

Bishop A H, Scudder J R 1990 The practical moral and personal sense of nursing: a phenomenological philosophy. State University of New York Press, Albany

Bisson J I, Cullum M 1994 Group therapy for bereaved children. Association for Child Psychology and Psychiatric Review and Newsletter 16: 3

Bjorck-Akesson E, Granlund M 1995 Family involvement in assessment and intervention: perceptions of professionals and parents in Sweden. Exceptional Children 61(6): 520–535

Black Sir Douglas (Chair) 1980 Inequalities in health: report of a research working group. DHSS, London

Black D 1996 Childhood bereavement. Distress and long-term sequelae can be lessened by early intervention. BMJ 312: 1496

Black K 1991 Campaigning against head lice in schools. Midwife Health Visitor and Community Nurse 27(1): 14

Black N 1992 The relationship between evaluative research and audit. Journal of Public Health Medicine 14(4): 361–366

Black P A 1995 Acne vulgaris. Professional Nurse 11(3): 181–183

Black S, Simon R 1980 The specialist nurse, support care and the elderly mentally infirm. Nursing Times, Community Outlook (Feb 14): 45–46

Blair G 1995 Starting to manage: the essential skills. Chartwell-Pratt, London

Bloom-Cooper L (Chair) 1992 Report of the Committee of Inquiry into Complaints About Ashworth Hospital. Command Report 2028-1. HMSO, London

Bloom-Cooper L, Haly H, Murphy M 1995 The falling shadow: one patient's mental health care 1978–1993. Duckworth, London

Boettcher M, Schiller R 1990 The use of a multidisciplinary group meeting for families of critically ill trauma patients. Intensive Care Nursing 6: 129–137

Bond S 1982 Communications in cancer nursing. In: Cahoon M (ed) Cancer nursing. Churchill Livingstone, Edinburgh

Bone M, Meltzer H 1989 The prevalence of disability among children. OPCS surveys of disability in Great Britain. HMSO, London

Boore J R 1996 Post-graduate education in nursing: a case study. Journal of Advanced Nursing 23(3): 620–629

Booth R 1992 Working for patients: further implications for nurse education. Nurse Education Today 12: 243–251

Borg L 1997 Pharmacological therapies for substance dependence. Current Opinion in Psychiatry 10(3): 225–229

Boseley S 1997 'Super' head lice beat the lotion. The Guardian, December 8, p 8

Bouley G, VonHofe K, Blatt L 1994 Holistic care of the critically ill: meeting both patient and family needs. Dimensions of Critical Care 13(4): 218–222

Bousfield C 1997 A phenomenological investigation into the role of the clinical nurse specialist. Journal of Advanced Nursing 25: 245–246

Bowey D, Caballero C 1996 A lead role. Nursing Times 92(30): 29–31

Bowlby J 1951 Maternal care and mental health. Monograph series, number 2. World Heath Organization, Geneva

Box J 1993 A family affair. Nursing Times 89(39): 38–39

Bradshaw A 1996 The legacy of Nightingale. Nursing Times 92(6)

Braye S, Preston-Shoot M 1995 Empowering practice in social care. Open University Press, Buckingham

Brett T 1987 A unit for psychopathic patients in Broadmoor Hospital. Medicine Science and Law 27(1): 21–31

Brett T 1991 The Woodstock approach: one ward in Broadmoor Hospital for the treatment of personality disorder. Criminal Behaviour and Mental Health 2: 152–158

Brett T 1992 The Woodstock approach: one ward in Broadmoor Hospital for the treatment of personality disorders. Critical Behaviour and Mental Health 2: 152–158

Breyer J, Kunin H, Kalish L, Patenaude A 1993 The adjustment to siblings and paediatric cancer patients – a sibling and parent perspective. Psycho-Oncology 2(3): 201–208

Briggs M 1997 Developing nursing roles. Nursing Standard 11(36): 49–53

British Market Research Bureau 1987 Everyday health care: a consumer study of self-medications in Great Britain. The British Market Research Bureau, London

British Paediatric Association 1991 Towards a combined child health service. BPA, London

British Paediatric Association 1993 Flexible options for paediatric care: a discussion document. BPA, London

British Paediatric Association 1995 Health needs of school age children. BPA, London

Brocklehurst N 1995 Specialist for sale. Primary Health Care 5(9): 8, 10, 12

Brook E 1986 Mental health and welfare rights: network directory. University of Birmingham, Birmingham

Brown H, Smith H (eds) 1992 Normalisation. A reader for the nineties. Routledge, London

Brown J 1990 Nurse training and education in mental handicap. An action plan. University of York, York

Brown J 1994 Analysis of responses to the consensus statement. University of York, York

Brown R 1995 Education for specialists and advanced practice. British Journal of Nursing 4(5): 266–268

Brown S 1992 Profession in teams. In: Thompson T, Mathais P (eds) Standards and mental handicap, keys to competence. Baillière Tindall, London, pp 371–385

Bullus S 1997 Childhood eczema: community care. Nursing Standard 12(6): 49–54

Burke L 1995 The new nursing teacher. Nursing Management 2(3): 24–26

Burke L 1997 Putting Working Paper 10 into practice: education and training. British Journal of Nursing 6(14): 817–823

Burke-Masters B 1986 The autonomous nurse practitioner: an answer to a chronic problem of primary care. Lancet 1266

Burnard P, Morrison P 1992 Aspects of forensic psychiatric nursing. Avebury Press, Aldershot

Burns N 1982 Nursing and cancer. Cancer beliefs, social expectations and health care. W B Saunders, Philadelphia

Burr S, Gradwell C 1996 The psychosocial effects of skin diseases: need for support groups. British Journal of Nursing 5(19): 1177–1182

Burrow S 1991 The special hospital nurse and the dilemma of therapeutic custody. Journal of Advances in Health and Nursing Care 1(3): 21–38

Burrow S 1992 The deliberate self-harming behaviour of patients within a British special hospital. Journal of Advanced Nursing 17: 138–18

Burrow S 1993 An outline of the forensic nursing role. British Journal of Nursing 2(18): 899–904

Busen N, Engleman S 1996 The CNS with practitioner preparation: an emerging role in advanced practice nursing. Clinical Nurse Specialist 10(3): 145–150

Butler K, Carr S, Sullivan F 1988 Citizen advocacy: a powerful partnership. National Citizen Advocacy, London

Butler L 1997 Effective campaigns for skin cancer prevention. British Journal of Dermatology Nursing 1(2): 10–12

Cain P, Hyde V, Howkins E 1995 Community nursing – dimensions and dilemmas. Arnold, London

Caine R M 1989 Families in crisis: making the critical difference. Focus on Critical Care 16(3): 184–189

Calkin J D 1984 A model for advanced nursing practice. Journal of Nursing Administration 14(1): 24–30

Callum C, Johnson K, Killoran A 1992 The smoking epidemic: a manifesto for action in England. Health Education Authority, London

Cancer Relief Macmillan Fund 1988 Published articles and knowledge of cancer in the UK. Cancer Relief Macmillan Fund, London

Cancer Relief Macmillan Fund 1994 Minimum standard of care for breast cancer. CRFN, London

Cancer Research Campaign 1994 Malignant melanoma factsheet 1994. CRC Promotions, London

Cancer Research Campaign 1995 Factsheet 22. CRC Promotions, London 1

Carlisle D 1990 Prisoners of the system. Nursing Times 86(47): 1–17

Carmichael A J 1995 Achieving an accessible dermatology service. Dermatology in Practice (Sept/Oct) 3(5): 13–16

Carper B A 1992 Fundamental patterns of knowing in nursing. In: Nicholl L H (ed) Perspectives on nursing theory. Lippincott, London

Carrier J, Kendall I 1995 Professionalism and interprofessionalism in health and community care: some theoretical issues. In: Owens P, Carrier J, Horder J (eds) Interprofessional issues in community and primary health care. Macmillan, London, pp 9–36

Carter Y, Thomas C 1997 Research methods in primary care. Radcliffe Medical Press, Oxford

Carton G 1991 Reducing violence in special hospital. Nursing Standard 5(17): 29

Casey A 1988 A partnership with child and family. Senior Nurse 8(4): 8–9

Casey A 1995 Partnership nursing: influences on involvement of informal carers. Journal of Advanced Nursing 22: 1058–1062

Casey N 1996 Editorial. Nursing Standard 10(43): 1

Cash C, Compston H, Grant J, Livesley J, McAndrew P, Williams G 1994 The preparation of sick children's nurses to work in the community (P2000 evaluation). English National Board, London

Castledine G 1983 The nurse for the job. Nursing Mirror (January 19): 63

Castledine G 1986 Clinical nurse specialists. Nursing Practice 1: 213–214

Castledine G 1991a The advanced nurse practitioner – Part 1. Nursing Standard 5(43): 34–36

Castledine G 1991b The advanced nurse practitioner – Part 2. Nursing Standard 5(44): 33–35

Castledine G 1992 The advanced practitioner. Nursing 5(7): 14–15

Castledine G 1993 Nurse practitioner title: ambiguous and misleading. British Journal of Nursing 2(14): 734–735

Castledine G 1995a Defining specialist nursing. British Journal of Nursing 4(5): 264–265

Castledine G 1995b Will the nurse practitioner be a mini-doctor or a maxi-nurse? British Journal of Nursing 4(16): 938–939

Castledine G 1996a Clarifying and defining nursing role developments. British Journal of Nursing 5(21): 1338

Castledine G 1996b The role and criteria of an advanced nurse practitioner. British Journal of Nursing 5(5): 288–289

Castledine G 1997 Framework for a clinical career structure in nursing. British Journal of Nursing 6(5): 264–271

Chaloner C, Kinsella C 1992 Caring with conviction. Nursing Times 88(17): 50–52

Chaloner C et al 1993 An alternative to seclusion? Nursing Times 89(18): 62–64

Champion R 1991 Educational accountability – what ho the 1990s. Nurse Education Today 11: 407–414

Champion R H, Burton J L, Ebling F J G 1992 Textbook of dermatology, 5th edn. Blackwell Scientific Publications, Oxford

Chapman C 1983 The paradox of nursing. Journal of Advanced Nursing 8: 269–272

Chappell A L 1992 Towards a sociological critique of the normalisation principle. Disability, Handicap and Society 7(1): 35–51

Chavez C W, Faber L 1987 Effect of an education orientation program on family members who visit their significant other in the intensive care unit. Heart and Lung 16(1): 92–99

Citizens' Advice Bureau 1985 Inside advice: the work of the CAB at Tooting Bec Hospital. CAB, London

Clare M 1997 My advice to patients with hand dermatitis. British Journal of Dermatology Nursing 1(4): 6–7

Clark D H 1958 A brief history of Fulbourn Hospital (unpublished). Fulbourn Hospital, London

Cleary J 1992 Caring for children in hospital: parents and nurses in partnership. Scutari Press, London

Clifton M, Brown J, Shaw I 1993 Learning disabilities and the specialist nurse. Targets for action. University of York, York

Clochesy M J, Breu C, Cardin S, Ruby B E, Whittaker A A 1993 Critical care nursing. W B Saunders, Philadelphia

Clore E R 1995 Natural and artificial tanning. Journal of Paediatric Health Care 9(3): 103–108

Cluzeau F, Littlejohns P, Grimshaw J, Hopkins A 1995 Appraising clinical guidelines and the development of criteria – a pilot study. Journal of Interprofessional Care 3: 227–235

Cluzeau F, Littlejohns P, Grimshaw J, Feder G P 1997 Appraisal instrument for clinical guidelines. St George's Hospital Medical School, London

Cochrane A 1972 Effectiveness and efficiency. Nuffield Provincial Hospitals Trust, London

Cochrane A 1989 Effectiveness and efficiency: Random reflections on health services. Cambridge University Press, Cambridge

Cohen D 1981 Broadmoor. Psychology News Press, London

Cohen P 1994 The loss adjusters. Nursing Times 90(9): 14–15

Cole A 1991 Advance to go? Nursing Times 87(7): 48–49

Community Care Act 1990 HMSO, London

Conroy M, Shannon W 1995 Clinical guidelines: their implementation in general practice. British Journal of General Practice 45: 371–375

Cook R 1998 Treatment of head lice. Nursing Standard 12(19): 49–55

Cooke D J 1989 Containing violent prisoners. An analysis of the Barlinnie Special Unit. British Journal of Criminology 29: 129–143

Cooper D B 1995 Habit-forming questions. Nursing Times 91(44): 36–37

Cooper D B 1997 Alcohol and alcohol problems. In: Hussein R G, Gafoor M (eds) Addiction nursing: perspectives on professional and clinical practice. Stanley Thornes, Cheltenham, ch 6, pp 57–65

Cooper M C 1988 Conventional relationships: grounding for the nursing ethic. Advances in Nursing Science 10(4): 48–59

Cordall J, Phipps R 1986 The changing face of Rampton. Nursing Times 82(3): 42–43

Cotterill J, Cunliffe W 1997 Suicide in dermatological patients. British Journal of Dermatology 137: 246–250

Cotton T, Locker A, Jackson L, Blamey R, Morgan I 1991 A prospective study of patient choice in treatment for primary breast cancer. European Journal of Surgical Oncology 17: 115–117

Couldrick A 1993 'Do you mean that Mummy is going to die?' Caring for bereaved children. Professional Nurse: 186–189

Couriel J, Davies P 1988 Costs and benefits of a community special care baby service. British Medical Journal 296(6628): 1043–1046

Coutu-Wakulczyk C G, Chartier L 1990 French validation of the critical care family needs inventory. Heart and Lung 19(2): 192–196

Cowe F 1996 Living wills: making patients' wishes known. Professional Nurse 11(6)

Cowley S, Casey A 1995 The language of community nursing. In: Littlewood J (ed) Current issues in community nursing: primary health care in practice. Churchill Livingstone, Edinburgh

Cox N, Walton Y, Bowman K 1995 Evaluation of nurse prescribing in a dermatology unit. British Journal of Dermatology 133: 340–341

Cranford R E 1995 Withdrawing artificial feeding from children with brain damage. British Medical Journal 311: 464–465

Cray L 1989 Initiating a family intervention program in a medical intensive care unit. Focus on Critical Care 16(3): 212–218

Crombie I 1996 The pocket guide to critical appraisal. BMJ Publishing Group, London

Crowther A G O 1996 Ethical issues. In: Hancock B (ed) Cancer care in the community. Radcliffe Medical Press, Oxford

Cullen C 1991 Caring for people. Community care in the next decade and beyond. Mental Handicap Nursing. HMSO, London

Cullum N 1994 The nursing management of leg ulcers in the community: a critical review of research. University of Liverpool, Liverpool

Curley W, Wallace J 1992 Effects of the nursing mutual participation model of care on parental stress in the pediatric intensive care unit – a replication. Journal of Pediatric Nursing 7(6): 377–385

Dale N 1996 Working with families of children with special needs. Partnership and practice. Routledge, London

Daley L 1984 The perceived immediate needs of families with relatives in the intensive care setting. Heart and Lung 13: 231–237

Dalley G 1992 Social welfare ideologies and normalisation: links and conflicts. In: Brown H, Smith H (eds) Normalisation. A reader for the nineties. Routledge, London, pp 100–111

Damant M, Martin C, Oppenshaw S 1994 Practice nursing: stability and change. Mosby, London

Darbyshire P 1994 Living with a sick child in hospital: the experiences of parents and nurses. Chapman & Hall, London.

Darke S, Swift W, Hall W, Ross M 1993 Drug use, HIV risk-taking and psychosocial correlates of benzodiazepine use among methadone maintenance clients. Drug and Alcohol Dependence 34, 67–70

David T, Boulton M, Olson A 1985 Meetings between experts, an approach to sharing ideas in medical consultations. Tavistock Publications, London, pp 173–178

Davies B, Hughes A M 1995 Clarification of advanced nursing practice: characteristics and competencies. Clinical Nurse Specialist 9(3): 156–160

Davis A, Hayton C 1986 Who benefits? The Rubery Hill Benefits Project. University of Birmingham, Birmingham

Davis B D 1993 An international approach to masters-level preparation for clinical nurse specialists. Journal of Advanced Nursing 18: 1429–1433

Davis B, Burnard P 1992 Academic levels in nursing. Journal of Advanced Nursing 17: 1395–1400

Davis-Martin S 1994 Perceived needs of families of long-term critical care patients: a brief report. Heart and Lung 23(6): 515–518

Dawkes K 1997 How to … treat scalp psoriasis. British Journal of Dermatology Nursing 1(1): 8–9

Deighan M, Boyd K 1996 Defining evidence based health care: a health care learning strategy. NT Research 1(5): 332–339

Department of Employment 1990 Employment Gazette, August 1990. London

Department of Health 1989a Education and training: Working Paper 10. HMSO, London

Department of Health 1989b Working for patients. Cm555. HMSO, London

Department of Health 1989c A strategy for nursing. HMSO, London

Department of Health 1991a The patient's charter: raising the standard. HMSO, London

Department of Health 1991b Welfare of children and young people in hospital. HMSO, London

Department of Health 1992a Citizen's charter. Cmnd 1599. HMSO, London

Department of Health 1992b The health of the nation: a strategy for health in England. HMSO, London

Department of Health 1993a The health of the nation key area handbook: cancers. DoH, London

Department of Health 1993b New world new opportunities. HMSO, London

Department of Health 1994a The challenges for nursing and midwifery in the 21st century – the Heathrow Report. HMSO, London

Department of Health 1994b Working in partnerships. HMSO, London

Department of Health 1994c Quality in cervical screening programme, EL (94) 33. DoH, London

Department of Health 1994d Nursing, midwifery and health visiting education: a statement of strategic intent. HMSO, London

Department of Health 1995a Circular (EL(95)114). HMSO, London

Department of Health 1995b Fit for the future: second progress report on the health of the nation. HMSO, London

Department of Health 1995c The health of the nation. A strategy for people with learning disabilities. HMSO, London

Department of Health 1996a Report of an independent review of drug treatment services in England. HMSO, London

Department of Health 1996b Primary care, delivering the future. HMSO, London

Department of Health 1997 The new NHS: modern, dependable. HMSO, London

Department of Health 1998a The new NHS. HMSO, London

Department of Health 1998b Our healthier nation – green paper. HMSO, London

Department of Health and Home Office 1992 Review of health and social services for mentally disordered offenders and others requiring similar services. Reed Committee Report. HMSO, London

Department of Health and Social Security 1974a Revised report of the working party on security in NHS hospitals. HMSO, London

Department of Health and Social Security 1974b Report of Committee of Inquiry into Pay and Conditions of Service of Nurses and Midwives. HMSO, London

Department of Health and Social Security 1976 Fit for the future. The report of the Committee on Child Health Services. (Chairman SDM Court). HMSO, London

Department of Health and Social Security 1979 Report of the Royal Commission on the National Health Service. HMSO, London

Department of Health and Social Security 1983 Mental Health Act. HMSO, London

Department of Health and Social Security 1984 Confidentiality of personal health information. DHSS circular DA (P4)25 + enclosures. DHSS, London

Department of Health and Social Security 1985 Data Protection Act: subject access to personal health information. DHSS DA(85) 23. DHSS, London

Department of Health and Social Security 1985 Local Government (Access to Information Act). HMSO, London

Department of Health and Social Security 1986a Neighbourhood nursing – a focus for care. Report of the Community Nursing Review. (Chair Cumberledge J) HMSO, London

Department of Health and Social Security 1986b Disabled Persons (Services, Consultation and Representation) Act. HMSO, London

Department of Health and Social Services 1991 Personal Health and Social Services (NI) Order. HMSO, London

Department of Health and Social Services for Northern Ireland 1991 People first. DHSS, Belfast

Department of Health and Social Services for Northern Ireland 1995 Review of policy for people with a learning disability. DHSS, Belfast

Department of Health and Welsh Office 1983 Code of practice, Mental Health Act 1983. HMSO, London

Department of Health, Nursing Division 1989 A strategy for nursing. HMSO, London

Department of Health, Special Hospitals Service Authority and the Central Office of Information 1989 Starting afresh. HMSO, London

Department of Health, Special Hospitals Service Authority 1992 Report of the Committee of Inquiry into Complaints about Ashworth Hospital. Cmnd 2028-1. HMSO, London

Department of Health Statistical Bulletin 1994 Drug misuse statistics for the six months ending 31st March 1993: England. Government Statistical Service, London

Department of Social Security 1994 Social security statistics 1994. HMSO, London

Disabled Persons Act 1995 HMSO, London

Disabled Persons (Services, Consultation and Representation) Act. HMSO, London

Douglas J W B 1975 Early hospital admission and later disturbance of behaviour and learning. Developmental Medicine and Child Neurology 17: 456–480

Dowling S, Barrett S, West R 1995 With nurse practitioners, who needs house officers? British Medical Journal 311: 309–313

Dowling S, Martin R, Skidmore P, Doyal L, Cameron A, Lloyd S 1996 Nurses taking on junior doctors' work: a confusion of accountability. British Medical Journal 312: 1211–1214

Dracup K 1993 Foreword. In: Clochesy M J, Breu C, Cardin S, Ruby B E, Whittaker A A (eds) Critical care nursing. W B Saunders, Philadelphia

Drummond D C, Edwards G 1990 Specialist versus general practitioner treatment of problem drinkers. Lancet 336: 915–918

Drummond D C, Tiffany S T, Glautier S, Remington B 1995 Addictive behaviour: cue exposure theory and practice. John Wiley, Chichester

Dryden S 1989 Care in the community. Paediatric Nursing 1(7): 19–20

du Boulay S 1984 Cicely Saunders – the founder of the modern hospice movement. Hodder and Stoughton, London

Dulfer S 1981 Danger: specialists at work. Journal of Community Nursing 5(1): 2

Dulfer S 1992 No holds barred. Nursing 5(4): 20–22

Duncan C 1997 Bug busters. Nursing Times 93(49): 46–47

Dunnell K, Cartwright A 1972 Medicine takers, prescribers and hoarders. Report of the Institute of Social Studies in Medical Care. Routledge and Kegan Paul, London

Dyck A, Fletcher J 1973 To live and to die: when, why and how. In: Williams R H (ed) Springer-Verlag, New York, pp 98–122

Dyer B 1996 Seeming parted. New Millennium, London

Dyregrov A 1994 Childhood bereavement: consequences for therapeutic approaches. Association for Child Psychology and Psychiatric Review and Newsletter 16(4)

Dyson J 1992 The importance of practice. Nursing Times 88(40): 44–46

Edwards V 1997 Dermatology care and the practice nurse – a primary role. British Journal of Dermatology Nursing 1(2): 5–7

Elgart M L 1993 Scabies: diagnosis and treatment. Dermatology Nursing 5(6): 464–467

Elliot B E, Luker K 1997 The experiences of mothers caring for a child with severe atopic eczema. Journal of Clinical Nursing 6: 241–247

Elsdon R 1995 Spiritual pain in dying people: the nurse's role. Professional Nurse 10(10)

Emerson E 1992 What is normalisation? In: Brown H, Smith H (eds) Normalisation. A reader for the nineties. Routledge, London, pp 1–18

Emmet E A 1984 The skin and occupational disease. Archives of Environmental Health 39: 144–149

English National Board for Nursing, Midwifery and Health Visiting 1990 Regulations and guidelines for the approval of institutions and courses 1990. ENB, London

English National Board for Nursing, Midwifery and Health Visiting 1995a Creating life-long learners. Guidelines for programmes leading to the qualification of Specialist Practitioner. ENB, London

English National Board for Nursing, Midwifery and Health Visiting 1995b Training needs analysis. ENB, London

English National Board for Nursing, Midwifery and Health Visiting 1996a Substance use and misuse: guidelines for good practice in education and training of nurses, midwives and health visitors. ENB, London

English National Board for Nursing, Midwifery and Health Visiting 1996b Annual report. ENB, London

English National Board for Nursing, Midwifery and Health Visiting 1996c Making it happen. ENB, London

English National Board for Nursing, Midwifery and Health Visiting 1997 Report on practice placement monitoring: children's nursing. ENB, London

Ennis B J, Emery R D 1978 The rights of mental patients. Avon Books, New York

Enthoven A 1991 National Health Service market reform. Health Affairs 10(3): 60–70

Ersser S J 1997 Dermatology nursing literature and the future of dermatology nursing. British Journal of Dermatology Nursing 1(4): 4–5

Ersser S J 1998 Annotated bibliography of the dermatological nursing literature. Oxford Brookes University, Oxford

Evershed S 1991 Special unit, C Wing, HMP Parkhurst. In: Herbst K, Gunn J (eds) The mentally disordered offender. Butterworth Heinemann, Oxford, pp 88–95

Expert Advisory Group on Cancer 1994 A policy framework for commissioning cancer services: Report by the Expert Advisory Group on Cancer to the Chief Medical Officer of England and Wales. EAGC, London

Fallowfield L, Roberts R 1992 Cancer counselling in the United Kingdom. Psychology and Health 6: 107–117

Faulkner A 1980 The student nurse role in giving information to patients. Steinberg Collections, RCN, London

Faulkner A 1996 Communicating with patients and relatives. In: Hancock B (ed) Cancer in the community. Radcliffe Medical Press, Oxford

Faulkner A, Maguire P 1994 Talking to cancer patients and their relatives. Oxford Medical Publications, Oxford

Fincham Gee 1992 A healthy skin: not as common as you think. RCN update. Nursing Standard 6(10): 9–14

Finlay A Y, Khan G K 1994 Dermatology life quality (DLQ1): a simple practical measure for routine clinical use. Clinical and Experimental Dermatology 19: 210–216

Firth P, Anderson P 1994 Teamwork with families facing bereavement. European Journal of Palliative Care 1(4)

Fitzpatrick J J, Kerr M E, Saba V K et al 1989 Translating nursing diagnosis into ICD code. American Journal of Nursing (April): 493–495

Flannagan 1954 The critical incident technique. Psychological Bulletin 51: 327–358

Forrester A D, Murphy P A, Price D M, Monaghan J F 1990 Critical care family needs: nurse–family member confederate pairs. Heart and Lung 19(6): 655–661

Forsdyke H, Watts J 1994 Skin care in atopic eczema. Professional Nurse 10(1): 36–40

Foundation of Nursing Studies 1996 Reflection for action – putting research into action. FNS, London

Fowkes F G R, Fulton P M 1991 Critical appraisal of published research: introductory guidelines. British Medical Journal 302: 1136–1140

Fox P 1995 Nursing developments: trust nurses' views. Nursing Standard 9(18): 30–34

Freichels A T 1991 Needs of family members of patients in the intensive care unit over time. Critical Care Nursing Quarterly 14(3): 16–29

Freismuth A C 1986 Meeting the needs of families of critically ill patients: a comparison of visiting policies in the intensive care setting. Heart and Lung 15(3): 309–310

Frick S, Pollock S 1993 Preparation for advanced nursing practice. Nursing and Health Care 14(4): 190–195

Friedman B D 1980 Coping with cancer: a guide for health care professionals. Cancer Nursing 3(2): 105–110

Friend B 1991 View from the top. Nursing Times 87(8): 24–25

Frost J 1994 Complementary treatments for eczema in children. Professional Nurse 9(5): 330–332

Fuller F B, Foster M G 1982 The effects of family/friend visits vs staff interaction on stress/arousal of surgical intensive care patients. Heart and Lung 11(5): 457–463

Gadow J 1983 Clinical subjectivity – advocacy for silent patients. Nursing Clinics of North America 24(2): 535–541

Gafoor M 1997a Polydrug users and nursing interventions. In: Hussein R G, Gafoor M (eds) Addiction nursing: perspectives on professional and clinical practice. Stanley Thornes, Cheltenham, ch 4, pp 36–44

Gafoor M 1997b Development of the role of the specialist nurse in substance misuse. Psychiatric Care 4(3): 132–134

Gates B 1994 Advocacy: a nurses' guide. Scutari Press, London

Gates B 1997 The nature of learning disability. In: Gates B, Beacock C (eds) Dimensions of learning disability. Baillière Tindall, London, pp 3–28

General Nursing Council 1957 Syllabus … for the certificate of mental nursing. GNC, London

General Nursing Council 1970 Syllabus … for the certificate of mental subnormality. GNC, London

General Nursing Council 1976 Syllabus … for the certificate in mental nursing. GNC, London

Ghodse A H 1995 Drugs and addictive behaviour: a guide to treatment, 2nd edn. Blackwell Scientific Publications, Oxford

Ghodse A H, Kelly S, Priestley J, Saunders V 1994 Addiction prevention in primary care. Annual report 1992–1993. Centre for Addiction Studies,

Department of Addictive Behaviour, St George's Hospital Medical School, University of London, London

Ghodse A H, McShane E, Priestley J S, Saunders V J 1996 Addiction prevention in primary care programme review. Department of Psychiatry of Addictive Behaviour, St George's Hospital Medical School, University of London, London

Gibbon B, Luker K 1995 Uncharted territory: masters preparation as a foundation for nurse clinicians. Nurse Education Today 15: 164–169

Gibson C 1991 A concept analysis of empowerment. Journal of Advanced Nursing 16(3): 354–361

Gibson C 1995 The process of empowerment in mothers of chronically ill children. Journal of Advanced Nursing 21(6): 1201–1210

Gibson J R 1997 Azelaic acid 20% cream and the medical management of acne vulgaris. Dermatology Nursing 9(5): 339–344

Gilbert T 1993 Learning disability nursing: from normalisation to materialism – towards a new paradigm. Journal of Advanced Nursing 18(5): 1604–1609

Gill A B 1993 Organ donation. In: Boggs RL, Wooldridge-King M (eds) AACN procedure manual for critical care, 3rd edn. W B Saunders, Philadelphia

Gilliss C L 1996 Education for advanced practice nursing. In: Hickey J V, Ouimette R, Venegoni S L (eds) Advanced practice nursing: changing roles and clinical applications. Lippincott, Philadelphia, ch 2

Glasman 1991

Glatt M 1955 A treatment centre for alcoholics in a public mental hospital: its establishment and its working. British Journal of Addiction 52: 55–89

Glover M 1998 The increased incidence of skin cancer in organ transplant recipients. Dermatology in Practice 6(1): 6–8

Godfrey C 1992 Alcohol in the workplace – a costly problem. Alcoholism. Centre for Health Economics, University of York, York, p 3

Godfrey C, Maynard A 1992 A health strategy for alcohol. Centre for Health Economics, University of York, York

Goding L 1997 Intuition and health visiting practice. British Journal of Community Health Nursing 2(4): 174–182

Goffman E 1961 Asylums. Pelican, Harmondsworth

Goffman E 1963 Stigma: notes on the management of spoiled identity. Prentice Hall, Englewood Cliffs NJ

Goodwin S 1992 Community nursing and the new public health. Health Visitor 65(3): 78–80

Gow M A, Ridgway G 1993 The development of a paediatric community nursing service. In: Glasper E A, Tucker A (eds) Advances in child health nursing. Scutari Press, London

Grant M, Hodgson R 1991 Responding to drug and alcohol problems in the community. World Health Organization, Geneva

Graves D, Nash A 1991 Macmillan nurse perceptions. Journal of District Nursing 10(1): 4–6

Gray W J 1974 Grendon Prison. British Journal of Hospital Medicine 12: 299–308

Green S 1985 Cancer: psychiatric aspects. In: Grossman G (ed) Advances in psychiatric care. Churchill Livingstone, Edinburgh

Greenhalgh L 1994 Well aware. Improving access to health information for people with learning difficulties. Milton Keynes General NHS Trust, Milton Keynes

Greer S 1984 Cancer: psychiatric aspects. In: Grossman G (ed) Advances in psychiatric aspects. Churchill Livingstone, Edinburgh

Griffiths J, Luker K 1994 Community nurse attitudes to the clinical nurse specialist. Nursing Times 90(17): 39–42

Griffiths P, Evans A 1995 Evaluating a nursing-led in-patient service. An interim report. King's Fund Centre, London

Gudjonsson G, Tibbles P 1983 Behaviour modification in an interim secure unit. Nursing Times 79(15): 25–27

Gunn J, Maden A, Swinton S 1991 Treatment needs of prisoners with psychiatric disorders. British Medical Journal 30: 338–341

Guzzo C 1997 Recent advances in the treatment of psoriasis. Dermatologic Clinics 15(1): 59–68

Hadley R, Clough R 1996 Care in chaos. Frustration and challenge in community care. Cassell, London

Hagemaster J, Handley S, Plumlee A, Sullivan E, Stanley S 1993 Developing educational programmes for nurses that meet today's addiction challenges. Nurse Education Today 13(6): 421–425

Hall V, Russell O 1985 Community mental handicap nursing – the birth, growth and development of the idea. In: Sines D, Bicknell J (eds) Caring for mentally handicapped people in the community. Lippincott, London, pp 38–47

Halm M A, Titler M G 1990 Appropriateness of critical care visitation: perceptions of patients, families, nurses and physicians. Journal of Nursing Quality Assurance 5(1): 25–37

Hames A, Stirling E 1987 Choice aids recovery. Nursing Times 83(8): 49–51

Hamilton H, O'Byrne M, Nicholai L 1995 Central lines inserted by clinical nurse specialists. Nursing Times 91(17): 38–39

Hammersley R, Cassidy M T, Oliver J 1995 Drugs associated with drug-related deaths in Edinburgh and Glasgow, November 1990 to October 1992. Addiction 90: 959–965

Hammond F 1995 Involving families in care within the intensive care environment: a descriptive survey. Intensive and Critical Care Nursing 1: 256–264

Hammond J 1983 Behaviour modification at Rampton Hospital. Nursing Times 79(39): 49–52

Hamric A B, Taylor J W 1989 Role development of the CNS. In: Hamric A B, Spross J A (eds) The clinical nurse specialist in theory and practice, 2nd edn. W B Saunders, Philadelphia, ch 3

Hancock B (ed) 1996 Cancer care in the community. Radcliffe Medical Press, New York

Harrell J S, McCulloch S D 1986 The role of the clinical nurse specialist: problems and solutions. Journal of Administration 16(10): 44–48

Harris R 1990 The advocacy alliance – a first attempt in the UK. Department of Psychology, St George's Hospital Medical School, University of London, London

Hartshorn C J, Ebert D, Scott G, Weaver L 1993 Individual and family response to the critical care experience. In: Hartshorn J, Lamborn M, Noll L M (eds) Introduction to critical care nursing. W B Saunders, Philadelphia

Hartshorn J 1993 Introduction. In: Hartshorn J, Lamborn M, Noll L M (eds) Introduction to critical care nursing. W B Saunders, Philadelphia

Haste F, MacDonald L D 1992 The role of the specialist in community nursing: perceptions of specialists and district nurses. International Journal of Nursing Studies 29(1): 37–47

Hattersly J 1995 The survival of collaboration and co-operation. In: Malin N (ed) Services for people with learning disabilities. Routledge, London, pp 260–273

Hawket S 1995 Policy issues and provision of cancer services. In: Richardson J, Wilson-Barnett J (ed) Nursing research in cancer care. Scutari Press, London

Hay R J 1993 Fungi and skin disease. Gower Medical Publishing, London

Head S 1988 Nurse practitioners: the new pioneers. Nursing Times 84(26): 27–28

Health Advisory Service (HAS) 1996 Children and young peoples: substance misuse services, the substance of young needs. HMSO, London

Healy P 1996 President of the BMA condemns the idea of generic workforce as 'nonsense'. Nursing Standard 10(39): 7

Heffline M S 1992 Establishing the role of the specialist nurse in post-anaesthesia care. Journal of Post-Anaesthesia Nursing 7(50): 305–311

Heginbotham C et al 1994 The report of the independent panel of inquiry examining the case of Michael Robinson. North West London Mental Health Trust, London

Heimlich H J, Kutscher A H 1970 The family's reaction to terminal illness in loss and grief. In: Schoenbert B et al (eds) Psychological management in medical practice. Columbia University Press, New York

Heller D R 1994 Ambulatory paediatrics: stepping out in the right direction. Archives of Disease in Childhood 70(4): 339–342

Helman C G 1994 Culture health and illness, 3rd edn. Butterworth-Heinemann, Oxford

Henneman E, Cardin S 1992 Need for information, interventions for practice. Critical Care Nursing Clinics of North America 4(4): 615–621

Henneman E A, McKenzie J B, Dewa C S 1992 An evaluation of interventions for meeting the information needs of families of critically ill patients. American Journal of Critical Care 1(3): 85–93

Hennessy D 1995 A changing health requires a changing workforce. In: Littlewood J (ed) Current issues in community nursing, primary health care in practice. Churchill Livingstone, Edinburgh

Herd R M, Tidman M J, Hunter J A A et al 1994 The economic burden of atopic eczema: a community and hospital-based assessment. British Journal of Dermatology 131(suppl 44): 34

Hickey M, Lewandowski L 1988 Critical care nurse's role with families: a descriptive study. Heart and Lung 17(6): 670–676

Hicks L E M, Lewis D J 1995 Management of chronic, resistive scabies: a case study. Geriatric Nursing 16(5): 230–237

Hill J 1997 Patient satisfaction in a nurse-led rheumatology clinic. Journal of Advanced Nursing 25: 347–354

Hillis G 1993 Diverting tactics. Nursing Times 89(1): 4–7

Hirschfeld M 1998 WHO priorities for a common nursing research agenda. International Nursing Review 45(1): 13–14

Hixon M E 1996 Professional development: socialisation in advanced practice nursing. In: Hickey J V, Ouimette R, Venegoni S L (eds) Advanced practice nursing: changing roles and clinical applications. Lipincott, Philadelphia, ch 3

Holmes P 1991 The patient's friend. Nursing Times 87(19): 16–17

Holmes S 1994 Development of the cardiac surgeon assistant. British Journal of Nursing 3(5): 204–210

Home Office 1992 Provision for mentally disordered offenders. Circular 66/90 (unpublished)

Home Office and DHSS 1975 Report of the Committee on Abnormal Offenders. Command Report 6244. HMSO, London

Hornby G 1994 Counselling in child disability. Skills for working with parents. Chapman & Hall, London

Hornby S 1993 Collaborative care. Interprofessional, interagency, and interpersonal. Blackwell Scientific Publications, London

Hospital for Sick Children, Great Ormond Street 1874 Minutes of a special meeting of the Joint Committee of The Hospital for Sick Children. 18th March

Hospital Information Service 1994 1994 directory of hospice and palliative care service. St Christopher's Hospice, 51–59 Lawrie Park Road, London SE26 6DZ

Houle C 1980 Continuing learning in the professions. Jossey-Bass, London

Houlton E 1988 In: Tiffany R, Webb P (eds) Oncology for nurses and health care professionals, 2nd edn. Harper and Row, London

House of Commons 1763 Report of Select Committee into Conditions in Private Madhouses. HMSO, London

House of Commons Health Select Committee 1997 Health services for children and young people in the community: home and school (third report). The Stationery Office, London

House of Lords Select Committee on Medical Ethics 1994 House of Lords Official Report on Parliamentary Debates (Hansard) 554: 83, 1344–1412

Hudson B 1995 A seamless service? Developing better relationships between the National Health Service and social services departments. In: Philpot T, Ward L (eds) Values and visions. Changing ideas in services for people with learning difficulties. Butterworth Heinemann, Oxford, pp 106–122

Hughes J 1997 Reflections on a community children's nursing service. Paediatric Nursing 9(4): 21–23

Hughes S 1993 Meeting a need. Nursing Times 89(39): 36–37

Hunsberger M, Mitchell A, Blatz S et al 1992 Definition of an advanced nursing practice role in the NICU: the clinical nurse specialist/neonatal practitioner. Clinical Nurse Specialist 6(2): 91–96

Hunt J 1995 The paediatric oncology community nurse specialist: the influence of employment location and funders on models of practice. Journal of Advanced Nursing 22(1): 126–133

Hunter J A A, Savin J A, Dahl M V 1989 Clinical dermatology. Blackwell, Oxford

Hunter L 1992 Applying Orem to the skin. Nursing 5(4): 16–18

Hunter R, MacAlpine 1974 Psychiatry for the poor. Dawsons, London

Hussey T 1997 Efficiency and health nursing ethics 4(3): 181–190

Hyde V 1995 Community nursing: a unified discipline. In: Cain P, Hyde V, Hawkins E (eds) Community nursing: dimensions and dilemmas. Arnold, London, ch 1, pp 1–26

Institute for the Study of Drug Dependence 1995 Drug use in Britain 1994. ISDD, London

International Council of Nurses 1996 Better health through nursing research. ICN, Geneva

Jackson R N 1988 Perils of pseudonormalisation. Mental Handicap 16(4): 148–150

Jarrold K 1995 Education and training in the new NHS. EL (95) 27. DoH, London

Jarvis T J, Tebbutt J, Mattick R P 1995 Treatment approaches for alcohol and drug dependence: an introductory guide. John Wiley, Chichester, p 211

Jasper M A 1994 Expert: a discussion of the implications of the concept as used in nursing. Journal of Advanced Nursing 20: 7869–776

Jay M 1997 The White Paper recognises that nurses have a critical contribution to make. Nursing Times 93(51): 3

Jenkins J, Johnson B 1991 Community nursing learning disabilities survey. In: Kelly P (ed) The community mental handicap nurse, specialist practitioner in the 1990's. Mental Handicap Nurses Association, Penarth, pp 39–54

Jeyasingham M 1997 National Eczema Society – 21 years of patient support and advice. British Journal of Dermatology Nursing 1(1): 10–12

Jezewski, M A 1993 Culture brokering as a model for advocacy. Nursing and Health Care 14(2): 78–85

Jobling R 1978 With and without professional nurses – the case for dermatology. In: Dingwall R, Macintosh J (eds) Readings in the sociology of nursing. Churchill Livingstone, Edinburgh, pp 181–195

Joint Council for Clinical Oncology 1993 Reducing delay in cancer treatment. Royal College of Physicians, London

Jowett S, Ryan T J 1985 Skin disease and handicap: an analysis of the impact of skin conditions. Social Science and Medicine 20: 425–429

Kalisch B J 1975 Of half gods and mortals: aesculapian authority. Nursing
Outlook 23(1): 22–28

Karani D, Wilshaw E 1986 How well informed? Cancer Nursing 9(5): 238–242

Kay B, Rose S, Turnbull J 1995 Continuing the commitment. The report of the
Learning Disabilities Nursing Project. Department of Health, London *(Copies
of this document, the resource package, and 'Meeting needs through targeting skills'
are available free of charge from: Mr J Turnbull, Dept. of Health, Room G20,
Wellington House, 135–155 Waterloo Road, London SE1 8UG)*

Kay J, Gawkrodger D J, Mortimer M J et al 1994 The prevalence of childhood
atopic eczema in a general population. Journal of the American Academy of
Dermatology 30: 35–39

Keating A 1996 Shared care – a new concept? Substance Misuse Bulletin 9(3): 1–2

Kegal L M 1995 Advanced practice nurses can refine the management of heart
failure. Clinical Nurse Specialist 9(2): 76–81

Kendrick K 1995 Ethical pathways in cancer and palliative care. In: David J (ed)
Cancer care. Prevention, treatment and palliation. Marie Curie Cancer Care.
Chapman & Hall, London

Kennedy J, Faugier J 1989 Drug and alcohol dependency nursing. Heinemann
Nursing, Oxford

Kenning D, Blackmore A 1996 Promoting sun knowledge in schools. Health
Visitor 69(6): 236–237

Kessel J 1978 The pattern and the range of services for problem drinkers. Report
by the Advisory Committee on Alcoholism. DHSS, London

King J B 1982 The impact of patients' beliefs on the consultation, a theoretical
analysis. Paper presented to the Colloquium of the Consultant. CIBA
Foundation 15–19 March. MSD Foundation, London

Kirchhoff T K, Hansen B C, Evans P, Fullmer N 1985 Open visiting in the ICU: a
debate. Dimensions of Critical Care Nursing 4(5): 296–304

Kitchener N, Riach G, Robinson T 1992 Suicide policies in secure environments.
Nursing Standard 6(31): 37–40

Kitson A (ed) 1993 Nursing: art and science. Chapman & Hall, London

Kitson A 1997 Using evidence to demonstrate the value of nursing. Nursing
Standard 11 (28): 34–39

Kitzman H J 1989 CNS and the nurse practitioner. In: Harmic A B, Spross J A
(eds) The clinical nurse specialist in theory and practice, 2nd edn. W B
Saunders, Philadelphia, ch 18

Klee H, Faugier J, Hayes C et al 1990 AIDS-related risk behaviour, polydrug use
and temazepam. British Journal of Addiction 85(19): 1125–1132

Kohl M (ed) 1975 Beneficent euthanasia. Prometheus Books, Buffalo NY, pp 233–236

Koller P A 1991 Family needs and coping strategies during illness crisis. Clinical
Issues in Critical Care Nursing 2(2): 338–345

Kosik S H 1972 Patient advocacy or fighting the system. American Journal of
Nursing 72: 694–698

Kosky J 1992 Queen Elizabeth Hospital for Children – 125 years of achievement.
John Brown (Printers), Nottingham

Kubler-Ross E 1970 On death and dying. Tavistock, London

Lalonde M 1974 A new perspective on the health of Canadians. Department of
Health and Welfare, Government of Canada, Ottawa

Lamanna L 1996 Be on the lookout for skin cancer. American Journal of Nursing
96(8): 16A, 16C–16D

Laxton M, Gray C J, Watts S M 1997 Teaching assertiveness skills to people with
learning disabilities: a brief report of a training programme. Journal of
Learning Disabilities for Nursing, Health and Social Care 1(2): 71–77

Layton A, Ibbotson S, Davies J, Goodfield M 1994 Randomised trial of oral
aspirin for chronic venous leg ulcers. Lancet 344: 164–165

Layzell S, McCarthy M 1993 Specialist or generic community nursing care for HIV/AIDS patients? Journal of Advanced Nursing 18: 531–537

Leeming J G, Elliott T S J 1995 The emergence of *Trichophyton tonsurans* tinea capitis in Birmingham, UK. British Journal of Dermatology 133: 929–931

Legemaate J 1985 Patient rights advocacy: the Dutch model. Paper presented at EFMH/MIND Congress, Brighton

Leino-Kilpi H, Suominen T 1997 Research in intensive care nursing. Journal of Clinical Nursing 6: 69–76

Leske S J 1991a Family interventions. AACN Clinical Issues in Critical Care Nursing 2(2): 181–184

Leske J 1991b Family centered critical care: an interview with Nancy Molter. Clinical Issues in Critical Care Nursing 2(2): 185–187

Leske J 1992 Needs of adult family members after critical illness: prescriptions for interventions. Critical Care Nursing Clinics of North America 4(4): 587–596

Lewis M 1989 Tears and smiles – the hospice handbook. Michael O'Mara Books, London

Leyden J J 1997 Therapy for acne vulgaris. New England Journal of Medicine 336(16): 1156–1162

Lichter I 1987 Communication in cancer care. Churchill Livingstone, pp 115–124

Lipman T 1986 Length of hospitalisation of children with diabetes: effects of a clinical nurse specialist. Diabetes Educator 14: 41–43

Lipson J G, Dibble S L, Minarik P A 1996 Culture and nursing care: a pocket guide. University of California, San Francisco Nursing Press, San Francisco

Littlewood J 1988 The work of the health visitor and district nurse in relation to the elderly, with specific reference to health promotion. PhD Thesis, South Bank University, London

Littlewood J 1991 Care and ambiguity: towards a concept of nursing. In: Holden P, Littlewood J (eds) Anthropology and nursing. Routledge, London

Littlewood J 1995a The UK primary health care in context. In: Littlewood J (ed) Current issues in community nursing: primary health care in practice. Churchill Livingstone, Edinburgh

Littlewood J 1995b Current issues in community nursing: primary health care in practice. Churchill Livingstone, Edinburgh

Lomax E M R 1996 Small and special: the development of hospitals for children in Victorian Britain. (Medical History, supplement No. 16). Welcome Institute for the History of Medicine, London

Luft S 1997 Specialist and advanced roles. In: Burley S, Mitchell E, Melling K, Smith M, Chilton S, Crumpling C (eds) Contemporary community nursing. Arnold, London

Lutzen K, Tishelman C 1996 Nursing diagnosis: a critical analysis of underlying assumptions. International Journal of Nursing Studies 33(2): 190–200

Lynch V 1993 Forensic nursing: diversity in education and practice. Journal of Psychosocial Nursing 31(11): 7–14

McCann G 1991 Involving the family. Nursing Times 87(39): 67–68

McCarthy J 1983 Taking liberties. Open Mind 2: 13

McClelland P B 1997 New treatment options for psoriasis. Dermatology Nursing 9(5): 295–304

McColl A, Smith H, White P, Field J 1998 General practitioners' perceptions of the route to evidence based medicine: a questionnaire survey. British Medical Journal 316: 316–365

McCorkle R, Benoliel JQ, Donaldson G, Georgiadou F, Moinpour C, Goodell B 1989 A randomised clinical trial of home nursing care for living cancer patients. Cancer 64(6): 1375–1382

McCoy K L, Bell K S 1994 Organ donation and the rural critical care nurse. American Journal of Critical Care 3(6): 473–475

McDougall J M 1994 The role of the neonatal nurse practitioner. Care of the Critically Ill 10(5): 207–209

McGee P 1993 Defining nursing practice. British Journal of Nursing. 2(20): 1022–1026

McGee P, Castledine G, Brown R 1996 A survey of specialist and advanced nursing practice in England. British Journal of Nursing 5(11): 682-685

McGrath M 1991 Multidisciplinary teamwork Aldershot. Avebury Studies of Care in the Community, Aldershot

McIver S 1993 Investing in patients representation. NAHAT, Birmingham

McIver S 1994 Establishing patient representation. NAHAT, Birmingham

McIvor D, Thompson J F 1988 The self perceived needs of family members with a relative in the intensive care unit (ICU). Intensive Care Nursing 4: 139–145

Mackay T 1989 A community nursing service analysis. Nursing Standard 4(2): 32–35 (This was written by J Carson but incorrectly attributed when published.)

Mackie C 1996 Nurse practitioners managing anticoagulant clinics. Nursing Times 92(1): 25–26

Macleod Clark J, Hockey J 1989 Further research for nursing. Scutari Press, London

McMurray A 1992 Expertise in the community. Journal of Community Health Nursing 9(2): 65–75

McNally S 1997 Participation in conferences: developing networks for users of learning disabilities services. Journal of Learning Disabilities for Nursing, Health and Social Care 1(2): 65–70

MacPhail H 1940 Mental nursing final examination questions and answers. Faber & Faber, London

McShane E 1997 Addiction nursing: a new direction in prevention. In: Hussein R G, Gafoor M (eds) Addiction nursing: perspectives on professional and clinical practice. Stanley Thornes, Cheltenham, ch 18, pp 162–169

McSweeney P 1996 Roles revamp. Nursing Standard 10(34): 25

Maguire P G 1976 The psychological and social sequelae of mastectomy. In: Howells J (ed) Modern perspectives in the psychiatric aspects of surgery. Churchill Livingstone, Edinburgh

Maguire P 1985 For debate: barriers to the psychological care of the dying. British Medical Journal 219: 1711–1713

Maguire P, Rutter E 1976 History taking for medical students. Deficiencies of performance. Lancet ii: 556–558

Maguire P G, Brooke M, Tate A, Thomas C, Sellwood R 1983 The effects of counselling on physical disability and social recovery after mastectomy. Clinical Oncology 9: 319–321

Maguire P G, Faulkner A 1988 How to do it. Improve the counselling skills of doctors and nurses in cancer care. British Medical Journal 297: 847–849

Maguire P G, Pentol A, Allen D, Tait A, Brook M, Sellwood R 1982 Cost of counselling women who undergo mastectomy. British Medical Journal 284: 1933–1935

Maguire P G, Tate A, Brooke M, Thomas C, Sellwood R 1980 The effects of counselling on the psychiatric morbidity associated with mastectomy. British Medical Journal 281: 1454–1456

Malin N (ed) 1995 Services for people with learning disabilities. Routledge, London

Mallik M 1997 Advocacy in nursing – a review of the literature. Journal of Advanced Nursing 25: 130–138

Malloy C 1989 Care of the family. In: Malloy C, Hartshorn J (eds) Acute care nursing in the home: a holistic approach. J B Lippincott

Maloney C, Preston F 1992 An overview of home care for patients with cancer. Oncology Nurses Forum 19: 75–80

Manley K 1996 Advanced practice is not about medicalising nursing roles. Nursing in Critical Care 1(2): 56–57

Manley K 1997 A conceptual framework for advanced practice: an action research project operationalising an advanced practitioner/consultant nurse role. Journal of Clinical Nursing 6: 179–190

Mansell J, Ericsson K (eds) 1996 Deinstitutionalisation and community living. Chapman & Hall, London

Manson D J, Knight K, Toughhill E, DeMaio D, Beck T, Christopher M A 1992 Promoting the community health clinical specialist. Clinical Nurse Specialist 6(1): 6–13

Mapperley Advice Project 1986 The first years work. Hyson Green Law Centre, Nottingham

Marlatt G A, George W 1984 Relapse prevention: introduction and overview of model. British Journal of Addiction 79: 261–263

Marlatt G A, Gordon J R (eds) 1985 Relapse prevention: maintenance strategy in the treatment of addictive behaviours. Guilford Press, New York

Marsh G N, Dawes M L 1995 Establishing a minor illness nurse in a busy general practice. British Medical Journal 310: 778–780

Martin C D, Crigger J N 1997 Ethical and legal issues in critical care nursing. In: Hartshorn J, Sole M L, Lamborn M L, Cullen N (eds) Introduction to critical care nursing, 2nd edn. W B Saunders, Philadelphia

Mason D, Knight K, Toughill E, DeMaio D, Beck T L, Christopher M A 1992 Promoting the community health clinic nurse specialist. Clinical Nurse Specialist 6(1): 6–13

Mason J K, Mulligan D 1996 Euthanasia by stages. Lancet 347: 801–811

Mason T, Lawson L 1992 Bipolar affective disorder. Nursing 4(47): 18–20

Mason T, Patterson R 1990 A critical review of the use of Rogers' model within a special hospital: a single case study. Journal of Advanced Nursing 15: 130–141

Mathias C G T 1985 The cost of occupational disease. Archives of Dermatology 121: 332–334

Mathias P 1992 Family vulnerability, support networks and counselling. In: Thompson T, Mathais P (eds) Standards and mental handicap, keys to competence. Baillière Tindall, London, pp 149–156

Mathieson A 1996 Anger at 'mini-doctor' jibe. Nursing Standard 10(5): 15

Maxwell V 1993 Look through the parents' eyes. Helping parents of children with a disability. Professional Nurse 9(3): 200–203

May C 1995 Patients' enquiries about cancer: nurses' coping strategies. Journal of Cancer Care 4: 101–104

Mayfield D, McLeod G, Hall P 1974 The Cage Questionnaire: validation of a new alcoholism screening instrument. American Journal of Psychiatry 131(10): 1121–1123

Maynard A 1991 Developing the health care market. Economic Journal 101: 1277–1286

Mead D 1996 Using nursing initiatives to encourage the use of research. Nursing Standard 10(19): 33–36

Meates M 1997 Ambulatory paediatrics – making a difference. Archives of Disease in Childhood 76(5): 468–476

Meehan S, Moore G, Barr O 1995 Specialist services for people with learning disabilities. Nursing Times 91(13): 33–35

Menard S W 1987 The clinical nurse specialist: perspectives on practice. John Wiley, Chichester

Mental Health Act 1959 HMSO, London

Mental Health Act 1983 HMSO, London

Mental Health Foundation 1996 Building expectations. Opportunities and services for people with a learning disability. MHF, London

Mervyn F 1971 The plight of dying patients in hospitals. American Journal of Nursing 71: 1988–1990

Millar J B 1987 A study to identify and describe the needs of families whose relative is critically ill in a general intensive care unit. University of Wales College of Medicine, MN, p 154

Millard A 1997 Evidence-based clinical guidelines – implementation plans in Scotland. International Journal of Health Care Quality Assurance 10(6): 236–240

Miller F 1991 Using Roy's model in a special hospital. Nursing Standard 5(27): 29–32

Miller M 1998 An interactive programme of learning events in mental health and illness. Outset Publishing, Sussex

Miller P, Plant M 1996 Drinking, smoking and illicit drug use among 15–16 year olds in the United Kingdom. British Medical Journal 313: 394–397

Miller W 1983 Motivational interviewing with problem drinkers. Behavioural Psychotherapy 11: 147–172

Miller W R, Sanchez V C 1993 Motivating young adults for treatment and lifestyle change. In: Howard G (ed) Issues in alcohol use and misuse by young adults. University of Notre Dame Press, Notre Dame

Ministry of Health 1959 The welfare of children in hospital: report of the Committee (Chairman Sir H Platt). HMSO, London

Ministry of Health, Central Health Services Council 1968 Psychiatric nursing: today and tomorrow. HMSO, London

Ministry of Health, Central Health Services Council 1971 The enrolled nurse. HMSO, London

Ministry of Health and Scottish Home and Health Department 1966 Report of the Committee on Senior Nursing Staff Structure. HMSO, London

Mitchinson S 1996 Are nurses independent and autonomous practitioners? Nursing Standard 10(34): 34–38

Modica M, Lund P Z, Bandfield M 1991 Responding to service models: a nurse practitioner training programme. Journal of Perinatal and Neonatal Nursing 5(3): 34–43

Molter C N 1979 Needs of relatives of critically ill patients: a descriptive study. Heart and Lung 8(2): 332–339

Monroe B 1993 Psychosocial dimension of palliation. In: Saunders C, Sykes N (eds) The management of terminal malignant disease. Edward Arnold, London

Monroe B, Kraus F 1996 Children and loss. British Journal of Hospital Medicine 56(6): 260–264

Moore K N 1995 Compliance to collaboration: the meaning for the patient. Nursing Ethics 2(1): 71–77

Morgan M, McCreedy R, Simpson J, Hay R J 1997 Dermatology quality of life scales – a measure of the impact of skin diseases. British Journal of Dermatology 136: 202–206

Morrall P A 1997 Professionalism and community psychiatric nursing: a case study of four mental health teams. Journal of Advanced Nursing 25: 1133–1137

Morris J, Royle G T 1987 Choice of surgery for early breast cancer; pre and post operative levels of clinical anxiety and depression in patients and their husbands. British Journal of Surgery 74: 1017–1019

Morris T, Greer S, White P 1977 Psychological and social adjustment to mastectomy. Cancer 40: 2381–2387

Morrison G 1996 Sun exposure and skin cancer development: nurses' attitudes. Nursing Standard 10(36): 39–42

Morse J M 1991 Negotiating commitment and involvement in the nurse–patient relationship. Journal of Advanced Nursing 16(4): 455–468

Moseley M J, Jones A M 1991 Contracting for visitation with families. Dimensions of Critical Care Nursing 10: 364–370

Muir Gray J 1997 Evidence based health care. Churchill Livingstone, Edinburgh

Mullins L 1996 Management and organisational behaviour, 4th edn. Pitman Publishing, London

Mundinger M O 1994 Advanced practice nursing – good medicine for physicians. New England Journal of Medicine 330(3): 211–214

Murphy S 1986 Family study and nursing research. Image: the Journal of Nursing Scholarship 18(4): 170–174

Murphy S A 1992 Validation of addictions: nursing diagnoses in a sample of alcohol abstainers 1 year post-treatment. Archives of Psychiatric Nursing 4(6): 340–346

Murray C, Thomas M 1996 Specialist practitioners: are they all the same? British Journal of Nursing 5(22): 1353

Murray C, Thomas M 1997 Advanced nursing practice: role or concept? British Journal of Nursing 6(9): 474

Naegle M A 1989 Targets for change in alcohol and drug education for nursing roles. Alcohol Health and Research World 13: 53–55

Nall M, Farber E 1997 World epidemiology of psoriasis. In: Farber E, Cox A (eds) Psoriasis. Proceedings of the Second International Symposium. York Medical Books, New York

Nash A 1993 A stressful role: specialist nursing. Nursing Times 89(26): 50–51

National Council for Hospice and Specialist Palliative Care Services 1995 Opening doors: improving access to hospice and specialist palliative care services by members of the black and ethnic minority communities. Occasional Paper 7

National Health Service Act 1946 HMSO, London

National Health Service Act 1977 HMSO, London

NHS and Community Care Act 1990 HMSO, London

National Health Service Executive 1995 Health authority drug misuse services 1995/6, HSG(95)26. HMSO, London

National Health Service Executive 1996a Child health in the community: a guide to good practice. HMSO, London

National Health Service Executive 1996b Primary care: the future. HMSO, London

National Health Service Executive 1996c Primary care: delivering the future. HMSO, London

NHS Health Advisory Service, DHSS Social Services Inspectorate 1988 Report on services provided by Broadmoor Hospital. HMSO, London

National Health Service Management Executive 1990 NHS trusts: a working guide. HMSO, London

National Health Service Management Executive 1992 Meeting the spiritual needs of patients and staff. HMSO, London

National Health Service Management Executive 1993 A vision for the future: the nursing, midwifery and health visiting contribution to health and health care. NHSME, London

National Institute of Drug Abuse 1980 The development approach to preventing problem dependencies. In: Glenn H S, Warner J W (eds) Community-based prevention specialist: participant manual. NIDA, Rockville MD, pp 133–153

Neagle M A 1989 Targets for change in alcohol and drug education for nursing roles. Alcohol Health and Research World 13: 53–55

Neame R L, Berth-Jones J, Kurinczuk J J et al 1995 Prevalence of atopic dermatitis in Leicester: a study of methodology and examination of possible ethnic variation. British Journal of Dermatology 132: 772–777

Neill S J, Muir J 1997 Educating the new community children's nurses: challenges and opportunities. Nurse Education Today 17(1): 7–15

Noble M A 1988 The critical care clinical nurse specialist: need for hospital and community. Clinical Nurse Specialist 2(1): 30–33

Norman A 1996 The contract culture: purchasers and providers. In: Twinn S, Roberts B, Andrews S (eds) Community health care nursing. Butterworth Heinemann, Oxford, pp 132–144

Normand C 1996 The search for evidence of effectiveness. NT Research 1(4): 249–250

North of England Study of Standards and Performance in General Practice 1992 Overview of the study (Report 50). Centre for Health Services Research, Newcastle upon Tyne

O'Brien J 1992 Developing high quality services for people with developmental disabilities. In: Bradley V J, Bersani H A (eds) Quality assurance for individuals with developmental disabilities. Paul Brookes, Baltimore

Office of Population Censuses and Surveys 1992 Annual mortality statistics. HMSO, London

Office of Population Censuses and Surveys 1994a Morbidity statistics from general practice 1991/92. Series MB5, No 3. HMSO, London

Office of Population Censuses and Surveys 1994b 1992 mortality statistics. HMSO, London

Office of Population Censuses and Surveys 1995 Social Survey Division. Results from the 1994 general household survey. HMSO, London

Ogden J 1994 Why we all need Macmillan nurses. Nursing Times (June): 90(25)

O'Hanlon M, Gibbon S 1996 Advanced practice. Nursing Management 2(10): 12–13

O'Malley S S, Jaffe A I, Chang G, Schottenfeld R S, Meyer R E, Rounsaville B 1992 Naltrexone and coping skills therapy for alcohol dependence. Archives of General Psychiatry 49: 881–887

Opeé T E 1971 Home care for sick children. British Journal of Hospital Medicine 5(1): 39–40, 43–44

Orem D 1985 Nursing: concepts of practice. McGraw-Hill, New York

Ovretveit J 1993 Co-ordinating community care. Multidisciplinary teams and care management. Open University Press, Buckingham

Owen G M 1983 Health visiting, 2nd edn. Baillière Tindall, London

Owen J, Black C 1996 Supportive and shared care. In: Hancock B (ed) Cancer in the community, Radcliffe Medical Press, Oxford

Oxman A, Cook D, Guyatt G 1994 Users' guide to the medical literature. Journal of the American Medical Association 272(17): 1367–1371

Parahoo K, Barr O 1996 Community mental handicap nursing services in Northern Ireland: a profile of clients and selected working practices. Journal of Clinical Nursing 5(2): 221–228

Parker E 1985 The development of secure provision. In: Gostyn L (ed) Secure provision: a review of special services for the mentally ill and mentally handicapped in England and Wales. Tavistock, London, pp 15–65

Parker H, Measham F, Aldridge J 1995 Drugs futures – changing patterns of drug use amongst English youth. Institute for the Study of Drug Dependence, London

Parkes C M 1990 Risk factors in bereavement: implications for the prevention and treatment of pathology. Psychiatric Annals 20(6): 308–313

Parkin D M 1993 Estimates of the worldwide incidence of eighteen major cancers in 1985. Int J Cancer 54: 594–606

Parkin D M et al (eds) 1992 Cancer incidence in five continents volume VI. IARC Scientific Publication No. 120, Lyon

Paton A 1994 (ed) A B C of alcohol. British Medical Journal Publishing, London

Patterson C, Haddad B 1992 The advanced nurse practitioner – common attributes. Canadian Journal of Nursing Administration 5(4): 18–22

Pennells M et al 1992 Bereavement and adolescence: a groupwork approach. Association of Child Psychology and Psychiatry Newsletter 14: 4

Pearson A 1983 The clinical nursing unit. William Heinemann Medical Books, London

Perkins E, Billingham K 1997 Working together to care for children in the community. Nursing Times 93(43): 46–48

Perkins P 1994 Caring for skin in the community. Practice Nurse 7(2): 96–99

Perkins P 1995 Safety under the sun. Practice Nurse 9(5): 361–363

Perkins P 1996 The management of eczema in adults. Nursing Standard 10(35): 49–53

Pettle S A, Britten C M 1995 Talking with children about death and dying. Child: Care, Health and Development 21(6): 395–404

Phillips M S 1983 Forensic psychiatry – nurses' attitudes revealed. Dimensions 60(9): 41–43

Philpot T, Ward L 1995 Values and visions. Changing ideas in services for people with learning difficulties. Butterworth Heinemann, Oxford

Pickering A 1997 Evidence-based health care – a resource pack. King's College School of Medicine and Dentistry, London

Pion I A 1996 Educating children and parents about sun protection. Dermatology Nursing 8(1): 29–36

Pitt R 1993 Who cares? Nursing Times 89(1): 27–29

Plant M, Single E, Stockwell T 1997 Introduction: harm minimisation and alcohol. In: Plant M, Single E, Stockwell T (eds) Alcohol – minimising the harm. What Works? Free Association Books, London, ch 1, pp 4–6

Pope John Paul II 1994 Evangelium vitae (Papal Encyclical). Catholic Truth Society, London

Pope S 1992 Fundamentals for a new concept of oncology nursing in the professional nursing programme. Cancer Nursing 15(2): 137–147

Poulton B, West M 1993 Effective multidisciplinary teamwork in primary health care. Journal of Advanced Nursing 18: 918–925

Price M 1993 Scabies – the 3000 year itch. Practice Nurse 6(8): 496

Price M J, Martin A, Newberry Y, Zimmer P, Brykczynski K, Warren B 1992 Developing national guidelines for nurse practitioner education: an overview of the product and the process. Journal of Nurse Education 31(1): 10–15

Pridham K 1990 Why clinical field study? Nursing Outlook 38(1): 26–30

Primary Care Act 1997 HMSO, London

Pritchard P 1995 Learning to work effectively in teams. In: Owens P, Carrier J, Horder J (eds) Interprofessional issues in community and primary health care. Macmillan, London, pp 205–232

Prochaska J O, DiClemente C 1983 Stages and processes of self change of smoking, and towards a more integrative model of change. Journal of Consulting and Clinical Psychology 51: 390–395

Prochaska J O, DiClemente C C 1986 Towards a comprehensive model of change. In: Miller W R, Heather N (eds) Treating addictive behaviours: process of change. Plenum Press, New York

Prochaska J O, DiClemente C C, Nocross J C 1992 In search of how people change: applications to addictive behaviours. American Psychologist 4(9): 1102–1114

Pullen F 1995 Advocacy: a specialist practitioner role. British Journal of Nursing 4(5): 275–278

Queen's Nursing Institute 1998 Go-ahead for first nurse-led pilot sites. Queen's Nursing Institute Letter 8(1): 4–5

Quinn S, Redmond K, Begley C 1996 The needs of relatives visiting adult critical care units as perceived by relatives and nurses Part 1. Intensive and Critical Care Nursing 12: 168–172

Ramos M C 1992 The nurse–patient relationship: theme and variation. Journal of Advanced Nursing 17(4): 469–506

Ramsey B, O'Reagan M 1988 A survey of the social and psychological effects of psoriasis. British Journal of Dermatology 118: 195–201

Rapley M, Baldwin S 1995 Normalisation – metatheory or metaphysics? A conceptual critique. Australia and New Zealand Journal of Developmental Disabilities 20(2): 141–157

Rassool G H 1993 Substance misuse: responding to the challenge. Journal of Advanced Nursing 18(9): 1401–1407

Rassool G H 1994 A multi-professional course in substance misuse. International Nursing Review 41(2): 53–56

Rassool G Hussein 1997a Addiction nursing– towards a new paradigm: the UK experience. In: Rassool G Hussein, Gafoor M (eds) Addiction nursing: perspectives on professional and clinical practice. Stanley Thornes, Cheltenham, pp 6–21

Rassool G Hussein 1997b Professional education and training. In: Rassool G Hussein, Gafoor M (eds) Addiction nursing: perspectives on professional and clinical practice. Stanley Thornes, Cheltenham, pp 217–226

Rassool G Hussein, Gafoor M 1997a Themes in addiction nursing. In: Rassool G Hussein, Gafoor M (eds) Addiction nursing: perspectives on professional and clinical practice. Stanley Thornes, Cheltenham, pp 3–5

Rassool G Hussein, Gafoor M 1997b Health education, prevention and harm minimisation. In: Rassool G Hussein, Gafoor M (eds) Addiction nursing: perspectives on professional and clinical practice. Stanley Thornes, Cheltenham, pp 170–179

Rassool G Hussein, McKeown O 1996 A review of the report on the education and training of health care in substance misuse: complacency or commitment? Journal of Substance Misuse 1: 114–115

Rassool G H, Oyefeso A 1993 The need for substance misuse education in health studies curriculum: a case for nursing education. Nurse Education Today 13: 107–110

Rassool G H, Winnington J 1993 Using psychoactive drugs. Nursing Times 89(47): 38–40

Rathbone W 1890 Sketch of the history and progress of district nursing from its commencement in 1859 to the present day. Macmillan, London

Rawaf S 1996 Substance misuse: a public health perspective. Psychiatric Care 3(1): 17–22

Rawson D 1994 Models of interprofessional work: likely theories and possibilities. In: Leathard A (ed) Going interprofessional. Working together for health and welfare. Routledge, London, pp 38–63

Rea J, Newhouse M, Halil T 1976 Skin disease in Lambeth. A community study of prevalence and use of medical care. British Journal of Preventative and Social Medicine 30: 107–114

Read S, Jones N, Williams B 1992 Nurse practitioners in accident and emergency departments: what do they do? British Medical Journal 305: 1466–1470

Representation of the People Act 1949 HMSO, London

Richardson G, Maynard A 1995 Fewer doctors? More nurses? A review of knowledge base of doctor–nurse substitution. University of York, York

Robards M F 1994 Running a team for disabled children and their families. Mac Keith Press, London

Robertson J 1958 Young children in hospital. Tavistock, London

Robinson D K, Mead M J, Boswell C R 1995 Inside looking out: innovations in community health nursing. Clinical Nurse Specialist 9(4): 227–235

Rodgers C 1983 Needs of relatives of cardiac surgery patients during the critical care phase. Focus on Critical Care 10(5): 50–55

Rodmell S, Watt A 1986 The politics of health promotion. Routledge & Kegan Paul, London

Roe Prior P, Watts R J, Burke K 1994 Critical care clinical nurse specialist in home health care: survey results. Clinical Nurse Specialist 8(1): 35–40

Rogers J 1990 Vision needed if training not to sink without trace. Health Manpower Management (March): 16–18

Rolfe G 1998 Education for the advanced practitioner. In: Rolfe G, Flubrook P (eds) Advanced nursing practice. Butterworth-Heinemann, London, pp 271–280

Rosenberg W, Donald A 1995 Evidence based medicine: an approach to clinical problem solving. British Medical Journal 310: 1122–1126

Ross T 1983 First in its field. Nursing Mirror 156(9): 19–21

Roth J A 1963 Timetables. Bobbs-Merrill, Indianapolis IN

Royal College of General Practitioners 1981 Health and prevention in primary care: 18. Prevention of arterial disease in general practice: 19. Prevention of psychiatric disorders in general practice: 20

Royal College of General Practitioners 1995 Morbidity statistics from general practice fourth national study 1991–92. HMSO, London

Royal College of Nursing 1964 The reform of nursing education. RCN, London

Royal College of Nursing 1975 New horizons in clinical nursing. RCN, London

Royal College of Nursing 1988 Specialities in nursing. RCN, London

Royal College of Nursing 1991 Standard of care: cancer nursing. RCN, London

Royal College of Nursing 1992a The role and function of the domiciliary community nurse for people with a learning disability. RCN, London

Royal College of Nursing 1992b Standards of care. Nursing people with a learning disability. RCN, London

Royal College of Nursing 1993a Standard of care: palliative nursing. RCN, London

Royal College of Nursing 1993b Evidence to the National Review of Mental Health Nursing. RCN, London

Royal College of Nursing 1994 Living wills: guidance for nurses (Nursing and Health Factsheet 4). RCN, London

Royal College of Nursing 1995 Standards of care for dermatology nursing. RCN, London

Royal College of Nursing 1996 Buying paediatric community nursing: an RCN guide for purchasers and commissioners of health care. RCN, London

Royal College of Nursing Cancer Nursing Society 1996a Guidelines for good practice in cancer nursing education. RCN, London

Royal College of Nursing Cancer Nursing Society 1996b A structure for cancer nursing services. RCN, London

Royal College of Nursing Paediatric Community Nurses Forum 1996 Evidence submitted to the House of Commons Select Committee on Health. RCN, London

Royal College of Paediatrics and Child Health, Association for Children with Life Threatening or Terminal Conditions and their Families 1997 A guide to the development of children's palliative care services. Royal College of Paediatrics and Child Health, London

Royal Marsden Hospitals NHS Trust 1994 Purchasing and providing cancer services: a guide to good practice. Royal Marsden Hospital NHS Trust, London

Ruane Morris M, Thompson G, Lawton S 1995a Designing a nursing model for dermatology. Professional Nurse 10(9): 565–566

Ruane Morris M, Thompson G, Lawton S 1995b Community liaison in dermatology. Professional Nurse 10(11): 687–688

Ruben S M, Morrison C L 1992 Temazepam misuse in a group of injecting drug users. British Journal of Addiction 87: 1387–1392

Rukholm E, Bailey P, Coutu-Wakulczyk G, Bailey W B 1991 Needs and anxiety levels in relatives of intensive care unit patients. Journal of Advanced Nursing 16: 920–928

Rumsfield J 1990 Sunscreens: what you and your patients should know. Dermatology Nursing 2(3): 139–147

Sabo K A, Kraay C, Rudy E, Abraham T, Bender M, Lewandowski W 1989 ICU family support group sessions: family members perceived benefits. Applied Nursing Research 2: 82–89

Sackett D 1997 Evidence based medicine. How to practice and teach EBM. Churchill Livingstone, New York

Sadler C 1996 Chinese herbs for eczema: risks and benefits. Community Nurse 2(5): 21–22

Safriet B 1992 Health care dollars and regulatory sense; the role of advanced practice nursing. Yale Journal of Regulation 9(2): 456-464

St Hill P 1996 Cultural/ethnic identity – West Indians. In: Lipson J G, Dibble S L, Minarik P A (eds) Culture and nursing care. UCSF Nursing Press, USA

Salussolia M 1997 Is advanced nursing practice a post or a person? British Journal of Nursing 6(16): 928–933

Sargeant L 1985 Clinical nurse specialist. Nursing Mirror 160(9): 24–25

Saunders C 1988 St. Christopher's in celebration (21 years of Britain's first modern hospice). Hodder & Stoughton, London

Saunders C 1991 The evaluation of the hospices. Parthenon Publishing Group and Free Inquiry 1991, 12(1)

Saunders C 1993 Some challenges that face us. Palliative Medicine 7(suppl 1): 77–83

Saunders-Wilson D 1992 Her Majesty's Prison: Grendon a maverick prison. Journal of Forensic Psychiatry 2(2): 179–183

Schultz A M, Daly B 1989 Differences and similarities in nurses' perceptions of intensive care nursing and non intensive care nursing. Focus on Critical Care 16(6): 465–471

Scottish Home and Health Department 1976 State Hospital Carstairs Report of Public Inquiry Edinburgh. HMSO, London

Selby M 1991 HMP Grendon – the care of acute psychiatric patients: a pragmatic solution. In: Herbst K, Gunn J (eds) The mentally disordered offender. Butterworth-Heinemann, Oxford, pp 96–103

Selzer M S, Vinokur A, Rooijien E V 1975 A self-administered Short Michigan Alcoholism Screening Test (SMAST). Journal of Studies on Alcohol 36(1): 117–126

Shanley E, Starrs T 1993 Learning disabilities. A handbook of care, 2nd edn. Churchill Livingstone, Edinburgh

Sheldon F 1994 Children and bereavement – what are the issues? European Journal of Palliative Care 1(1)

Shepherd D 1995 Learning the lessons: mental health inquiry reports published in England and Wales between 1969–1994 and their recommendations for improving practice. Zito Trust, London

Shindler A 1992 Loss. Bereavement Care 11(3)

Shuldham C 1996 Introducing an integrated nursing research programme. Nursing Standard 10(18): 42–43

Simpson T 1991 Critical care patients' perceptions of visits. Heart and Lung 20(6): 681–688

Sines D 1995a Impaired autonomy – the challenge of caring. Journal of Clinical Nursing 4(2): 109–116

Sines D 1995b Community health care nursing. Blackwell Science, London

Sines D, Barr O 1998 Professions in teams. In: Thompson T, Mathias P (eds) Standards and learning disabilities, 2nd edn. Baillière Tindall, London, pp 343–346

Sloman D 1995 Home economics. Health Service Journal 2(Nov): 26–27

Smith F 1995 Children's nursing in practice: the Nottingham model. Blackwell Science, Oxford

Smith J, Hughes A, Wiles R 1996 Loddon NHS Community Trust: paediatric community nursing team – service evaluation. College of Health, London

Smith S, Pennells M 1993 Bereaved children and adolescence. In: K Dwivedi (ed) Group work with child and adolescence. A handbook. Jessica Kingsley, London, ch 14

Sobell L C, Sobell M B, Toneatto T, Leo G I 1993 What triggers the resolution of alcohol problems without treatment? Alcoholism: Clinical and Experimental Research 17: 217–224

Social Services Inspectorate 1991 Comprehensive assessment and care management. Practitioner's guide. HMSO, London

Sole M L, Hartshorn C J 1997 Overview of critical care nursing. In: Hartshorn J, Sole M L, Lamborn M L, Cullen B N (eds) Introduction to critical care nursing, 2nd edn. W B Saunders, Philadelphia

Sontag S 1991 Illness as metaphor AIDS and its metaphor. Penguin Books, London

South Bank University 1992 MSc interprofessional health and welfare studies. South Bank University, London

South Bank University 1997a BSc (Hons) nursing and social work studies. South Bank University, London

South Bank University 1997b Context of community nursing. South Bank University, London

Soutter J, Bond S, Croft A 1994 A strategy for caring for families in bereavement. Nursing Times (27 July)

Sparancino P 1992 Advanced practice: the clinical nurse specialist. Nursing Practice 5(4): 2–4

Spowart K 1993 Management of eczema in children. Paediatric Nursing 5(8): 9–12

SMAC – Standing Medical Advisory Committee 1980 Terminal care – report of a working group (Chairman, Eric Wilkes). HMSO, London

SMAC – Standing Medical Advisory Committee 1984 Acute services for cancer: Report of a working group. HMSO, London

SMAC – Standing Subcommittee on Cancer of the Standing Medical Advisory Committee 1991 Quality assurance in radiotherapy. Health Publications Unit, Heywood, Lancs

Stafford R 1991 The evolution of the specialist. Nursing Times 87(16): 39–40

Starr P 1982 The social transformation of American medicine. Basic Books, New York

Stern R S 1994 Epidemiology of skin disease in HIV infection. Journal of Investigative Dermatology 102: 34S–37S

Stevens J 1997 Improving integration between research and practice as a means of developing evidence-based health care. NT Reasearch 2(1): 7–15

Stilwell B 1982 The nurse practitioner at work. Nursing Mirror 78(3): 1799–1803

Stone L 1995 Dermatitis in the elderly. Community Nurse: Nurse Prescriber (Feb): 5–7

Stone L 1997 The local application of drugs. In: Trounce J (ed) Clinical pharmacology for nurses, 15th edn. Churchill Livingstone, New York, ch 26

Stone L A, Lindfield E M, Robertson S 1989 A colour atlas of nursing procedures in skin disorders. Wolfe Medical, London

Strang J 1993 Drug use and harm reduction: responding to the challenge. In: Heather N et al (eds) Psychoactive drugs and harm reduction: from faith to science. Wurr Publishers, London

Strang J, Clement S 1994 The introduction of community drug teams across the UK. In: Strang J, Glossop M (eds) Heroin and drug policy – the British system. Oxford University Press, Oxford

Strang J, Farrell M 1989 HIV and drug misuse: forcing the process of change. Current Opinion in Psychiatry 2: 402–407

Tackling Drugs Together: a strategy for England (1995–1998) 1995 HMSO, London

Tait A 1995 Describing breast care nurses. In: Richardson A, Wilson-Barnett J (eds) Nursing research in cancer care. Scutari Press, London

Tatman M 1994 Wise decisions: developing paediatric home care teams. Royal College of Nursing, London

Taylor H 1983 The hospice movement in Britain; its role and its future. Centre for Policy on Ageing. Nuffield Lodge Studio, London

Taylor M 1992 A simplified biology of cancer. In: Hiller T, Bailey L, Paterson S (eds) Preventing cancers. Open University Press, Milton Keynes

Taylor P, Roberts D 1997 Skin cancer prevention. Nursing Standard 11(50): 42–45

Taylor-Brown J, Acheson A, Farber J M 1993 Kids Can Cope: a group intervention for children whose parents have cancer. Journal of Psychosocial Oncology 11(1): 41–53

Thiboutot D 1997 Acne: an overview of clinical research findings. Dermatologic Clinics 15(1): 97–109

Thomas J 1994 Parents. In Hill L (ed) Care for dying children and their families. Chapman & Hall, London

Thomas S 1997 Developing the primary care led NHS. Journal of Community Nursing 11(6): 8–11

Thornes R 1987 Where are the children? (Prepared on behalf of 'Caring for Children in the Health Services'.) Action for Sick Children, London

Thornes R 1988 Parents staying overnight with their children in hospital. (Prepared on behalf of 'Caring for Children in the Health Services'.) Action for Sick Children, London

Thornes R 1991 Just for the day. (Prepared on behalf of 'Caring for Children in the Health Services'.) Action for Sick Children, London

Thornes R 1993 Bridging the gaps: an exploratory study of the interfaces between primary and specialist care for children within the health services. (Prepared on behalf of 'Caring for Children in the Health Services'.) Action for Sick Children, London

Tierney A 1998 Nursing research in Europe. International Nursing Review 45(1): 15–19

Tiffany R 1984 The Marsden experience. Nursing Mirror 159(21): 28–30

Tingle J 1997 Clinical guidelines: legal and clinical risk management issues. British Journal of Nursing 6(11): 639–641

Titler G M, Walsh M S 1992 Visiting critically ill adults: strategies for practice. Critical Care Nursing Clinics of North America 4(4): 623–632

Tomlinson Sir Bernard 1992 Report of the Inquiry into London's Health Service, Medical Education and Research. HMSO, London

Townsend J, Frank H O, Fremont D et al 1990 Terminal care and patients' preference for place of death: a prospective study. British Medical Journal 301: 415–417

Tripp-Rumer T, Brink P 1985 Cultural brokerage. In: Bukchek G, McCloskey J (eds) Nursing interventions: treatments for nursing diagnosis. W B Saunders, Philadelphia

Trnobranski P H 1994 Nurse practitioner: redefining the role of the community nurse? Journal of Advanced Nursing 19: 134–139

Turnbull R 1994 Use of wet wrap dressing in atopic eczema. Paediatric Nursing 6(2): 22–26

Turner S 1995 Living wills help doctors and patients work together. BMA News Review 21(4): 16

Turton P, Barnett J 1981 In: Simpson J, Levitt R (eds) Going home: a guide for helping the patient on leaving hospital. Longman, London

Twinn S, Buttigieg M, Daucey J 1992 Responding to the challenges – working with opportunities. Health Visitor 65(3): 84–85

Twycross I R G 1980 Hospice care: redressing the balance in medicine. Journal of the Royal Society of Medicine 73: 474–481

Tyne A, O'Brien J 1981 The principles of normalisation. CMH/CMHERA, London

UK Association of Cancer Registries 1994 Cancer registry handbook. UKACR, London

United Kingdom Central Council for Nursing, Midwifery and Health Visiting 1984 The code of Professional Conduct. UKCC, London

United Kingdom Central Council for Nursing, Midwifery and Health Visiting 1986 Project 2000: a new preparation for practice. UKCC, London

United Kingdom Central Council for Nursing, Midwifery and Health Visiting 1990a Post-registration education and practice project (PREP). UKCC, London

United Kingdom Central Council for Nursing, Midwifery and Health Visiting 1990b Discussion paper on post-registration education and practice project. UKCC London

United Kingdom Central Council for Nursing, Midwifery and Health Visiting 1991 The report of the post-registration education and practice project. UKCC, London

United Kingdom Central Council for Nursing, Midwifery and Health Visiting 1992a Code of professional conduct, 3rd edn. UKCC, London

United Kingdom Central Council for Nursing, Midwifery and Health Visiting 1992b The scope of professional practice, 3rd edn. UKCC, London

United Kingdom Central Council for Nursing, Midwifery and Health Visiting 1993 Final draft report on the future of professional education and practice. UKCC, London

United Kingdom Central Council for Nursing, Midwifery and Health Visiting 1994a The future of professional practice. The council's standards for practice following registration. UKCC, London

United Kingdom Central Council for Nursing, Midwifery and Health Visiting 1994b The Council's standards for education and practice following registration. Programmes of education leading to the qualification of specialist practitioner. UKCC, London

United Kingdom Central Council for Nursing, Midwifery and Health Visiting 1994c The future of professional practice – position statement on policy and implementation. UKCC, London

United Kingdom Central Council for Nursing, Midwifery and Health Visiting 1996a Guidelines for professional practice. UKCC, London

United Kingdom Central Council for Nursing, Midwifery and Health Visiting 1996b Issues arising from Professional Conduct Committee. UKCC, London

United Kingdom Central Council for Nursing, Midwifery and Health Visiting 1996c PREP – the nature of advanced practice – an interim report. UKCC, London

United Kingdom Central Council for Nursing, Midwifery and Health Visiting 1997a Post-registration education and practice and you. UKCC, London

United Kingdom Central Council for Nursing, Midwifery and Health Visiting 1997b Standards for the preparation of teachers of nursing, midwifery and health visiting. UKCC, London

United Kingdom Central Council for Nursing, Midwifery and Health Visiting 1998 Standards for records and record keeping. UKCC, London

United Kingdom Central Council for Nursing, Midwifery and Health Visiting 1998a Higher level practice (Specialist practice project phase II). UKCC, London

United Kingdom Central Council for Nursing, Midwifery and Health Visiting 1998b A higher level of practice: the UKCC's proposals for recognising a higher level of practice within the post registration regulatory framework. UKCC, London

Van der Weyden R 1994 Changing attitudes to sun exposure. British Journal of Nursing 3(5): 765–769

Vanderpool H Y 1978 The ethics of terminal care. Journal of the American Medical Association 239(9)

VanGott L M, Tittle B M, Moody E L, Wilson E M 1991 Analysis of a decade of critical care nursing practice research: 1979 to 1988. Heart and Lung 20(4): 394–397

Vargo N L 1991 Basal and squamous cell carcinomas: an overview. Seminars in Oncology Nursing 7(1): 13–25

Volpicelli J R, Altermen A I, Hayashida M, O'Brien C P 1992 Naltrexone in the treatment of alcohol dependence. Archives of General Psychiatry 49: 876–880

Voluntary Euthanasia Society 1992 Your ultimate choice. Souvenir Press, London

Wade B, Moyer A 1989 An evaluation of clinical nurse specialists: implication for education and the organisation of care. Senior Nurse 9(9): 11–16

Wadsworth M E J, Butterfield W J H, Blaney R 1968 Without prescription. Office of Health Economics, London

Wagner J L, Power E J, Fox H 1988 Technology-dependent children: hospital vs home care. United States Congress, Office of Technology Assessments. J B Lippincott, Philadelphia

Walk A 1961 A history of mental nursing. Journal of Mental Sciences 446(107): 1–17

Wallace P, Cutler S, Haines A 1988 Randomised controlled trial of general practitioner's intervention in clients with excessive alcohol consumption. British Medical Journal 297: 663–668

Walsh P 1995 Speaking up for patients. Nursing Times 81(18): 24–26

Warren A N 1993 Perceived needs of the family members in the critical care waiting room. Critical Care Nursing Quarterly 16(3): 56–63

Watson H E 1992 A study of the effectiveness of brief intervention for problem drinkers in acute hospital setting (unpublished PhD thesis). University of Strathclyde, Glasgow

Watson M, Denton S, Baum M, Greer S 1988 Counselling breast cancer patients – a specialist nurse service. Counselling Psychology Quarterly 1(1): 23–31

Watts M J 1997 Psoriasis. Professional Nurse 13(2): 101–106

Weisman A D 1979 Coping with cancer. McGraw-Hill, New York

West R 1997 Getting serious about stopping smoking. A review of products, services and techniques. A report for No Smoking Day

Weston J 1975 Whither the 'nurse' in nurse practitioner? Nursing Outlook 23(3): 148–152

While A E, Citrone C, Cornish J 1996 A study of the needs and provision for families caring for children with life-limiting incurable disorders. Department of Nursing Studies, King's College, London

White R 1985 Political regulators in British nursing. In: White R (ed) Political issues in nursing past, present and future. John Wiley, Chichester, ch 2

White S J 1997 Evidence-based practice and nursing: the new panacea? British Journal of Nursing 6(3): 175–178

Whitfield L 1998 A second bottom line. Health Service Journal (26 Feb): 16

Whiting M 1988 Community paediatric nursing in England in 1988. MSc Thesis, University of London

Whiting M 1995 Nursing children in the community. In: Campbell S, Glasper A (eds) Whaley and Wong's children's nursing. CV Mosby, London

Whiting M 1996 Directory of community children's nursing services. Royal College of Nursing, London

Whiting M 1997 Community children's nursing: a bright future? Paediatric Nursing 9(4): 6–8

Whiting M, Godman L, Manly S 1994 Meeting needs: RSCNs in the community. Paediatric Nursing 6(1): 9–11

Whyte D, Baggaley S, Rutter C 1995 Chronic illness in childhood: a comparative study of family support across four diagnostic groups. Physiotherapy 81(9): 515–520

Wide M 1996 A partnership in caring. A guide for professionals who work with families that support a person with a learning disability. United Response, London

Wilkinson P 1995 A qualitative study to establish the self-perceived needs of family members of patients in a general intensive care unit. Intensive and Critical Care Nursing 11: 77–86

Wilkinson S 1991 Factors which influence how nurses communicate with cancer patients. Journal of Advance Nursing 16(6): 677–688

Wilkinson S 1995 Communication. In: David D (ed) Cancer care prevention, treatment and palliation. Chapman & Hall, London

Wilkinson S, Maguire P, Tate A 1988 Life after breast cancer. Nursing Times 84(40): 34–37

Willard C 1996 The nurse's role as patient advocate: obligation or imposition. Journal of Advanced Nursing 24: 60–66

Williams H C 1997 Dermatology. In: Stevens A, Raftery J (eds) Health care needs assessment: the epidemiologically based needs assessment reviews, 2nd series. Radcliffe Medical Press, Oxford

Williams H C, Pembroke A C, Forsdyke H et al 1995 London-born black Caribbean children are at increased risk of atopic dermatitis. Journal of the American Academy of Dermatology 32: 212–217

Williams H C, Pottier A, Strachan D 1993 The descriptive epidemiology of warts in British schoolchildren. British Journal of Dermatology 128: 504–511

Williams H C, Strachan D P, Hay R J 1994 Childhood eczema: a disease of the advantaged? British Medical Journal 308: 1132–1135

Williams P 1995 Residential and day services. In: Malin N (ed) Services for people with learning disabilities. Routledge, London, pp 79–110

Williams P, Schoulz A 1982 We can speak for ourselves. Souvenier Press, London

Wilson-Barnett J 1985 Learning from specialists. Nursing Mirror 160(2): 20–21

Wilson-Barnett J, Beech S 1994 Evaluating the clinical nurse specialist: a review. International Journal of Nursing Studies 31(6): 561–571

Winder A E, Hlam J R 1978 Therapy of the cancer patient's family: a new role for nurses. Journal of Psychiatric Nursing and Mental Health Services 16: 22–27

Winsor A S, Croney S D, Midgely G, Smith C H 1997 An epidemic of tinea capitis in London. Poster, British Association of Dermatologists, Harrogate

Wolfensberger W 1972 A Balanced multi-component advocacy/protection scheme. NIME/CAMR Publications, Toronto

Wolfensberger W 1983 Social role valorisation: a proposed new term for the principle of normalisation. Mental Retardation 21(6): 234–239

Wolfensberger W, Thomas S 1994 Obstacles in professional human services culture to the implementation of social role valorization and community integration of clients. Care In Place 1(1): 53–56

Woods L P 1997 Designing and conducting case study research in nursing. NT Research 2(1): 48–56

Worden I W 1991 Grief counselling and grief therapy. Tavistock, London

World Health Organization 1987 Manual for community health care workers. WHO, Geneva

World Health Organization 1993 Expert Committee on Drug Dependence, 28th report. WHO, Geneva

World Health Organization 1994 World health statistics annual – 1993. WHO, Geneva

World Health Organization/International Council of Nurses 1991 Nurses responding to substance abuse. WHO/ICN, Geneva

Wright D, Digby A 1996 From idiocy to mental deficiency. Routledge, London

Wright K, Haycox A, Leedham I 1994 Evaluating community care. Services for people with learning difficulties. Open University Press, Buckingham

Wright S 1986 Building and using a model. Edward Arnold, London

Wright S 1992 Advances in clinical practice. British Journal of Nursing 1(4): 192–194

Young E 1998 Food, additives and cutaneous reactions. Dermatology in Practice 6(1): 18–20

Young E, Stoneman M, Petruckevich et al 1994 A population study of food intolerance. Lancet 343: 1127–1130

Zazpe C, Margall A M, Otano C, Perochena P M, Asiain C M 1997 Meeting needs of family members of critically ill patients in a Spanish intensive care unit. Intensive and Critical Care Nursing 13: 12–16

Index